John Smeaton

A narrative of the building and a description of the construction of the Edystone Lighthouse with stone

John Smeaton

A narrative of the building and a description of the construction of the Edystone Lighthouse with stone

ISBN/EAN: 9783337149970

Printed in Europe, USA, Canada, Australia, Japan

Cover: Foto ©Andreas Hilbeck / pixelio.de

More available books at **www.hansebooks.com**

A

NARRATIVE OF THE BUILDING

AND

A DESCRIPTION of the CONSTRUCTION

OF THE

EDYSTONE LIGHTHOUSE

WITH STONE:

TO WHICH IS SUBJOINED,

AN APPENDIX, giving some Account of the LIGHTHOUSE on the SPURN POINT,

BUILT UPON A SAND.

BY JOHN SMEATON, *CIVIL ENGINEER*, F.R.S.

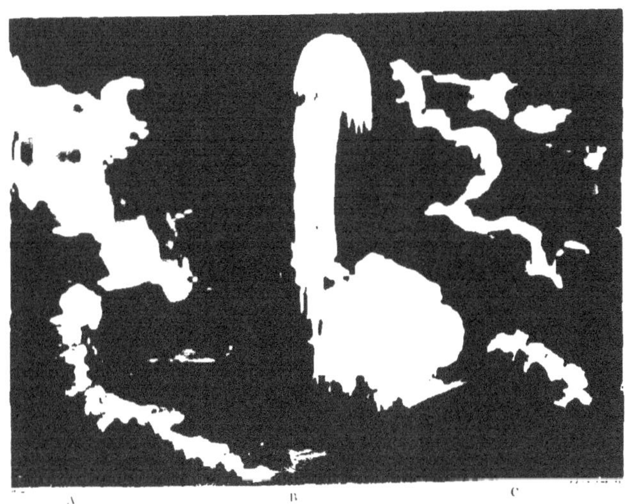

The MORNING after A STORM at S.W.

Advertiſement to the Reader.—The Length of Time the Work has been in Hand, and the great Number of Avocations that has unavoidably occurred to the Author during the Progreſs thereof, has neceſſarily ſubjected it to many Inconveniences. For, the greateſt Part of the Work having been printed before the finiſhing Parts could be prepared for the Preſs, each could only be compiled with that Degree of Information which the Author had at the Time. Hence the Diſtance of *Edyſtone* from the *Ramhead* is ſaid, in the Book, and Plate Nº 3 (engraved in 1785) to be *Ten* Miles; whereas the *corrected* Diſtances, Plate Nº 18, Fig. 11, give that 9¼ Miles nearly; as deduced from the *Trigonometrical* Survey, which was *laſt* computed.

Again, while the Preface was in the Preſs, conceiving *that* to be the *laſt* Opportunity of Correction, and haſtily taking the Meaſure of the Line WE (Nº 18 Fig. 11) inſtead of that of FE, an Error was announced to be in Page 197, which was indeed right before: The laſt Line of *Addenda* to the Preface ſhould therefore be *expunged*.

TO THE

K I N G.

S I R,

FROM the ambition natural to man, all authors are deſirous, that their works ſhould be placed in the moſt favourable point of view. This motive alone would have urged me to ſolicit permiſſion to lay mine at the feet of my Sovereign; a Sovereign whoſe reign has been marked by the moſt rapid and diſtinguiſhed progreſs, in the arts, in commerce, and in the moſt ſublime as well as the moſt uſeful diſcoveries, altogether ariſing from YOUR MAJESTY's immediate protection and encouragement.

To be allowed to approach YOUR MAJESTY, and mix my tribute with others of ſo much higher importance, is a moſt flattering diſtinction. It is further my particular felicity, that the tribute I offer is of ſuch a nature as to accord with the ſcope of YOUR MAJESTY's private ſtudies.

The very cloſe manner in which the model of the Edyſtone Lighthouſe was examined by YOUR MAJESTY, ſoon after the building itſelf was completed, has left the moſt laſting impreſſion upon my mind, of the critical knowledge which YOUR

MAJESTY has acquired in the art of building; and the earneſt attention YOUR MAJESTY was then pleaſed to beſtow upon the ſubject, has emboldened me, at this diſtant period, to preſent it once more to Your conſideration.

It certainly requires an apology, that I have not more early acquitted myſelf of a work, that then ſeemed to engage YOUR MAJESTY's curioſity; the delay, however, as it has given me time to mature my thoughts, and has afforded proof of the ſtability of the ſtructure, may poſſibly render the book more worthy of acceptance: and it will be a further excuſe, that I can with truth ſay, I have ever ſince been employed in works, tending to the immediate benefit of YOUR MAJESTY's ſubjects; and indeed ſo unremittingly, that it is not without the greateſt exertion, that I am enabled, even now, to complete the publication.

I have it not in my power to preſent YOUR MAJESTY with a fine piece of writing, or of drawing; neither literature, nor the fine arts, having been much the objects of my ſtudy; but I humbly ſubmit to YOUR MAJESTY, a plain account of the conſtruction of a plain and ſimple building, that has nevertheleſs been acknowledged to be, in itſelf, curious, difficult, and uſeful; and as ſuch, I truſt, worthy of obſervation.

I have the honour to be,

SIR,

YOUR MAJESTY's

Moſt dutiful ſubject,

and moſt obedient ſervant,

J. SMEATON.

P R E F A C E.

HAVING in ſome part or other of the following work, delivered the whole of what I would wiſh to ſay relative to the building, the hiſtory, and the deſcription of the *Edyſtone Lighthouſe*, I have little to offer by way of *Preface*, but what regards myſelf; or, my reader.

WHEN I re-commenced the compoſition of this work, in the year 1784; as I had then written ſeveral eſſays in the *Philoſophical Tranſactions*, in which I had been happy enough to make myſelf underſtood; I did not ſuppoſe it a matter of difficulty to give a diſtinct account of the progreſs and ſtructure of the *Edyſtone Lighthouſe*. I conſidered the account of every operation as a ſeparate eſſay; and conceived, that by joining them all together, I ſhould produce the book I meant to write. The motive to this undertaking will be found fully explained, in the latter part of the following Introduction; but the time it has taken, and the difficulties I have met with, have been, beyond all compariſon, greater than I expected.

THE *Introduction* was the eſſay with which I began; but this Preface being written after every conſtituent part of the work is gone through, I now find reaſon to change my firſt opinion, and am convinced, that to write a book, *tolerably* well, is not a light or an eaſy matter; for, as I have proceeded in this work, I have been leſs ſatisfied with the execution. In truth I have found much more difficulty in *writing*, than I did in *building*; as well as a greater length of time, and application of mind, to be required. I am indeed now older by 35 years, than I was when I firſt entered upon the enterprize; and therefore my faculties are leſs active and vigorous; but when I conſider that I have been employed full ſeven years, at every opportunity, in forwarding this book; having all the *original draughts* and materials to go upon; and that the production of theſe original materials, as well as the building itſelf, were diſpatched in half that time, I am almoſt tempted to ſubſcribe to the ſentiment adopted by Mr. Pope, that

"*Nature's chief Maſterpiece is writing well.*"——Roscommon.

It is true that I have not been bred to *literature*, but it is equally true, that I was no more bred to *mechanicks*; we muſt therefore conclude that the ſame mind, has, in reality, a much greater facility in ſome ſubjects, than in others. How I am to ſucceed as a writer, is yet to be tried, and I ſhall readily ſubmit to the deciſion of the impartial *Public*. I can ſay with great truth, that I have taken much pains, and have left nothing undone, that appeared neceſſary to the full information of my reader upon the ſubject: and I hope, that however I may be defective otherwiſe, I have not fallen ſhort of an *explanation*, to thoſe whoſe leiſure, and patience, may give them leave to go regularly through the *detail*.

AS it is not a kind of work, that I could expect to find intereſting to many readers, I have printed but a ſmall edition in point of number; which renders it neceſſary to lay a heavier *tax* upon the *curioſity* of thoſe, who may be inclined to acquaint themſelves with the ſubject, than I could have wiſhed; at the ſame time, if the whole edition were ſold, it will a good deal fall ſhort of reimburſing my expences. Could I have publiſhed within four or five years of the completion of the Lighthouſe, the performance was then ſo much talked of, that I ſhould certainly have ventured to have printed a conſiderable impreſſion; but the novelty having yearly worn off, down to the preſent time, the expectation muſt now be rated very low; eſpecially if it be conſidered, that moſt part of my readers were then unborn: and, the greateſt real praiſe of the edifice, being *that nothing has happened to it*, nothing has occurred to keep the talk of it alive. The public curioſity, therefore, will be with more difficulty excited afreſh.

PERHAPS

P R E F A C E.

PERHAPS I ought to make an apology for the largeness and fineness of my paper, as an article apparently enhancing the expence.——When I have seen a set of fine prints, produced with great labour and cost, spoilt as [illegible] *pictures*, by being folded into a book, I could not but much regret it: and, the expedient of binding up the prints into a separate book, while the *letter-press* matter is of a different size, I can only look upon as the necessary choice of two *evils*: for, I suppose it must be unhandy, and disagreeable, to have the book upon one shelf, and the prints belonging to it on another. On this account, I intended from the beginning, to bring my prints within the compass of half a sheet of imperial paper, and to have the letter-press work of the same size *, though the paper should be coarse.——I therefore made choice of a sample of an ordinary paper of the imperial size, and engaged my friend Mr. WHATMAN to make me the quantity: but he, willing to shew himself a patron of the work, gave me a paper of the best fabric, at the same price I must have paid for the coarse. To Mr. WHATMAN therefore my reader is obliged for the superior goodness of the paper.——I do not however mean to pass the supposition upon my reader, that the prints, I either meant, or have been able, to procure, are of that *delicacy* as in themselves to demand all the attention I have had towards them. They are in reality little more than *geometrical lines*, drawn to explain *geometrical* and *mechanical* subjects. If any of them puts on the appearance of any thing further, it is to render it more *explanatory* and *descriptive*. They are in reality not meant as *pictures*: but yet, if a right line or circle, is drawn upon paper, it will appear a right line or circle, if the paper is *flat*; but let that piece of flat paper be folded into one, two, or more *angles*, the natural appearance of the figures is destroyed; and figures, that are in themselves complex, are rendered still more so. By this treatment, good prints are in reality spoilt, and bad ones rendered still worse. I am therefore rather surprized, that the learned have not much attended to this matter.

AS I speak, and even write a *provincial language*, and, as I have already mentioned, was not bred to letters, I am greatly obliged to my friends in the country †, for perusing and abundantly correcting my manuscript: and last of all, to my friend Dr. BLAGDEN, who has been so obliging as to overlook the greatest part of the *printed proofs*, with much advantage to the work. I say the greatest part; as in justice to him, I must observe, I was obliged to send several of the sheets to the press, without his seeing them. Whenever therefore a more than ordinary deficiency occurs in point of diction, my reader may conclude that sheet never went to Dr. BLAGDEN.

IF I am asked why, being so slenderly equipped as a writer, I set about it at all; and did not wholly commit it to some other person? My answer is, that I consider this, as of the nature of a *commentary*; and that in an executive matter of *art*, the artist must write for himself; as he only can feel the force of his subject, so as to give it energy. I do not apprehend it to be of the *nature* of a commentary that the style should be polished; only that it should explain the subject, in the most *easy* and *familiar* manner. If I have failed in this last respect, I have fallen short of my hopes and wishes.——It is possible some discordancies may be met with on a strict perusal, notwithstanding the care and pains I have bestowed.——As it is, I commit it to its fate; having no presage it will be used worse than it deserves.

* One of my plates, indeed, somewhat exceeds the *imperial* in size; but that was not the case, when it was engraven, in the year 1762: which seems to shew, that the size of this paper is somewhat lessened since that time.

† Mr. [illegible], formerly my *colleague* in the *Derwentwater* Receivership: and after him the Reverend Mr. MICHELL, well known to [illegible]

SOME [illegible] mentioned as relative to the *present* time, that would now properly refer to the *past*; it may be of use to the reader to [illegible] hindrance, this work has been in a course of printing ever since the year 1786.

[illegible] Table of Contents, the following *Errata* have occurred:

Page	Line	For	Read
168,	l. 37, 38,	*for* N° 12, 14, and 16,	*read* N° 12, and 15.
175,	17,	(§ 19)	(§ 17, and 21.)
197,	26, col. 2,	14½ miles,	14 miles 1 furlong.

CONTENTS.

CONTENTS

Of the several Sections; being an EPITOME *of the Work.*

INTRODUCTION.

Page 1. PHAROS the most celebrated Lighthouse of Antiquity. General *Description* and dimensions.—Size of its base uncertain. *Distance* at which it could be seen.—Compared by *Josephus* to the *Phasael* at *Jerusalem*.

P. 2. Apparent *mistake* of Josephus relative to the *size* of the *Pharos*. Reconciled.—Pharos built by *Sostratus*. His *inscription*; by *permission* of *Alexander* according to *Pliny*.—Otherwise intimated by *Lucian*.—Lucian's *invective adopted* by *modern* Historians; but rejected.—The Reasons.

P. 3. The Pharos *cost* 800 *Talents*. Their value *uncertain*.—*Destroyed*; the occasion and time uncertain; yet subsisting complete in the 12th century.—By *Abulfeda*'s account, about 400 years ago, it was reduced in height; since then destroyed. Most probably by an earthquake. Subsisted 1600 years.

P. 4. Other Lighthouse *Towers* have obtained the same appellation.—The *Tour de Cordouan* upon the French Coast, the most remarkable of the modern ones.—Finished in 1610 by *Lewis de Foix*, a French Architect.—Built upon a *bare rock* 500 fathoms long and 250 broad. Liable in storms to a *great Surf*.—Its *foundation* described.—Surrounded by a *circular wall*. Not a place of defence.—Principal dimensions of its *elevation*.—*Accommodation* for the *Lightkeepers*.

P. 5. *Architecture* highly finished. The *rooms* described in the first and second story.—Third story described.—Original *Lantern*.

P. 6. Decoration of the *King's Apartment*.—Different Orders of Architecture in the Building.—*Architect reproved*, by *Belidor*, for using a profusion of ornaments. Vindicated.—Lantern *damaged* by the original Fires. *Taken down* and fire kindled below. Found there *inadequate*, and restored.—The *New Lantern*.

P. 7. *Reflectors* applied to the new Lantern.——EDYSTONE *Lighthouse* an object of public curiosity. *Awakened* by the Completion of the present building in 1759.—*The Model* shewn to their present MAJESTIES and several of the *Royal Family*.—The Author *requested* to *publish* an *Account* of his proceedings.—His reason for complying therewith.

P. 8. Progress made in 1763. Reasons why discontinued till 1783.—Proposes beginning with a description of the Rocks; and of the former buildings thereon.

BOOK I.

CHAP. I. *Containing a* general Account *of the* Edystone Rocks.

§. 1. *Rocks* described as in Nature *independent* of any building.

2. *Name*. Its probable origin.

3. Course of the *Tides*.

4. *Situation*, with respect to the Coast——to the *Rambead*, the *Start*, and *Lizard* Points.

5. *Situation* respecting the *Bay of Biscay*, and the *Atlantic Ocean*.

6. The *violence* of the *Sea* augmented on these Rocks by their particular *Form* and *Position*.

7. Effect of the *Ground Swell* augmented by an *upright Face*, naturally formed on the Rock.

8. Further augmented by the *particularity* of the *Tide*.

9. *Flow* of the Tide upon the *Rock*.

10. A *rocky Bottom* extends considerably from the Rocks, a cause of *Impediment* in the mooring of a proper *Attendant Vessel*.

11. *Component Matter or Substance*. A peculiar species of *Laminated Granite*, in Cornwall called a *Killas*.—Elastic.

12. *General directions*. Time and flow of the *Tides*. Proper time of setting forward from *Plymouth*, for visiting the *Edystone*.

CHAP. II. *Concerning the Construction of the Lighthouse upon the Edystone, built by Mr.* WINSTANLEY.

§. 13. A Lighthouse upon the Edystone desireable.

14. First attempted by Mr. *Winstanley*.

15. Peculiarity of Winstanley's *genius*—prompted him not only to attempt difficult enterprizes, but in a difficult mode.

16. Erections by Winstanley on the Edystone.

17. A *Narrative of the Building*, begun in 1696, and more than four years in hand.—Many difficulties, as the Sea in *calm Weather* would *mount* and fly more than 200 Feet.

§. 18. The *first Summer* spent in making twelve holes, and fixing twelve *great Irons* into the Rock.

19. The *second Summer* in making a *solid Body* or round Pillar.

20. The *third Season*, the Pillar enlarged at its Foundation, and the *Superstructure raised* to 80 Feet high. Lodged therein soon after Midsummer.—Great Distress by a Storm. Finished the Building and put up the Light the 14th November 1698.

21. The *fourth Year*, finding that in the Winter the Sea had buried the Lantern at times, though above 60 Feet high; he encompassed the former Building with a new work, took down the upper part, and raised it to 120 Feet high; and yet in time of Storms the Sea appeared to fly 100 Feet higher than the Vane.

22. Besides the Narrative—Winstanley gives the *Situation* of the Lighthouse; and some *Account* of the Edystone Rocks.

23. A further Account of the *Rocks* and of the *Tides*.

24. An Orthographic *Elevation* from Winstanley's Perspective.—*Literal* References.—Critical Observations.

25. Great *Merit* in Winstanley not only to undertake but *achieve* what had been generally deemed *impracticable*. An *Anecdote*.

26. In 1703 *Repairs* wanted, and Mr. *Winstanley* went off to superintend the same.—An Anecdote.—A violent *Storm* arose, the Lighthouse and all therein *perished*.

27. Extracts from a Book intitled the STORM.—Describes the Loss of the Lighthouse, and of Mr. Winstanley.—The *Model* of it in Essex *broke* to pieces at that time.—A *Virginia* Ship lost soon after.

CHAP. III. *Account of the Second Lighthouse built on the Edystone by Mr.* RUDYERD.

§. 28. The great *utility* of Winstanley's Lighthouse.—Desireable to have one there. Not impracticable.—An Act passed in 1706, and the Work begun the same year.

29. The Privilege and Duties vested in the Corporation of the *Trinity House, Deptford Strond*. A Term granted to Captain *Lovel*.

30. Captain *Lovel* engaged Mr. *John Rudyerd* to be his Engineer, then a *Silk Mercer* on *Ludgate Hill*, assisted by Mr. *Smith* and Mr. *Norcutt*, Shipwrights.—Mr. *Rudyerd* endeavoured to avoid the Errors of his Predecessor, by aiming at *Simplicity*.

31. Mr. Rudyerd compleated his Design and published a *Print* with Explanations.

32. An *Orthographic Elevation* from the Print.

33. Mr. Rudyerd did not *distinguish* himself by any *After*-work. The Print seems taken from some *previous* Drawing.

34. Mr. Rudyerd's Description of the *Situation*, and general Construction of his *Building*.—The upright Timbers described as composing the *outside Shell*, different from the real Number.

35. Proposes cutting the inclined surface of the Rock into *Steps*—executed imperfectly.

36. Method of forming *Dovetail* Holes for fixing his *Iron Branches*.

37. Method of running in those Iron Branches with *Lead*.

38. Method of establishing a solid *Basement* of *Wood*. Situation of the Branches.—In Number 36.

39. Method of *keying* and fixing the Branches. A material Improvement. Winstanley's less perfect.

40. Rudyerd, besides the Fastenings of his *Timber* Work described, applied the great Principle, *Weight is most effectually resisted by Weight*.

41. *Strata* or Courses of *Cornish Moorstone* inlaid.

42. *Tonnage* of the *Stone*; and Description of the *Courses* of *Wood*. Particular Courses furnished with *Compass Timbers*.—Places of the Compass Timbers. *Wellhole* for the Stairs described. Reference to the Plans of the Moorstone Courses. *Upright* Bars.

43. The Ascent to Rudyerd's Entry Door by an *Iron Ladder*.

44. *Wellhole* for the Stairs and Passage in the 2d Set of Moorstone Courses. Their Tonnage.—3d Set of Moorstone Courses. Their Tonnage. Timber Courses up to the Store Room Floor.

45. Height of the Store Room Floor. From the Rock to this floor, denominated *The Solid*.

46. Floor of Rudyerd's *Store Room* as high as Winstanley's *State Room*; regulated by the Height of the *unbroken Waves*.

47. Application of the *upright Bars*. The Connection after.

* 42. P. 25. Mode of building the *Rooms* above the Solid to the *Balcony Floor*.

* 43. P. 25. The *Main Column* a simple Frustum of a *Cone*. General Dimensions.

* 44. P. 25. Method of *joining* the *upright timbers* by *Scarfs*. The

* The Numbers to which an *Asterisk* is prefixed, have been by mistake repeated; the *Page* is therefore added.

dimensions. Caulked with Oakum.—The whole a piece of *Shipwrightry*; the Architect considered as *Shipwright*. Its tonnage.

§. * 47. P. 25. The windows and doors, like the *Port-holes* of ships. Two projecting parts beyond the *Frustum*; the *Cornice* at top—and the Knee at bottom.

* 48. P. 26. Description and dimensions of the *Lantern*; and height of the *Light*.—*Weight* and *bulk* of this *Lighthouse*.

* 49. P. 26. The *Rock represented* in the *plate* as it *appeared* in 1756; and its *Seating*, as it *stood* previous to its Demolition in 1755.—*Technical* description.

49. Use of the *Rollers* and *Rails*.—No Cranes used as in *Winstanley's*.—The Chink in the Rock pointed out, where one of *Winstanley's Crane* Chains was found fast in the storm of 1703.

49. Useful *instruction* as to *Engineers* to be drawn from this Building.

50. *Temporary Light* fixed by Rudyerd. The Manner of it.—The Building finished in 1709.

51. *Accidents* that arose in the course of this Building.—Behaviour of *Lewis* XIV.

52. Account of *materials* used in the Construction of this Building.

CHAP. IV. *Containing subsequent Transactions and Occurrences from finishing Mr.* Rudyerd's *Lighthouse to the total demolition thereof.*

§. 53. About 1715, Captain *Lovel* being *deceased*, his property therein sold, and purchased by Messrs. *Weston*, *Noyes*, and *Cheetham*, in Shares.

54. House needed no material *Repairs* till 1723. *Worms* then discovered in the Timbers. Mr. *Holland* appointed to make the necessary *Repairs*.

55. Experiments on *sheathing* the Timbers with Copper, &c.—Found not fully to answer.

56. *Storm* in 1744 tore away 30 *pieces* of the *Uprights*. Repaired by Mr. *Jessop*.—Mr. Holland promoted to be *King's Builder* at *Deptford*, recommended Mr. *Jessop*.

57. The House attended originally by two men, a difficulty arose. Afterwards attended by three.—This furnished a seasonable relief.

58. *Anecdote* of *Lightkeepers* living together *without speaking*.—*Anecdote* of a man's commencing Lightkeeper to avoid *Confinement*.

59. Fatal *Catastrophe* of this Building.—Recital of particulars.

60. How the Building caught *Fire*, not certainly known; but began in the *Cupola*.—The Author's *Conjectures*. Began 2d December at two in the morning, one of the Lightkeepers exerted himself to quench the Fire. Frustrated by want of water. Singular instance of receiving *melted Lead* into his *Stomach*.

61. The fire seen from the Shore, and a fishing boat sent off by Mr. *Edwards*.—The men found retreated to the Cave in the Rock, to save themselves from the falling Fire.

62. Landing on the Rock impracticable. Contrivance to take off the men. One of them ran away as soon as landed.—The sufferer by the lead sent home to be taken care of.

63. Efforts of Mr. *Telcher*, Collector of the Light Duties, and his Son. Landing impracticable. The fire communicating itself to the solid, and not likely to be stopped there.

64. *Admiral* West, Commander of the *Fleet* in *Plymouth Sound*, sent out a Boat with an *Engine*, and attended by Mr. Jessop the Surveyor. Remarkable incident to the boat.—The Engine *broke*, and further attempts *baffled*.

65. The only remaining hopes from a *change* of the wind. Reasons why.—Became one great body of *red hot matter*. Burnt for five days.

66. *Henry Hall*, who had received the *Lead*, put under the care of an eminent *Surgeon*, for some days *grew better*, taking his medicines and swallowed other things; but died on the 12th.—On opening the *stomach*, a piece of *solid lead* was taken out.

67. An account of the *Case* transmitted by the Surgeon to the *Royal Society*. At first *disbelieved*.—*Experiments* on *Animals*, tried by the Surgeon, in support of his character. *Animals* found to *sustain* the operation.—These Experiments corroborated by the testimony of others.—The Surgeon censured for *Cruelty* to Animals.—*Vindicated*.

68. Suggestions of some, how some part of the Building might have been saved. The expedient in the Author's opinion could not have been successful, nor any other practicable.—Nothing, as it would seem, could have saved it, but a *Storm*.—Its *duration* 49 years.

BOOK II.

An Account of preparatory Matters towards building the present Lighthouse *upon the* Edystone Rock, *with* Stone.

CHAP. I. *Containing the proceedings from the destruction of Mr.* Rudyerd's *Lighthouse in December* 1755, *to Mr.* Smeaton's *departure from* London *to* Plymouth, *in March* 1756.

§. 69. The Proprietors having the Remainder of a Term of more than *half a Century*, strenuously apply themselves towards re-building. *Difficulties* arose and stated. An *Act* to empower Mrs. *Hussilegger* to sell part of her property.—Three eighth Shares represented by the *Westons*. A fortunate Circumstance.—Considered it not as a Work for a general undertaker in the building way; but for some one of a natural *mechanic* genius.

§. * 60. P. 38. Mr. Weston considered the *Royal Society* as likely to furnish or recommend a proper person.—Applied to Lord *Macclesfield*, then President; who recommended the Author. Then in the Country, and unknown to Mr. *Weston*.—Pointed out a friend to write to him, —The Author wrote to by Mr. *B. Wilson*, that he was made choice of to rebuild the *Edystone Lighthouse*. The Author conceiving this Building to have been of Stone, could not imagine it could be *totally* destroyed by fire.—Desired further information. Answered, that it was a *total demolition*; and he was *absolutely chosen* to this work.

* 61. P. 39. Returns to *London*. An interview with Mr. *Weston*; *papers*, *plans*, and *models* of the late Structure *explained* by Mr. Weston. —Great *bias* in favour of the *old building*. A question suggested. Answered satisfactorily.

* 62. P. 39. The *Plans* and *Models* being *sent* to the Author, were attentively considered. Not *sufficient* to make out the *precise plan* of any of the preceding Architects. Had been compiled from occasional observations.—Hence led to consider those *preconceptions* the Author had formed, of its being a *Stone Structure*. An *interview* desired with the *Body* of the *proprietors* upon a *leading* question.

* 63. P. 40. The *Author* states the *advantages* of a *Stone building*. The *proprietors* the *certainty* of *success* in one of the *same* structure as the last. Universally believed the *safety* of the late Building was owing to its *Compliancy*.—The objections answered; and reduced to a *simple Question*.—Determined in a satisfactory manner.

* 64. P. 41. The Author's *reasoning*, on the difference in structure of *Stone* and *Wood*. An *Enlargement* of the *base* very eligible.

* 65. P. 42. The figure of the *Bole* of an *Oak* furnished an *idea*. *Reasoning* upon its *figure*. The *Column* of greatest *Stability*.—References to a *figure*.

* 66. P. 42. *Bond* of the *Stone* to the *Rock*, and to one another.—*Cramping* considered. Objections. Of great Consequence, by all possible means, to *save time* upon the *Rock*.—*Dovetailing* considered. *Sparingly* practised in *Masonry*. An idea, taken from a method sometimes practised, of fixing the *Kirbs* of the *walking paths* in *London Streets*.—Sketch of the method. An Example from *Belidor* of a sort of *upright dovetail* Stones, in the floor of the great Sluice at *Cherbourg*.—The idea of *Dovetailing* maturated.

* 67. P. 43. *Fair Section* made out for a *Stone* Building.—The *sloping* of the *Rock advantageous* to the strength of the foundation.

* 68. P. 44. Another *interview* proposed with the *Proprietors*.—On exhibiting those *original Sketches*, they declared their entire *satisfaction*; and proposed they might be shewn to the *proper Boards*: and, if *they approved*, to prepare for *execution*.—In the Author's opinion, matters not *ripe* for this. He ought to see the Rock, and take real *Dimensions*, to enable him to make a *working model*. Approved by the Proprietors: and that it should have the *same* general *form* and Conveniencies as the last.

CHAP. II. *Containing an Account of the Proceedings and Occurrences on Mr.* Smeaton's *first Journey to* Plymouth, *in the Spring of the Year* 1756.

§. * 69. P. 45. Arrival at *Plymouth*. Interview with Mr. *Jessop*, who appeared likely to answer the Character the Author had had of him.—Openings of his proposal of a *stone building*, and Mr. *Jessop's Objections*. —The late House in a state of *decay* by the *worm*.

70. Wind not favourable to go out to the Rock. Waited on Commissioner *Rogers*. Directs Artificers to make *Tools* for *trial* of the Rock.

71. The 2d of April *failed* out *near* the Rock. Viewed it, but could not land.

72. 2d *Voyage*, April the 5th. Landed and staid 2½ hours. General Observations.—Traces of *Winstanley's Irons*.—Observations on *Rudyerd's* Iron *Branches* and *Steps*.—Upper part of the Rock *damaged* by the *fire*. —Tried the *workableness* of the *Rock*.

73. No appearance of *Impracticability* of a *stone building*. A more safe and *certain* way of *landing* highly *desirable*.—Often difficult, after a vessel had delivered her Cargo, to get out again from the *Gut*.—An *attending vessel* in company, necessary.

74. April 9th. Wind favourable, went out at Midnight, but obliged to return.—No prospect of success at sea till the 14th.—Looked out for a *Work-yard*. Its necessary *properties*.—No place to be had in or about *Plymouth*.—*Emparcombe* the work-yard used by *Rudyerd*; *not suitable* to a stone building.—*Millbay* the most *likely* situation.

75. Excursion to see the *Moorstone* at *Hingstone Downs*. *Manner* of *working* it.—*Price*.—Rendered low by the *regularity* of its *splitting*.

76. April 14th. The 4th *Voyage* proved unfavourable to land. An hard gale; *bore away* to the Harbour of *Fowey*.—This Harbour described. —*Mistakes* concerning it.—*Fowey*, or *Foy Harbour* the *Key* of the *Edystone* service.

77. Went to *Lanlivery*. Found *Walter Treleven*, who wrought *Moorstone* for *Rudyerd*. Described the manner. The Moorstone here different from that of Hingstone Downs, and more suitable to the Author's purpose. Manner of its carriage by Land.—Walking Paths of *Westminster Bridge* chiefly from hence.

78. Blew hard till 19th. Went out the 5th *time* for Edystone. A calm;

* Those Numbers to which an Asterisk is prefixed, and the Page added, have been also, by mistake repeated.

anchored

anchored 4 miles from it, succeeded by an hard gale, and with difficulty regained Plymouth.—Hence the *Expediency* of a *store vessel* to be moored near the Rock appeared to the Author. Approved by Mr. Jessop, who recommended a particular construction for that purpose. If a *floating Light* was *moored there*, it might answer both purposes.

§. 79. A piece of *Portland Stone* cut out of the *King's Dock*, that had been *perforated* by a kind of small *shell-fish*; like wood with the Worms.—Pieces of *Marble* Rock found to be perforated in a *similar manner*. *Portland* Stone *not* eligible for the *outside* of the Lower works of the Edystone.—This *stone* likely to last longer than *Wood*; but the Author's ideas not confined to *an age or two*.—Those *Perforations* chiefly confined to *low Water* Mark. Unnecessary to run any *risque*, *Moorstone* being *undeniable*.

80. April 22. The 6th *Voyage*. *Landed* on the Rock before 6 Morn. Staid till Noon. Operations interrupted by the *Ground swell*. Relanded at 2, and staid till 9 at Night.—Boat laid in the *Gut* all Night. Next Morn landed at 5, and went on till 11. Obliged to retreat by a *Ground Swell*, which was *succeeded* by an *hard gale* of wind. Observations on its effects till 5; then returned.

81. *Account* of the *Operations* on the Rock. *Instrument* for taking *certain points* of the Rock.—Construction and use of the Instrument.—*Improvements* in this Apparatus.—Thirty-five *primary points* herewith determined. Manner in which *many more* were *deduced* from those *originals*. The *measures* hence deduced *laid down* to a *scale*.

82. The 7th *Voyage* unsuccessful in landing. *Bore away* to *Falmouth*.—*Excursion* from thence to *Constantine*. Interview with Mr. *Box* a Moorstone worker there.—A capital workman, but had chiefly applied to small works.—Author determined to use *Portland Stone* for the *inside* works; and on account of the difficulties of *carriage*, to *reduce* the size first intended of the Granite Pieces.—Returned by way of the Edystone; not landing, returned to Plymouth.

83. Report of 40 *fish prize ships* in Plymouth, to be *sunk* near the *Edystone*.—The weather appearing favourable, the Author proceeded to sea; but this *Attempt* rendered *fruitless*, by a change of weather. On return waited on the *Commissioner*; and *remonstrated* against this measure: he proposed to consult *Adm. Mostyn*, who commanded at *Plymouth*. Delays dangerous. The Author wrote to a proprietor, who applied to the *Admiralty* to give other orders. Next day saw *Adm. Mostyn*, who then *relieved* him from his *Apprehensions*.

84. Weather bad till May 14. The Author in this interval turned his thoughts on the subject of *facilitating* the *Landing*; and on the proper *mode* of carrying on the *works* upon the *Rock*.—An *expedient* described by Mr. *Jessop*.—Mr. *Jessop* a man of *judgment*, but not of *invention*.—Approved the Author's plan. Substance of Letters to the Proprietors thereupon.

85. A stone building consisting of a *greater tonnage*, would take more time than if of wood. *Ineligible* to take a *greater time* in the whole than formerly. *Expedition* must therefore be procured by *Art*. The means pointed out.—Further means. A *store vessel* and *two sets* of workmen.—Mode of *payment*, such as to make it their *interest* to do their best.—Plan for carrying on the *works*, and management of the *workmen*.

86. May 11th, the 9th *Voyage* commenced. *Practicable*, but *hazardous*, to go into the *Gut*.—The Author considers how to remedy this inconvenience.—To *level* the *Sugar Loaf* Rock, in itself a *great work*. The use of *Transport Buoys* and a *Windlass* of a *new* contrivance * seemed applicable.—Approved by Mr. Jessop, who suggested Improvements.

87. Landed at 7 Morn, and staid till 11; obliged to quit on account of rain; but the most material measures now obtained.

88. May 15th, the 10th *Voyage*, landed at 11¼M. Quitted at 2¼A. All observations now completed.

CHAP. III. *Containing transactions and occurrences during the Author's return from* Plymouth *to* London, *in May* 1756.

§. 89. The Author in his return to London visited the quarries that were likely to furnish *Freestone* to Plymouth.

90. The quarries at *Beare* in *Devonshire*. Account thereof.

91. Visited *Portland*. Recommended to Mr. *Roper*, Agent at Portland for . . . . *Tucker*, Esq. of *Weymouth*.

92. First object of Curiosity the *Portland Quarries*. Description of the *Strata*.—The *Portland Cap*.—Manner of *working* the *Merchantable* Beds into *Blocks* for Sale.

93. Description of the *Carriages* for the Stone, and method of using them.

94. The best *Freestone* to be had here, in any quantity, *rough scappelled*, but not *hewn*.

95. The *Pier* for Shipping adjoining to *Weymouth Road*.—Portland *Lighthouses* visited.—The *Strata* of this Island, various, and curious to the Naturalist. The most striking *curiosity* to the Author was the *Portland Beach*. Renders it doubtful whether Portland is *properly* an *Island*. The *Beach* described.—Seemed to the Author not to have had its origin at a very remote period.—*Loose* in its component parts, but *not shifting*; and rests on a *Blue Clay*.

96. The Author not having met with a full account of the *Beech*, was willing to give such a one, as the time employed on this visit would allow; to excite the able Naturalist to a more full investigation. A singularity obtains in the *manners* and *customs* of the *Portland Quarrymen*.

97. Settled with Mr. *Roper* and determined; the best mode would be to send *Moulds* to direct the *Scappelling*. Proceeded to view the *quarries* at *Purbeck*.

§. 98. The *Peninsula* commonly called the *Island of Purbeck*. *Cone Castle*. The *Mortar* examined.

99. *Swanage* the principal town. The *quarries* viewed, and the *Strata* described.—Manner of working them. Strata of *Marble* raised here; such as seen in many of our old *Cathedrals*. The *Paving Stone* from hence having for many years past supplied the *London Markets* wholly; now come at with *more difficulty*.

100. Strata called *Purbeck Portland*; quarries chiefly near *St. Alban's Head*. Manner of working, and qualities.—Departed from hence to *London*.

CHAP. IV. *Containing Transactions in* London, *after* the Author's *first Journey to* Plymouth.

§. 101. The Author attended the Proprietors. Account of Proceedings, as already related. The *leading Question*, whether to rebuild with Stone entirely, or entirely with Timber; or partly with both. *Time*, a *principal* consideration; that *stated* as relative to the different modes. An *Estimate* not practicable for the whole business; as the greatest part of it would be widely open to Accidents. But whichever mode the proprietors chose, the Author would endeavour to perform in the most substantial manner and at the least possible expence.

102. *Unanimously* determined to *rebuild* with *Stone*; and in the very *best manner*. Reasons for *waving* their own *immediate interest*, in this determination.

103. The Author could not think himself justified in suppressing these Reasons.

104. A *Stone Building* being *resolved upon*; the Author was directed without loss of time to prepare such models and designs, as should fully explain the proposition to themselves; and to those Boards, they should think it right to consult. The *Time* and *Means* left to the Author.

105. *Good effect* of leaving him *unfettered*.—*Main object* to digest such a *scheme* as should go *progressively* on, according to opportunities, *without* derangements. With this view, having got sufficient dimensions, applied himself to the making an *accurate model* of the *Rock*. The time spent in a *mature digestion*, likely to be more than saved by avoiding *unnecessary work*.—A first principle, to cut the *rock as little as could be helped*. For this end a second *model* was necessary, to shew the manner of applying the new work thereto.—The Author determined to make both these *models* with his *own hands*.

106. His reasons, for executing these models *himself*.—In other matters he availed himself of the hands of others. The *Purchase tackle*.

107. Viewed the *Neptune Buss*, then fitting out for a *floating light*; chiefly to judge whether applicable as a *store vessel*, in the building service. Description of her.—Observed that if situated in a certain position she might answer that double purpose.—*Declaration* of a Proprietor thereon.

108. The 13th July, the *two models* executed by the Author *exhibited to the Proprietors*.

109. Being fully considered, by the *Proprietors*, they declared their *entire approbation* of the whole of the Author's proposition; and desired him to explain the scheme to the *Admiralty* and *Trinity House*; and adjourned their Meeting to the 17th, in expectation of those Exhibitions being over.—The Board of *Admiralty* appointed the 15th, when the Author *attended*, and met with their *thorough approbation* of his scheme.—The 17th no appointment received from the Trinity House; and the Season fast advancing, the Proprietors *determined* the Author should set out for *Plymouth* on Monday morning the 19th of July.

110. During this absence from Plymouth a constant *correspondence* with Mr. *Jessop*. Final *Instructions* from the *Proprietors*.—One of the Proprietors delegated their Agent, in corresponding with the Author, and managing affairs.

111. The Author set out according to appointment for Plymouth.

112. The *original* Designs and Models, except that of the *Rock* as the Author *found* it, *differ* from the Building, as it now *stands executed*; yet is sufficient to explain the mode of the Building. *Concise* Explanation of several *Plates*.

B O O K III.

Containing an Account of Proceedings from the Commencement *of the* Work *upon the* Rock *in* 1756, *to the beginning of the second Season in June* 1757.

CHAP. I. *Narrative of the* Progress *of the Work done upon the* Edystone, *from (the* Author's) *Arrival at* Plymouth *in July* 1756 *to the time of mooring the* Neptune Buss.

§. 113. Arrival at *Plymouth*, 23d July 1756. Met Mr. *Roper* at *Dorchester*. Found *Hancock's* Sloop and other Vessels properly prepared by Mr. *Jessop*.—*Neptune Buss* arrived, and lay in *Stonehouse Creek*. Not likely to be applied to the use intended. *Sloop* got ready for *temporary service*. Weather now unsuitable, and had been so for some time past.

* Author finds, in 1789, that *windlasses* on this *principle* have been used in the *Severn Barges* time immemorial.

§. 114. Weather still unfavourable till 3d August. Mr. *Thomas Richardson* appointed *Foreman* of one of the Companies. *William Hill* of the other. Mr. *Jessop*, general *Assistant*. *Wages* settled.—Mr. *Delacombe* agreed with for Half an Acre of Ground for a *Work-yard* at *Mill Bay*. Mr. *Hamilton* arrived as *Clerk* to the works.

115. The 3d August *1st Company* went out. Wind became contrary; and the Author was rowed to the Rock in the *Yawl*, and began to fix the *Center*, and *Lines* of the work. After which, obliged to return with the Sloop to *Cawsand Bay*.—The Weather becoming more unfavourable, returned to Plymouth.

116. The 5th, went out again, came to an anchor, and *attempted* to *moor* the Sloop, but obliged to *desist*. The Company *landed* and *worked* four hours with good effect.—The 6th, worked both Morning's and Evening's tide. Got nearly the whole of the work laid out.

117. Reasons for not using *Gunpowder* in performing this work.

118. The 7th being *Saturday*, the *Companies changed* upon the *Rock*.—The *Lines* on the Rock *completed*. Distribution of the seamen.

119. Settled weather attended with *Land* and *Sea Breezes*. The advantage thereof.

120. The work pursued *without interruption* till the 15th of August.

121. *Cable* found greatly *damaged* by the *sharpness* of the *Rocks* at bottom. Place of the *Moorings shifted*.

122. The 13th August, vessel fitted out by the *Trinity House* as a *Floating Light*, exhibited the same. The *ground cable* again *cut* by the Rocks. One-third of the *work* of this Season now *dispatched*. *Extraordinary Wages* made last week, by the *favourable weather*. *Position* of the *Floating Light*. Judged two *miles* to the *westward* of the Rock. Of no use to the artificers, unless to shelter them when *driven westward*, by *distress of weather*.

123. Sunday the 15th, a *rough sea* obliged the hands to *slip* their *Moorings* and bring the sloop into *Cawsand Bay*. Returned on Tuesday Morn, but weather still unfavourable. This day the 1st *draughts* for stone sent to *Portland*. This afternoon the *sloop* came again into *Cawsand Bay*. Lay there till Thursday. Then again went out, but obliged to return. *Companies* changed in *Cawsand Bay*.—*Hill's* Company *attempted* to go out, but obliged to put back. Sunday got out; laid hold of the moorings, and landed; but after half an hour obliged to quit.—Next night the sloop's *ground cable* being *again cut*, obliged to go into *Cawsand Bay*.

124. The Author next day received *order* from the *Proprietors* to make use of the *Neptune Buss*. Adapted her to the service with little alteration.—The 27th, wind and weather moderate, *Hill and Co.* again went out in the *Sloop*. The *Buoys* being gone, they came to an anchor. Enabled to make short tides. The *Moorings recovered* by *sweeping*. Sloop again moored. August 29th, *Buss cleared* of unnecessary stores, and made ready. Wind, though moderate, unfavourable for carrying out the Buss. Richardson's Company *rowed out* in the Yawl and *changed* upon the Rock.

125. 31st. *Buss brought out* of Stonehouse Creek. Warped to one of the *King's Buoys* in *Hamoaze*. Sept. 1st, Wind not in favour, endeavoured to make a *Tack*, but the vessel would *not stay*. Came to an anchor.—Next day wind fair; but being moderate, and the *Buss* an *heavy Sailer*, made but little way. Came to an anchor in the evening 2½ miles from the Rock. Dispatched *sharp tools* to the *Company* at work.—Friday 3d, got the vessel *out* and were assisted by Richardson's Company in *warping* her to her birth; *proceeded to moor*.

126. The chain *Moorings described*.—Mode of mooring as originally intended. A necessary *alteration* in the mode.

127. Manner of *laying down* the *Moorings* described.—*Safe completion* of this business.

128. September 4th. *Work examined*, and judged *one half*, for this *season*, to be completed.—The *sloop* brought home.

CHAP. II. *Sequel of the* Operations *upon the* Rock, *of the first Season of* 1756.

§. 129. The Buss being *satisfactorily moored*; nothing now to hinder but bad weather.—*Draughts* sent to *Portland* for the *foundation* Courses.

130. Companies worked *regular tides* from 27th August to 14th September. Manner of preparing *wooden moulds* for the exact cutting of the Stones.—*Moulds* necessary to every *different size* and shape of Stone.

131. A *West India Ship* and a *Man of War's Tender* saved from driving upon the N. E. rock.—Manner of *splitting Stones* by the *Key and Feather*. *Winstanley's Chain* released.

132. Sept. 14th and 15th, an hard Gale at S. W. The first since the Buss was moored, and was found to ride perfectly easy. The work examined by the Author *and the state of it described*.

133. Unsettled weather. Work further examined. *Difference* of *Level* of the *foundation Courses*. The *Yawl* having *parted* her grapling rope, and *left her grapling* in endeavouring to weigh it; occasioned the expedient of the *Transport Buoy*, before suggested, to be *put in use*.

134. The 2d Oct. an *hard gale* of wind brought *Richardson* and Co. *home* in the *Yawl*, having no sharp tools. Hill and Co. prevented going out.—The 4th, the *seamen wanting provisions*, and the weather continuing bad, *came home* in the *little Yawl*, with an *Oar* for a *Mast* and a *Blanket* for a *Sail*. This evening Hill and Co. got out.

135. The season far advanced. The Author forms a scheme to avoid *weighing* the *Buss's chain Moorings*.—Approved by Mr. *Jessop*, who suggests Improvements.

136. The 13th, the *Great Yawl* broke *adrift* in a hard gale of wind.—Only 23½ *hours worked* in *October*. Little wanting but *levelling*.—*Cause of the Cable damaged* by the Rocks, and repaired.

137. Nothing to hinder the Commencement of *setting* the *stone foundation* next Season. Richardson's ordered to return at the end of their week, though they were not relieved by the other Company. Instance of great *difference* of the *weather* at *Edystone* and at *Plymouth*. Both Buoys of the mooring anchors *broke loose*.

§. 138. *Machinery*, &c. of the *Work-yard* got *ready* for use. Experiments on the *Strength* of the *Tackle*.

139. A better appearance of weather in November. *Hill's* Company went out. The Author went off with a carpenter, &c. to make *wooden moulds* from the Rock. Prevented by weather. Having landed, reports the state of the works.

140. The 12th Nov. the *Buoy Chain completed*. *Experiment* of its Strength. Edystone Boat sent out with *Provision*; but returned without being able to get out. Attempted again the 15th without success; and this evening the *Buss arrived* in *Millbay*. Since Oct. 2, the work had amounted only to 38½ hours.

141. *Buss's Bottom* become very *foul*, was cleaned, and again prepared for Sea.

142. The Author with proper Assistants sailed the 21st November. Retarded by an accident; and the slow sailing of the Buss even when clean.—*Bridle Cable* being *hard laid*, and stiff by the water, came in very tardily. Somewhat damaged by the Rocks. The 22d at 3 morning, the *Swivel* got *above water*; and the *Buoy Chain attached* thereto. The *fore lock* clinched by the Author.—Fresh of wind obliged the Edystone Boat to go home. Circumstances hindered the *quitting* the *moorings* till 3 A.

143. The *wind* become *unfair* for *Plymouth*, steered for *Fowey*.—Night *dark* and stormy, *missed* the *Harbour*. *Breakers* ahead. By great Exertion the *vessel got about*. Heaved down by stress of wind, *gunnel frequently under water*. Company in great *Jeopardy*. Concluded to stand out to Sea. *Escaped the Rocks*, but *split* their Sails, the Main Sail excepted.

144. Tuesday, 23d, at break of Day, obliged to *cut* the only remaining *yawl adrift*. *Wore* the vessel, and stood in for the Land; which saw about noon, and judged the *Lizard*. Discerned Land right ahead, which proved the *Land's End*, but upon the *Weather Bow*. Evening more *moderate*, bent *fresh sails*, and made an *Attempt* to get into *Mounts Bay*.—*Stood off* the Land during the Night; and at Two on Wednesday morning *wore* the vessel. *Saw Land* soon after day-light, which proved the *Land's End*, still more to *Windward* than the day before. Came to an *Anchor*. Wind fresh right from the Land. A *Consultation* on Measures. *Resolved* to attempt to make *Scilly*.

145. Saw a *vessel* from the East, which *bore down* upon them, and proved to be the *White Hart* of *Pool*, bound for *Guinea*. Could get no relief from her; but learnt the Course for *Scilly*. Prepared for sailing for those Islands, very early the next morning.

146. Thursday 25th, at two morning, began to *heave in* the *Cable*; while doing, the wind ceased, and a *breeze in favour* sprang up, which enabled the Company to steer for *Plymouth*. At four on Friday morning *abreast* of *Ram Head*, and at six at an *Anchor* in *Plymouth Sound*.

147. The relation of the work of the Season completed.—Concludes with the *commendation* of a *deserving* seaman. *Safety* of the vessel and Company, in the late Adventure, principally due to the activity and alertness of *John Bowden*.

CHAP. III. *Containing the Transactions of the* Winter *of* 1756, *and of the following* Spring 1757, *to the Commencement of the* Outwork *of the ensuing Season.*

§. 148. The most interesting *facts related*, without strictly conforming to Time.—Mr. *William Tyrrel* chosen *foreman* of the *Work-yard*.

149. *General design* and *contrivance* of the *Work-yard* explained.—Proper to use as *large Stones* as the *situation* and *service* would admit.

150. *Modern Buildings* in general composed of *Stones* rather *small* than large. The Reason thereof. Advantages of large pieces.

151. The *size* of Stones most *proper* for the *Edystone* work pointed out.—*Stones* of a *Ton* and upwards, not to be managed in the *Work-yard* without *Machinery*; or an *increase* of *Labour*.—Reasons for *trying* every *course* to its *neighbour*.

152. Vessels arrived with *Stone* from *Portland* in *December* 1756. The *Masons began* to work. *Difficulty* in getting the *Moorstone* brought home on account of its *size*. Dispatched a *vessel* from *Plymouth* with proper *Tackle*.

153. *Moorstone* though hard yet *friable*, and difficult to bring to an *Arris*. Necessary to do the *principal part* of the work at *home*. *Mode* of *Agreement* for doing a certain part in the country. The *Prices* agreed for.—*Reasons* for employing *more* than *one Contractor*.

154. Construction of *additional vessels* necessary for the service of the ensuing year. The service best performed by *small vessels*.—*Size* of *vessels* pointed out.—The number.

155. *Yawls*: the *sort* pointed out.—A large yawl purchased. The smaller made at *home*. Why to be *preferred* for the Edystone service, to those made at *Deal*. *Drawing* of a *Yawl* preserved; and referred to, and the larger *Boats described*, which answered the service.

156. The importance of obtaining *Cement*, the most *perfect* that it was possible to make. *Nothing* of the *resinous* or *oily* kind could possibly *answer* in this situation. Only such as would become *hard*, without being *ever dry*.

157. The Author resolves to *winter* at *Plymouth*, and go through a course of *Experiments* on *Cements*.

158. A *Journey* to the *West*, the spring of the year 1757. The *Church* of *Lostwithiel* viewed, that had suffered much by *Lightning*.—Its *damages described*.

159. The Author went out to the Edystone to get the *Moulds* made of the *Work* upon the *Rock*. Viewed the work, but could not land.

The

The *Moorings* in good order.—Several other attempts; but could not land till 23d April. The *Moulds* then got in *part made*; but hindered *from proceeding* by a neglect of the carpenter. *Completed* on the 30th.

§. 160. The work of the Moulds for the foundation *rendered inconvenient* by being denied the use of the *public rooms*.

161. Much *hindrance* last season by our *seamen* being frequently detained by the Men of War's cutters to *impress* Seamen. The Author suggests a *remedy*.

162. The *Vessels* from *Portland* with *Stone* for the Edystone, detained by *fear of French privateers*; and an *order* from the *Admiralty* for a *Convoy* obtained thereupon.

163. The *Stone* in Millbay *Work-yard* being all *wrought up*, Masons employed in quarrying *Marble* for *Cubes* for inlaying between the Courses. The Tinners employed in *boring holes* through the Stones for *Trenailing* them down. 300 *Trenails* purchased.

164. A *Combination* among the workmen, and *William Hill*, one of the *foremen* of the Rock Companies, *discharged*.

165. The *premium* per *hour* given the last season proposed to be *reduced*; *agreed* to by the workmen.

166. The Commanding Officer of the *Fleet* at Portsmouth being applied to, for a *Convoy* for the Stone from *Portland*; regular *Answers* were received, yet *no Convoy* ever attended this service.

167. *Five fathoms* of large *Chain* for the Moorings arrived from London in May. *Prepared to begin* the *Work* of the *Season*, as soon as weather permitted; but previous to the relation of it, the Author proposes to give an *Account* of his Experiments on *Cement*.

CHAP. IV. *Containing* Experiments *to ascertain a complete Composition for* Water Cements; *with their results.*

§. 168. The common *Tarras* Composition recognized. Some assertions of Workmen concerning Mortar *unsupported*.—*Salt water* by them *disapproved*.—The Author's reasoning thereupon.

169. Enquiry into the effect of *Limes* being *imperfectly burnt*. *Great waste* hereby in works at large; but did *not hinder* the Author's *Experiments*.

170. *Method* of making *Mortar* for trials.

171. *Common Lime* and Sand would not stand the *Water Test*.

Question 1st. Concerning *Lime* from Stones of different *hardness*.—The *Investigation*. Comparison of *Chalk Lime* with that of *Plymouth marble*.

Quest. 2d. Concerning the difference of *salt* and *fresh water* for making *Water Mortar*.—The *Investigation*.

Quest. 3d. Difference resulting from different *qualities* of *Limestone*.—*Investigation*. That of *Aberthaw* in *Wales* approved.

172. The *notion* of Workmen examined concerning *repeated beatings* of Mortar.

Quest. 4th. If *tarras mortar* is better by *repeated beatings*. *Investigation* with *Aberthaw* lime.

173. *Shell Lime* for water building examined.

174. *Plaster* of *Paris* for water building examined.

175. Lime of *Bridistow* in *Devonshire* examined.

176. *Chemical* examination of *Lime Stones* proposed.

177. *Method* of the Chemical Analysis of Lime Stones.

178. Trial of *White Chalk*, Plymouth *Marble*, and *Plaster*. *Aberthaw* Lime Stone tried, and also *Bridistow*.

179. *Pure Limes* not the best for water building. The *best* generally contain *Clay*.

180. *Tarras*, its *properties* recounted, and not answerable where subject to become *dry*.

181. Another *property* of *Tarras unfavourable* for some uses. *Terra Puzzolana* recommended by *Belidor*, and some *procured* for *trial*.

182. *Puzzolana tried* and approved; and *best* with *Aberthaw* lime.

183. The *best method* of making *Grout*, or liquid Mortar, *necessary* to be known; and proposed to be examined.

184. *Investigation* of the best method of making *Grout*.—*Plaster* for this purpose tried and *rejected*.

185. Some *account* of *Tarras* and *Puzzolana*.—Method of the *Preparation* of *Tarras* in *Holland* for use.

186. *Puzzolana* described. In great quantities near *Mount Vesuvius*. That used for the Edystone from *Civita Vecchia*. That from Naples of an *inferior* quality.

187. *Tarras* and *Puzzolana* agreeing in several obvious properties, other *similar substances* tried, but without success.

188. Composition of *Edystone mortar* being determined: enquiry how and where to procure the Lime. That of *Watchet* recommended; to which place the author determined to take a *journey*.

189. *Journey* to *Watchet*. Saw *specimens* of work done with that Lime, and that of *Aberthaw*.

190. *Watchet Pier* satisfactory as to the Mortar work. Manner in which the Strata of *Lyas* Stone lie. Those used for burning into Lime are got from the *sea shore*.—Then but *little demand* for this Lime, and the reason.—A quantity burnt to ascertain the *bulk* and *weight*. The *mode* of *package* agreed upon and described.

191. *Blue Lyas* Stone of *Watchet* described; *White Lyas* analysed. *Unfit* for water works.

192. Author proposes an *Account* of what has *occurred* to him on this subject *since*.

Limes since examined.

193. That of *Barrow* in *Leicestershire*.

194. *White Lyas* of *Somersetshire* compared with *Clunch* Lime of *Sussex*; a species of *Chalk* described, containing *Clay*, and good for *Water building*. The Lime of *Dorking* in *Surry* esteemed of the same kind.

§. 195. *Sutton* Lime of *Lancashire*. The Stone analysed and described. Good for *Water building*.

196. *Gray Lime* of *Berryton* near *Petersfield*, *Hampshire*, a *Chalk* Lime containing *Clay*, like the Clunch. A *Water Lime*.—A *Water Lime* of the Chalk kind also near *Guildford*.

Blue Lyas Limestone at *Lyme* in *Dorsetshire*, also esteemed good *Water Lime*.—*Table* containing the *results* of Water Limestones *examined*.

197. Trials for a *succedaneum* for *Tarras* or *Puzzolana*; Smith's *forge* scales found *equal* in quality, but not to be had in quantity.

198. *Minion* described. *Inferior* to *Puzzolana*.—A particular *Red Stone*, found *equal* to *forge Scales*, but could not find it in quantity.

199. Means of *increasing the quantity* of good water Mortar.

200. The use of *Sand* in Mortar.

201. The proportion of increase of *bulk* of Mortar by different quantities of *sand*.

202. Pursuit of the subject and introduction of *Pebbles*.

203. Trial of *Clay* in the Composition of Mortar, *hurtful*.

204. *Stones* naturally *flat-bedded* recommended for Water building.

205. *Flat backing* recommended in preference to *rough rubble*.

206. *Table* containing 20 Compositions of *Water Mortar* suited to different situations and circumstances.

Observations on the Table——in seven different Heads.

B O O K IV.

An Account of the Proceedings of the Construction *of the* Stone Work, *&c. upon the* Rock, *from the beginning to the finishing of the Building. With after occurrences.*

CHAP. I. *Containing an Account of the* First Year's Building *upon the* Rock.

§. 207. 3d June, 1757, sailed out of Plymouth Sound to *begin* the *work* of the *season*. A *Difficulty* arose in getting up the *Moorings*. The manner of *obviating* it described.—Some *danger* attending this operation, was performed by the Author. The *Buoys* successfully *moored*.

208. The *Fender Piles*, the *Shears*, and *Windlass*, and the *Transport Buoy* fixed.

209. The *first Stone* landed, got to place and fixed, Sunday the 12th June, 1757. Next day the *first Course completed*.

210. The 14th, the *second Course began*. A *fresh Gale* arose, obliging the Workmen to quit the Rock.—Things *secured* in the best manner possible. The *Gale increasing*, impracticable to get out of the Gut, otherwise than by passing the *Sugar Loaf*. Yawls could not both *recover* the *Buoy*. The *Sea-horse Yawl* made her way Westward to the *floating Light*.—An hard *struggle* to the *light Yawl* to regain the *Buoy*.—Next morning the wind shifted, and the *Weston*, obliged to *quit* the *Transport buoy* and get into Port. Afternoon the *Sea Horse* Yawl got back in *safety*, from the floating Light.

211. The *Work proceeded* with. The 18th, hands again obliged *suddenly* to quit the Rock; and the Weston to go into Port.—Several disasters described. The most considerable, the *loss* of several *pieces* of *Stone*.—The Author *returned* to Plymouth, to expedite the forming of other Stones instead of those lost.—In carrying out the Stones, a *Gale of Wind* arose, obliging the vessel to run into *Fowey harbour*.

212. The 30th June the IId *Course closed*; and the IIId begun.—A new *Tool contrived* for getting up *lost Stones*.—Further progress reported.

213. Weather unfavourable.—Afternoon of the 5th July the work *renewed*; and pursued the next day. In the night the *Charming Sally* of Biddeford *wrecked* upon the Rocks, though the Weather was fine.

214. The 12th, the IIId *Course completed*, and the IVth begun. A sudden violent *gust of wind*, which as *suddenly ceased*.

215. Company *driven home* in bad weather for *want of provision*. An *alarming accident*; but without hurt to the people.—*Seamen pressed* from a vessel laden at *Portland* with *Stone* for the Edystone; but *discharged* by an order from the *Admiralty*.

216. Various interruptions; yet July 31, *Course* IVth *completed*, and the Vth begun. 5th August the work visited and Vth *Course completed*. A *Cramp applied* to remedy an accidental defect. An *additional* Boat called *The Assistant*, *Samuel* [illegible], Master, brought out her *first Cargo* of Stone; a gale of wind arose, obliging her to seek an harbour. The *Edystone Boat* also came out. *Lime* and *Puzzolana* being much *wanted*, an *Expedient* contrived to get a cask of each from on Board her. Course VI begun.

217. A *Meridian* traced on *Course* 6th. The Sea for the first time *never* having *washed over* the *work* at *high water*, this opportunity was taken to *repair* the *Pointings*. The method thereof; and observations.

218. The 9th of Aug. four vessels arrived from Portland with stone. The 11th, the VIth *Course* completing the basement was *closed* in. *Recapitulation* of this part of the work.

219. Method of *setting and fixing* the *Stones* described.

220. Further descriptions.

221. Method of making the *mortar*. *Simple Machinery* used for *bedding* the stones.

222. Further detail of the manner of setting. Application of *Wooden Wedges*.

§. 223. *Oaken*

§. 22[illegible]. [illegible] and described. The manner of *Grouting*.

2[illegible]. [illegible] VIth *course*. The method of fixing it described, [illegible]

22[illegible]. [illegible] the Author.

22[illegible]. [illegible] of the method of proceeding with Course VII, [illegible]

227. [illegible] landing the stones.

228. [illegible] the Rock [illegible] by Mr. [illegible]. Manner of [illegible] described. Those cubes might possibly have been [illegible] but in such a situation, nothing should be omitted.

229. The Author's reasons for using the *Joggles*, in *preference* of other [illegible] the work.

230. This B[illegible] intended to be a *Column* of proportionably *equal* [illegible] upon it.

231. Mr. [illegible] returned the 18th to Plymouth, leaving the Author [illegible] Course VII wholly closed. An *hard gale* arose, while working with [illegible] the Rock. Things put in the best posture. The weather [illegible] the Author returned to Plymouth. On the 28th it came [illegible].—The 29th, the Author looked out with his Telescope, and missed the *Shears*; next day confirmed; and went out to [illegible] the works, leaving orders for new Shears. The *Shears* and [illegible] gone; and also two of the *largest Stones* which had been *left* [illegible] upon the work. *Damages* to the *Windlass* and its frame. The *Buss* rode well.

232. *Richardson* sent word the 1st Sept. that the two large *Stones* could be [illegible]. The 3d, the *new Shears* set up, and the work [illegible] that had been interrupted by bad weather since the 18th.—The method of *getting up the Stones* described.

233. The weather favourable. *Course* VII *completed*. Mr. *Weston*, accompanied by the Author, went to see the 1st *stone* of the VIIIth *Course laid*; which performed, Mr. Weston returned.—The season continuing favourable, the VIIIth *Course completed* in *five days*; and on the 20th, the IXth far advanced, when the works were again interrupted by bad weather.

234. During the late favourable time, there had been uncommonly [illegible] *Tides*, which produced an *hindrance* in *shipping the Stones*. An *expedient* made use of by Mr. *Jessop*. A *malevolent intention* to retard the progress of the work *brought to Light*.

235. On the 26th the work recommenced. A *great Swell* in the *Gut* from *Easterly Winds*. Great *difficulty* and *hazard* in landing the Stones, necessary to complete the IXth Course.

236. [illegible] of going into and out of the *Gut* described.

237. [illegible] *state and progress* of the works *considered*. Being the *Eve of October*, resolved to put a *period* to the *outwork* of the Season.—The *Shears* and [illegible] taken down. An *imminent danger* escaped in getting the [illegible] on Board.

238. October 1st, the *Neptune Buss* prepared to cast off her *Moorings*. The Author, attended by Mr. Jessop and the Masons, *revisit the Rock*; and [illegible] every thing that appeared amiss. Returned to Plymouth with the Companies. The *Buss* came in the next day, and laid up for the winter.—An *incident* described.

CHAP. II. *Comprehending the Account of Transactions from* (the Author's) *leaving Plymouth in October* 1757, *to the conclusion of the working Season of* 1758.

§. 239. Tempestuous weather till March. The *great Buoy* on the Moor[illegible] *carried away*. A reward offered for recovery of the Moorings. *New Chains* bespoke.

240. The proceedings proposed to be laid before the Board of *Trinity House*. A day appointed.—The Author's work and propositions received [illegible] *Approbation* of that honourable *Corporation*.—A set of *Mooring Chains* [illegible] by that Board, and the Author desired to *acquaint them* with his *future proceedings*.

241. The *sweeping* for the moorings proving *unsuccessful*, the Author took a *Journey* to *Plymouth* to expedite that operation.

242. Reports the progress of the works at *Mill Bay*. *Express* arrives to carry him back to attend the *House* of *Commons*. *Consultation* with Mr. *Jessop* and the Seamen about the *sweeping*. *Expedients* proposed.

243. Author returned the 30th. One of the *Anchors hooked*, and *secured*. The 2d May, went out to weigh the Anchor; got it to the surface, but a fresh gale coming on, obliged them to lower it to the bottom.—Bad weather till the 11th.—In this interim a further *expedient* proposed; [illegible], and the *Buss*, after some difficulties, *moored*.

244. The Author *landed* on the Rock. Reports the *Condition* of the Work, after the Winter. All well; except the *Fender Piles*, all gone.

245. The 14th May, the *Portland Stone Work* all *finished* in the Work-[illegible]. The [illegible] *new Fender Piles* fixed, as also the *Shears*, *Windlass*, and [illegible]. The Boats loaded with Stone, and the first went out to [illegible]. All being *ready to begin*, an unforeseen *disaster* re-[illegible] works for some time.

246. The Author attended to lay the *first stone* of *this year*, but pre-[illegible] the 16th to the 23d May; when without any [illegible] and a fresh Gale obliged her to [illegible]. A *Buoy* being placed on the western anchor, [illegible]

247. [illegible] weather [illegible] 3d June. The *Buoy* of the *Anchor* then [illegible] with the *Buss*. Enquiry made at the [illegible], and two *fishing Boats* in sight.—[illegible]ed, and continued, but *without* [illegible]

248. [illegible] of the *Polperro Fishermen*. [illegible] *search* made, which [illegible] cut up for *Crab Pots* and [illegible]

§. 249. Frequent attempts to recover the Moorings; and notwithstanding a Declaration from the Seamen, that they would *not return* till they had succeeded, yet all endeavours proved *abortive*.

250. The *Chain* lately *made* in *London* arrived; and the *Corporation's Chain* from Falmouth repaired. The 1st July, the Buss failed with the *new Ground Tackle*. Was moored, and the work recommenced. Consolation for the late Disasters.

251. On the 5th July the Xth *Course completed*; but the XIth, being interrupted by bad weather, not till the 18th.

252. The 8th Aug. the *Fundamental Solid* completed, with the XIVth Course. The *Well hole* for the Stairs to be now begun, the difference of Construction described.

253. The *Entry* and *Well hole* begun with the XVth *Course*; and the weather proving good, on the 20th the XVIIIth *Course* was *completed*; which finished the *Entry* and *Doorway*. An *Accident* happened, which might have been *fatal*; but without material Damage.

254. A succession of bad weather, so that *the solid* was not *completed*, till the 24th Sept. In this interval an accident happened, by which the *Workmen* were *detained* upon the Rock, being the *only one* of the kind.—One Leg of the Shears was also unfixed by hard weather, but in this state of the Building, they could not fall: nor was any damage done, which accounts for a former accident mentioned § 232.

255. A *wish* to complete the 1st room, and make the *Building useful* to keep a *Light* thereupon, induced the Author to proceed beyond the *present* period with the Building this Year. The practicability as well as utility thereof set forth. Also the method of performing it. The proposal communicated to the *Trinity House* and the *Proprietors*.

256. The 26th Sept. *Course* XXV, being the *first* of the *Superstructure*, completed. Mode of Construction *very different* from the former. Account of it, and particularly of the *Joggles*.—*Joint Stones* necessary. Described.—Cramps necessary.

257. Method of applying the *Cramps*.

258. The 30th Sept. *Course* XXVIII, being the *first Chain Course*, was completed; as was the 2d *Chain Course*, XXIX, the next day.—The *reason* of the *Chain Courses*.—Preferable to *Cramps*, and taken from a like Construction in the *Dome* of *St. Paul's*.—Method of *leading* in the Chains.—Extreme *precaution* allowable in such a Situation, where *time* is *not* materially *lost*.

259. Oct. 2d, the *Center* for the *first floor* set up. Described. All the Stones for the floor got into, and upon the building; but, in making this Effort, the *Boat Weston* had a *narrow Escape* from a Gale arising. The Author returned to Plymouth, went out again the 5th, and saw the two first Stones of the Floor set. The *Shears* and *Windlass taken down*, as being done with this Season.—Broken weather till the 7th; *materials* arrived for *covering* the Building, and *stores* for *furnishing* the same. The floor proceeded with, but foul weather appearing, every thing put in the best posture of defence.—The Author returned to Plymouth, leaving *Orders* with Mr. *Jessop*. A *Storm* ensued.

260. Next Morning, Oct. 9th, the Author *looked out* with his *Telescope*, but the Air being very hazy, could discern the House and the Sea *breaking over it*, but *nothing* of the *Buss*. The afternoon somewhat less hazy, but no appearance of the *Buss*; which created *Apprehensions*.—The 10th, Air more clear; distinct view of the Building. The *Buss really gone*. This a day of *double regret*, as it brought the Author a *negative* upon his proposal, for exhibiting a Light from the House during the Winter, § 255.

261. The same Evening at 10, Mr. *Jessop* returned to Plymouth from *Dartmouth Harbour*, where the *Buss* lay. Described the particulars of this *Storm* since the 8th.—The 11th, *John Bowden* sent to Dartmouth to take *Charge* of the *Buss*. Every thing prepared for the Author to go out the next Morning with a set of Workmen, to do what they could in *securing things* against the *Winter*. A *Gale of Wind* at *East* came on, which rendered it to no purpose to attempt to go out.—This continuing for several days, brought home the *Buss* on Friday the 13th, and on Sunday came on a Storm, and a continuance of bad weather. The Author left the necessary orders, and departed for London the 25th Oct. 1758.

CHAP. III. *Containing an Account of the Transactions of the* Fourth *and* last Year's Work, *to the finishing of the Building in the Year* 1759.

§. 262. The *Lantern*, *Balcony Rails*, &c. made in *London*. Bad weather at Plymouth, which was terminated by a *violent Storm*; so that the works on the Rock could not be visited till *March*. *Transport Buoy gone*, as well as the *Buoy* on the *Moorings*, and the South *Fender Pile*. All the *work* of the Building *firm* as it was left; and the *Triangle standing*, with the Stone suspended; yet a large Stone washed from the top.—Seamen swept for the Moorings. A further *expedient* proposed, and *Rewards* offered, but *all ineffectual*. A new *Chain ordered*; and an old Chain and *Anchors* procured.

263. *Iron Pillars* for the Lantern, cast by Mr. *Prickett*. *Copper Sash Frames*, by Mr. *Kinnan*. *Lantern framed*, and *Balcony Rails* made by Mr. *Broadbent*.

264. The Author repeatedly attended the *Trinity Board*, who expressed their approbation of his proceedings. *Consulted* upon the proposal of an *Optician*, respecting the *figure* of the *glass* of the *lantern*.

265. The Author arrived at Plymouth 22d June; found all the *stone work prepared*, and all in forwardness. A violent *Storm* the 13th had damaged the *Neptune Buss*. Repaired, and with the Seamen then in Search of the Moorings. Five of the *best hands* demanding more *wages discharged*.—A *Bridle Cable* and *Plumb*, *requested* by the Seamen, and *prepared*.—

ERRATA.

Page.	Line.		FOR	READ
25	17	— —	§. 42 — — — — —	§. 49. N.B. This, with the numbers of the five following Sections, are by mistake *repeated*; and would be well to be distinguished by an * as *printed* in the table of Contents.
28	14	— —	60 — — — — —	70. N.B. This also, with the numbers of the nine following Sections, are by a similar mistake *repeated*; the * is therefore to be applied as in the Contents.
4[illegible]	—	[illegible] Title	FIRST PROCEEDINGS *towards* REBUILDING.	FIRST JOURNEY *to* PLYMOUTH. N.B. This running Title should also have been prefixed to pages, 47, 49, and 51.
[illegible]	19	— —	— — — —	78. This number wants prefixing to this Section.
[illegible]	6	[illegible] —	— — — — —	103. This number to be prefixed.
7[illegible]	[illegible]	— —	1st of Aug. — — — — —	5th of August.
[illegible]	[illegible]	— —	Thursday — — — — —	Tuesday.
1[illegible]	—	[illegible]	SEQUEL *of the first Season's* OUTWORK — —	*Transactions of the First* WINTER.
1[illegible]	[illegible]	— —	3[illegible] — — — —	309.

INTRODUCTION.

INTRODUCTION.

THE building of Watch Towers, now called *Lighthouſes*, for the direction of mariners, has doubtleſs, from the obvious utility thereof, had its riſe in the earlieſt ages; and in ſeveral inſtances has been the object of royal magnificence. None however was ſo much celebrated amongſt the ancients, as the *Pharos* of *Alexandria*, which has been accounted one of the ſeven wonders of the world. This famous tower was built by the PTOLEMIES kings of *Egypt* and ſucceſſors of ALEXANDER; it is ſuppoſed to have been finiſhed about 283 years before the Chriſtian era, that is, 2070 years ſince, and had the name of *PHAROS* from the iſland; upon a rock at the eaſtern end of which it was built, ſo that its walls were waſhed by the ſea. It was a ſquare edifice of a white hard ſtone, and was built in a ſtyle aſtoniſhingly ſuperb. According to the *Nubian* Geographer, a writer of the 12th century*, its height was 300 cubits; that is, 547 feet Engliſh meaſure; and a fire upon the top of it was conſtantly kept burning in the night, to light ſuch ſhips as ſailed near theſe dangerous coaſts, which are ſaid to be full of ſands, and ſhelves of rocks: and according to JOSEPHUS†, it could be ſeen at the diſtance of 300 *ſtadia*; that is 41½ *Engliſh* miles‡.

THE ſize of its baſe is not ſo well aſcertained; and indeed, as a Lighthouſe, it is not ſo material. A ſcholiaſt on LUCIAN takes upon him to aſſert, that it was a *ſtadium* in baſe! but this muſt have been a random ſtroke; as it would make the *Pharos* to have been greater in *bulk* than the great *Pyramid*, and therefore in that reſpect taking place of it as one of the *Wonders*. The ſame ſcholiaſt alſo aſſerts, that it could be ſeen at the diſtance of 100 miles; but this is quite impoſſible: for a tower 547 feet high, cannot be ſeen above 29 miles from the ſurface of the ſea; the reſt of the diſtance mentioned by JOSEPHUS, muſt be obtained by an elevation of the obſerver's eye above the ſea; which at the height of 111 feet, would enable him to gain a ſight of the fire upon the tower at the diſtance of 300 *ſtadia*: and an elevation of this kind we may very well ſuppoſe to be afforded from the tops of the maſts of their largeſt ſhips, eſpecially when lifted up upon the top of the waves of the ſea: whereas to ſee the fire at the diſtance of 100 miles would not only require the tower itſelf to be 560 *yards* in height; but the obſerver's eye to be elevated as much: a ſituation which does not ſeem afforded in this flat country.

JOSEPHUS in another place, ſpeaking of a magnificent building called the *Phaſael* at *Jeruſalem*§, ſays it was 40 cubits in length and breadth, and about 90 cubits in height; and in its appearance reſembled the Tower upon the *Pharos*, which gave a light to thoſe who were ſailing to *Alexandria*: but in its *circuit* it was *much bigger*.——According to this account the Pharos could not be ſo much as 73 feet

* Geog. Nub. p. 94. *Paris* Latin Edit. 1619.

† Joſeph. Bell. Judaic. l. iv. ch. 11.

‡ It perhaps may not be amiſs to obſerve, that this reduction of the ancient meaſures to thoſe of *England*, is on the ſuppoſition that the *Egyptian* cubit, and which I underſtand was likewiſe the cubit uſed all over *Paleſtine*, *Aſia Minor*, &c. conſiſted of 21,888 inches nearly; as has been aſcertained from the pillar ſtill remaining on an iſland in the *Nile*, upon which the cubits ſuppoſed to be marked thereon 2000 years ago, are ſtill uſed for the original purpoſe of meaſuring the height of its inundations. For though the *Nilometer* now ſtanding is ſaid to have been erected in the 8th or 9th century by OMAR, yet it is ſuppoſed to be an exact copy, in the upper part at leaſt, of the ancient one. And there is ſtill the leſs doubt that this was the true meaſure of the cubit, as this remarkable circumſtance has been noticed concerning it; that 400 of thoſe cubits making a *ſtadium*, 500 ſuch *ſtadia* make a degree of the meridian; agreeing with ſufficient exactneſs to the modern meaſures, to ſhew that this meaſure of the cubit was not a mere arbitrary aſſumption; but intended to be the 200,000th part of a degree: The baſe of the great *Pyramid*, being a *ſtadium* of this meaſure.

§ Joſeph. Bell. Jud. l. v. ch. 3.

in base, so that if the walls of it were 20 feet in thickness upon the ground, the clear hollow area it would contain could be only 53 feet square; a space in appearance (though there may be supposed rooms above each other) unequal to the containing a *garrison*, that CÆSAR is said to have thrown into it; that by commanding the narrow passage by it into one of the harbours, he secured by his ships the necessary supplies *.

It however is not difficult to conceive how in this article JOSEPHUS might be mistaken, with regard to the relative bulk of the *Pharos*; for as he describes the *Phasaël*; viz. that after rising a considerable part of its height upon a large base, it was contracted on all four sides, by a broad platform with battlements round it; and that in the middle of this area there rose up a second building to a considerable height further; and as this description entirely agrees with that which the *Nubian* Geographer gives of the Pharos; it is probable the resemblance JOSEPHUS had in view, was chiefly this of the outward form: now if JOSEPHUS had been in use to see the *Phasaël* in the neighbourhood of *Jerusalem*, and the *Pharos* at a distance only; its height being in appearance lost by distance, he would suppose the circuit of its base to be less, in proportion to the less *apparent* bulk of the Pharos; for, if the *Pharos* was in reality double the *Phasaël* in bulk (as it probably might have been) yet as it was more than three times the height of the Phasaël, JOSEPHUS would be liable to have been deceived in the comparison of bulk or *circuit*; unless he had measured them both, or judged otherwise than from distant views.

THIS magnificent structure, called even by CÆSAR *wonderful*, was the work of SOSTRATUS of *Cnidus*: and we are informed by PLINY †, that PTOLEMY very nobly permitted the name of the architect to be inscribed upon the building; who accordingly cut the following inscription upon the solid stone. SOSTRATUS THE CNIDIAN, THE SON OF DEXIPHANES, TO THE GODS PRESERVERS, FOR THE BENEFIT OF THOSE WHO USE THE SEA.

LUCIAN it seems has dropped a passage that has given a different turn to this business; which I should not have mentioned, had it not been to rescue the great architect from so invidious an aspersion. LUCIAN, though a satirist, and joker of those times, in the present case seems very grave; for in teaching his pupil the art of writing history, he bids him not to look out to please his cotemporaries, but to write for future times; and as an example bids him consider what the *Cnidian* artist did ‡. When he had finished the work, he engraved his own name upon the stone, and smearing it over with mortar, he engraved upon that, the name of the king who then reigned; knowing that would happen, which did happen; that in a short period of years, the letters falling off with the mortar, there would come to view the inscription before set forth.

This account of the matter, though resting upon the single authority of LUCIAN, yet accords with that propensity of human nature, to lower all great characters, so much better than that of PLINY, that it seems currently adopted by the modern compilers of ancient history §; and indeed the story tells well enough in common conversation; yet as it appears to contain the evident marks of falsity, arising from the impracticability thereof, I have therefore no doubt but that PLINY's account is the truth.

Let us for a moment imagine the work to be done in modern *London* instead of ancient *Alexandria*: Can any one conceive it possible to get so many letters engraved of so large a size, and so deep, as to be suitable to so lofty a building; without its being known to several persons concerned in the execution; and in consequence soon getting to the ears of the king? Besides, it would not be easy to make use of any plaster or partial coating, the surface and colour of which could not be distinguished from that of the stone, in those critical examinations, that a public building of such *eclat* would unavoidably undergo upon its first completion. In reality the king could have little doubt of his own name being celebrated to poste-

* Cæsar Com. de Bell. Civ. l. iii. sect. 112. † Plin. l. xxxvi. chap. 12. ‡ Lucian de scribend. hist. § 52.

§ See *Dissertation sur le Phare d'Alexandrie*, par MOUNTFAUCON. Acad. Royal des Inscriptions et Belles Lettres. Vol. vi. p. 577, dated 7th Jan. 1721.

rity

rity as the finiſher of ſo great and uſeful a work; this being generally aſcribed to PTOLEMY PHILADELPHUS, the ſame who founded the *Alexandrian* Library.

IN reſpect to the expence of it, all ancient authors agree that it coſt 800 *talents*; but as modern authors differ very greatly in the value of thoſe talents; and we are furthermore at a loſs to judge what proportion ſubſiſted betwixt the value of *work*, and that of *money* in thoſe times, compared with our own; we are as much unable to compare its coſt, as we are its real bulk, with any of the ſtructures of modern times *.

AN edifice of ſo great a ſize, ſo well built, and of ſuch durable materials, as this building is deſcribed to have conſiſted of, one might very well have expected to be exiſting at this day: but this is not the caſe; there is indeed ſtill a Lighthouſe, but of a much more humble form, riſing out of the midſt of an irregular caſtle or garriſon, kept in this iſland, and which is now called *Farion.*——Upon what occaſion this famous building was deſtroyed or met its deſtruction, hiſtory is, as far as we know, totally ſilent: but the *Nubian* Geographer mentioned before, ſpeaks of it, not only as a building ſubſiſting in his time, but in perfect good condition: for, he ſays, there is nothing like it in the whole world, for the fineneſs of the edifice, or the ſtrength of its ſtructure; for, beſides that it is built of the hardeſt *Tiburtine* ſtones, theſe ſtones are alſo joined together with melted lead, and ſo firmly connected that they cannot be looſened from one another; for the ſea beats againſt the very ſtones wherewith it is built, upon the north ſide †.

ABULFEDA an *Arabic* writer who lived in the 14th century, amongſt the ſtupendous monuments of *Egypt* ‡, deſcribes the *Pharos* as being 180 cubits high; that is 120 cubits leſs than it had been deſcribed by former authors; and particularly the *Nubian* Geographer, who ſeems the moſt particular, and beſt founded: ſo that whether ſome decay happening in the upper works (where indeed it was moſt likely to happen) had occaſioned its height to be reduced, as the leaſt expenſive mode of repair; or that ABULFEDA meaſured by ſome other cubit than the ancient one; or that he has ſpoke of the dimenſions at random, or by hearſay, is now uncertain: but ſtill, as the lower and moſt ſolid parts were remaining about 400 years ago, it is evident that ſome extraordinary fate muſt have happened to it ſince that time; which cannot be accounted for merely by the neglect of it, conſequent upon the ruin of that empire. To have pulled it down would have been a work of ſo much labour, that even a wanton deſire of deſtruction would have been foiled in the attempt: and it is ſcarce poſſible to ſee that the demolition thereof could anſwer any real purpoſe. Nor can we ſuppoſe that it has been undermined by the ſea's gaining upon the rocks it was built upon; as thoſe are ſaid to be of *granite*. It ſeems therefore the moſt likely that it has been deſtroyed by the ſhake of an earthquake, at the ſame time producing a ſubſidence: and to this, the obſervations of modern travellers give ſome ſort of countenance; as it is ſaid that the foundations or ruins of art, are ſtill ſeen amongſt the rocks of the iſland *Farion*, under the ſurface of the water. At any rate we have authentic teſtimony of this ſtupendous tower's having ſubſiſted for a period of 1600 years §.

* The computations of the value of thoſe 800 talents in Engliſh money, by different authors, differ no leſs than from 330,000 to 50,000 pounds ſterling.

† The height of 300 cubits mentioned by this author, he leaves in no doubt, as to their being the ancient cubit; becauſe, he alſo ſays, the height of this building is 100 *ſtatures* of man; ſo that taking the cubit, as before, at 21,888 inches, the ſtature of man will come out 5 feet 5 ⅔ inches; agreeable to the ſtature of the *Egyptians*, which is ſaid to be rather low than tall.

‡ ABULFEDA's deſcription of *Egypt* tranſlated from the Arabic into Latin by *Profeſſor* MICHAELIS.

§ ABULFEDA mentions, that there was formerly, viz. about the beginning of *Mahomedaniſm*, in this Lighthouſe, a *Speculum* formed of *Chineſe ſteel*, in which the ſhipping could be ſeen in the port of *Conſtantinople*; but of which it was deprived by the intriguing practices of the *Chriſtians.*——That ſuch a Speculum *might* be formed, and erected with ſuch *intent*, is not to be diſputed: but *Conſtantinople* being diſtant from *Alexandria* no leſs than 700 miles, as it was impoſſible for an obſerver at the former to ſee the Pharos, ſo it was as impoſſible for a perſon on the Pharos to ſee any thing at Conſtantinople; it being equally impoſſible that any thing could be ſeen by reflexion, which an obſerver at the Speculum could not ſee by a direct view: and therefore if ſuch a *Speculum* ever exiſted, its removal may be accounted for, without having recourſe to the *intriguing arts* of Chriſtians, or others; namely by its not *anſwering the end* for which it was made.

FROM

FROM this Lighthouse, as the most celebrated, structures of this kind have generally obtained the same name; as the *Faro di Messina* and others: but the most remarkable amongst the moderns is the *Tour de Corduan* situated near the coast of *France*, upon a small island near the mouth of the river *Garonne* in the bottom of the bay of *Biscay*.

THIS LIGHTHOUSE was begun above 200 years ago, in the reign of HENRY II. of *France*; was 26 years in building; was finished in the reign of HENRY IV. in the year 1610; and was the work of LOUIS DE FOIX a celebrated *French* architect.

THE *island* upon which it is built is dry at low water, and wholly covered with the tide at high water. It is a bare rock, the upper surface of which, except its natural asperities, is nearly level, and at low water is about 500 fathoms in length, from north to south, and 250 fathoms in breadth from east to west. It is surrounded with detached rocks, which giving a resistance to the seas, they break upon them in blowing weather, with an horrible noise: and the access to this tower is rendered very difficult by the great *surf* that generally breaks upon it; so that nothing larger than boats of three tons burthen can approach it with safety; and that only by one passage of sixty fathoms wide, reaching within 100 fathoms of the tower, where there is a sand, upon which the boats ground at low water.

ON the level rocky surface above described, and nearly in the middle of the island, the building is founded; and the base fills a circle of no less than 135 feet in diameter, *English* measure.——Upon the whole extent of this base, the work is carried up entirely solid with masonry (except the opening of the stone stairs) to the height of eight feet, or thereabouts, which I suppose to be nearly on a level with the surface of the sea at high water. A cavity is then left in the middle of the area, of above 20 feet square, to form the cellar, and a fresh water cistern; this rises eight feet more, including the arches that cover it. The remainder of the area is built up quite solid with masonry (except the opening before mentioned) to the level of the top of the arches; the whole there making one regular floor or platform; but as the outside surface is built sloping, or *battering* (as it is termed) from the perpendicular, the diameter of the greatest circle is there reduced to 125 feet.——The stone stair-case begun, and carried up in the solid, from about four feet high above the rock, to the platform already described, is on the east side, being that next the shore. The ascent from the rock to the beginning of the stone stairs, is on the outside, by a wooden ladder, and the entry is shut by strong wooden doors, on the outside.

Within the circumference of this platform, at the distance of 12½ feet, is drawn a circle of 100 feet diameter; and the space of 12½ feet between the inner and outward circles, limits the thickness of a circular wall; which is carried up somewhat battering on the outside, and perpendicular within, to the height of 12 feet, being 11 feet thick at the top; which circular figure, renders this wall, which in itself is so stout, still more able to resist the action of the western seas, in like manner as the parapet of a *Mole*.——There seems in the whole building no idea of defence against the attacks of an enemy; yet to defend the entry against small thieves and plunderers, a lodgment, in fortification called a *Machicoulis*, is built upon the wall over the stairs.

IN the middle of this clear area of 100 feet diameter, the base of the tower is begun upon a circle, the diameter of which is 50 feet; and the building is carried up from thence, by diminishing stories, to the height of 115 feet; at which level is the base of the lantern, which originally was of stone, and domed over; the doming being supported upon eight stone pillars or *mullions*, with openings between them for the passage of the light; and it was finished above, with small spire-like ornaments.

THERE being according to this description a space of 25 feet between the inside of the circular wall, and the outside of the tower; this space is in part occupied by several small rooms, which were built within the parapet, and served as lodgings for four light-keepers; and also for store-houses, for the reception of the different articles necessary for their own maintenance, as well as for the light itself: so that

that the light-keepers having nothing to do in the ſeveral other apartments of the tower (the cellar excepted) but to go up a circular ſtair-caſe, carried up (partly in the thickneſs of the wall, and partly on the outſide) from the level of the platform, to the commencement of the lantern; the different apartments of the tower are by that means preſerved clean, and free from incumbrance.

THOSE different ſtories and apartments being highly finiſhed, and ornamented within and without, a further deſcription of a ſubject but little known in *England*, will I doubt not be agreeable to my reader.——There are four different ſtories that principally diſtinguiſh themſelves on the outſide, and are ornamented with columns, of different *orders*. Thoſe of the baſe ſtory are *Doric*, the next ſeem to be a ſpecies of the *Ionic*, the third are *Corinthian*, and the uppermoſt, which ornament the lantern, are of the *Compoſite* order.

THE principal room on the ground floor is a great Hall of 22 feet ſquare, by 20 feet high, to which are annexed two wardrobes, and other conveniencies; the whole arched over. Above this, on the firſt floor is the *king*'s apartment, comprehending a grand *Saloon* 21 feet ſquare, and 20 feet high; a *Veſtibule*, two wardrobes, and other conveniencies, which are arched over with flat elliptical arches. The next floor above, or ſecond chamber floor, is taken up by the *Chapel*, where maſs is performed, as often as the weather will permit the officiating prieſt to attend. This is a circular room covered with a dome, the internal diameter of which is 31 feet; its height from the floor to the top of the cornice of the *Corinthian* pilaſters, wherewith the inſide of the chapel is ornamented, is 22½ feet, and the dome being higher than hemiſpherical, makes the whole height near 40 feet. The inſide of the dome is a rich *Moſaic*, and receives light from eight *luthern* windows regularly diſpoſed. There is alſo a circular opening in the crown of the dome, of four feet diameter, not open to the ſky as that of the *Pantheon*; but being ſurrounded with a circular baluſtrade, and covered with the inferior lantern, it will have much the ſame appearance as the dome of *St. Paul*'s, when looking up from the floor on the inſide.

The diameter of this third ſtory, or inferior lantern, is 14 feet within. It is ſurrounded with a circular parapet, forming a *Balcony* round it; the internal diameter whereof is 21 feet, and it forms the *cap* of the ſolid ſtone cover of the dome of the chapel. This lantern is enriched on the outſide with eight Corinthian *Pilaſters*, applied to the eight ſupporting pillars, or mullions, between which are eight glazed windows, 2½ feet wide, and ſeven feet high. The inſide, which in this ſtory is leſs ornamented than it is without, is 20 feet up to the ſquare; and being covered with an hemiſpherical cupola, its whole height is 27 feet; and it is cloſed with a ſolid ſtone arch, which ſerves as a baſement to the lantern for the light.——The lantern juſt deſcribed ſeems deſtined to no particular uſe; ſerving only to give, by an agreeable figure, and a juſt gradation of diminution, the required *Elevation* of the principal *light*: it may however be conceived to be of occaſional uſe; for being glazed, a lamp or lamps, candles, &c. may be placed in any of its windows, at pleaſure, and give a full light in any direction, for any particular ſervice for which it may be wanted.

The original lantern for the *light* was of a diameter ſomewhat exceeding five feet clear, within, and nine feet without; and, as already ſaid, was externally ornamented with eight pillars of the *Compoſite* order. The unglazed openings between the ſupporting pillars, being but little bigger than the ſolid mullions, thoſe openings therefore could ſcarcely exceed twelve inches wide in the *clear*. The height of this lantern was 17 feet to the top of the cupola, which was of ſtone; and there, a perforation was left in the middle of it about 18 inches in diameter, by which the ſmoke of the fire might aſcend into another little turret of 2½ feet external diameter; and paſs out of its openings, which ſomewhat reſembled *pigeon-holes*. This little turret was capped over with a ſolid ſtone cupola, upon which a ſmall ſtone ſpire or pinnacle was erected, that terminated the whole at the height of 31 feet above the floor of the lantern of the light. The total height of the building therefore was 146 feet *Engliſh* meaſure, above the baſe of the tower; and 162 feet above the ſurface of the rock.

BESIDES the ornaments already described, the king's apartment was decorated with the arms of *France*, and also with the busts of HENRY II. and HENRY IV. in niches: likewise with a figure in stone representing MARS, with his proper attributes; and a female figure in stone, holding a palm in one hand, and a crown in the other. The bust of the architect LOUIS DE FOIX was placed in the chapel: to which the busts of LOUIS XIV. and of LOUIS XV. were added in the year 1735.

I have here described the ornamental parts as being of the *Greek* and *Roman* orders, to which indeed they the most nearly refer; but a number of ornamental parts and mouldings, derived from the *Gothic* architecture, are intermixed; such as turrets, pinnacles, &c. the composition of the whole is however in a style really grand and striking.

M. BELIDOR, from whose description and draughts* I have extracted what relates to this tower, seems to blame the architect; and much to lament that so great a profusion of ornaments should have been bestowed upon so inhospitable a place †. But here it seems to me, that M. BELIDOR somewhat mistakes the matter. Had this building been erected at the cost of private adventurers; their endeavours no doubt ought to have merited the approbation of their fellow citizens, though they had contented themselves with merely doing what was *necessary*; provided they had not stopped short of doing that in the *best way*: but as this work appears to have been undertaken and carried on by a Series of *Kings*, who probably had the *Pharos* of *Alexandria* in view; the *Tour de Cordoüan* must have been intended by them, not only as a work of public utility, but as a work of *Magnificence*: for, according to Mr. POPE, " 'tis only *use* " that sanctifies expence."

TO the above account it is necessary to add, that the fire made in the lantern was of *oak wood*, deposited in a kind of large *chafing-dish*, elevated about six feet above the floor of the lantern; and that the bulk of the fire must necessarily exceed the bulk of the mullions; otherwise, when a mullion interposed to the eye of the spectator at a distance, he would perceive little, or rather, would not be able to perceive any light: this, in consequence produced a larger bulk of fire than otherwise might have been necessary; so that after the period of a century from the finishing of the building, it was found, that the fire had *calcined* the inside of the walls, and to prevent its falling ‡, the *French* court ordered the lantern to be taken down in the year 1717, and the fire to be lighted *below*.——The change however had not long subsisted before the whole marine complained of their not being able to see the light at sea, at the distance of *two* leagues §, as they used to do: and in the year 1720 this occasioned M. LE COMTE DE TOULOUSE, Admiral of France, and M. LE MARECHAL D'ASFELD, Director of the Fortifications, to give the superintendence of this tower to M. BITRI, Engineer in Chief at *Bourdeaux*; who diligently applied himself to establish the light at its ancient height, and to remove the inconveniencies of the former; one of the most material, being the bulkiness of the *stone* mullions, which stopped a great part of the light that the fire gave.

HE therefore contrived, upon the platform which was the base of the former, to erect a lantern or cage of *iron*, consisting of four principal pillars, and supporting a cupola above, which was finished with a large ball, and a *vane*, 36 feet above the platform; and was compleated in the year 1727, with all the success that was expected; after the public had shifted with having the fire below for the term of ten years. ‖

* [illegible] *Hydraulique*, Tom. iv. page 151.

† [illegible] fâcheux, qu'un aussi bel édifice soit placé dans le lieu le plus ingrat du monde, qui ne méritoit point assuré- [illegible] qu'on y a faite; mais voilà comme en usent assez ordinairement, ceux qui ne sont qu' architectes; qui mettent dans [illegible] par-tout, sans trop se soucier de remplir l'objet principal." BELIDOR, Tom. iv. p. 152.

‡ [illegible] it appears that this tower is built of a calcareous freestone, such as *Portland, Bath Stone*, &c.

§ [illegible] BELIDOR, Tom. iv. p. 153.

‖ [illegible], that this entire change of *principle* in the re-construction of the lantern, took place many years after [illegible] the *Edystone*.

THERE

THERE is one thing defcribed of this new lantern, that fhould not pafs unnoticed; as it was I apprehend, the firft attempt of the kind. The lantern being entirely open, the fmoke could efcape on all fides: inftead therefore of compofing a funnel in the upper works as before, or forming an hollow cupola internally; the area of the great circle of the cieling of the cupola, was made the bafe of an inverted cone, whofe *Apex* projected downwards about three feet: the entire floping furface of this cone was then covered with tin plates, which becoming fo many reflecting furfaces, ferved to increafe the light of the fire, and made it to be perceived at a greater diftance *.

THE CONSTRUCTION of a Lighthoufe upon the *Edyftone Rock*, has from its very origin, been confidered as one of the artificial wonders of this kingdom: and fo great was the curiofity of the public, at the completion of the prefent building, in the year 1759; and fuch were the numbers, by the interceffion and recommendation of friends, that for fome years after, flocked daily to fee the model; that, to avoid having the whole of my time confumed in fatisfying their curiofity, I found myfelf under a neceffity of deputing Mrs. SMEATON, to fhew and explain the model. I was honoured alfo with the command of his *prefent* MAJESTY, to fhew and explain the fame to himfelf, and our GRACIOUS QUEEN: when his MAJESTY fhewed fuch a degree of attention to, and criticifm thereon, as I have fcarcely met with from any of his fubjects. It was alfo exhibited to the late PRINCESS DOWAGER OF WALES, and the DUKE OF CUMBERLAND, at their efpecial requefts; and the late DUKE OF YORK was pleafed to honour the works themfelves with his infpection, while they were carrying on at *Plymouth*.

The feeming avidity that the public fhewed to be made acquainted with the detail of the conftruction of this building, concurred with other confiderations, that I will prefently mention, in determining me, to liften to the wifhes of my friends, in publifhing an account thereof; together with fuch matters, as in point of utility or curiofity related thereto, and might be acceptable: but nothing more effectually weighed in my mind, than the earneft requeft of the gentlemen who employed me in the work itfelf; and more efpecially as this was ftrengthened by the fame requeft, from feveral gentlemen of the *Trinity Houfe*; that I might publifh an account of my proceedings; together with as much as I had learnt concerning the former buildings; to the end, that if any future unforefeen accident fhould unhappily caufe the deftruction of the prefent edifice, pofterity might not be at a lofs for the difcovery of the errors and imperfections both of the prefent and former buildings; fo as to avoid or purfue the principles already followed, as the improved *genius* and fkill of the age fhould judge to be moft expedient.

It is indeed as natural for me to wifh, there may never be any occafion to refort to this treatife for *that* End; as it would be prefumptuous to fay there never could. He only who firft created the atoms, can afcertain what is the *full* extent of thofe powers, that may poffibly be combined, towards the deftruction of the mafs; but with refpect to myfelf, it would furely be more creditable that the building fhould be permanent, than that it fhould be faid to be well contrived, and the means of its reftoration well defcribed: and further, though the fituation of this building is fo peculiar, that there may not in the whole world be an occafion of erecting a ftructure *perfectly fimilar*; yet I have myfelf always found, that exact accounts of buildings which were in any degree remarkable, and actually executed, were much more inftructive to my mind, than *fyftematical* writings †: and when a new method of operation, or a new

* We are told by the fame author, that in *fact* it had this effect; but it would have been more fatisfactory if we had been told, how *long* it continued to have that effect: as a reflecting furface placed directly above the fire, and expofed to the fmoke, muft be expected in a little time to get fuch a tarnifh, as could not eafily be rubbed off: and it may be a further *query*, whether the fuperiority of the light, might not altogether proceed from the leffening of the interpofing folids, and from their having a fire grate containing 225 lb. *French* weight, of *pit coals*, which are faid to be laid on at once, and to laft the whole night; in lieu of a much fmaller fire of *oak wood*; (which though it gave a great flame for the time, yet is faid fcarcely to have lafted three hours) rather than from the reflection of the *tin plates*.

† Previous to my entering upon the building of the *Edyftone Lighthoufe*, I perufed PRICE's account of *Salifbury Cathedral*, and the *Parentalia* of Sir CHRISTOPHER WREN, with particular fatisfaction: and though another ftone for the bafe for the ftatue of CZAR PETER may not be wanted, amongft all the monarchs of *Europe*, yet the account given of that *great* operation by CARBURI, cannot but infpire every artift that reads it, with new ideas, accompanied by a wifh that it had fallen to his own fhare to execute the fame.

Idea

Idea is once ſent forth, it is impoſſible to ſay, to how many good purpoſes it may by ingenious men be applied.

IN conſequence of my determination to publiſh; ſome progreſs was made in the preſent work, between the time of compleating the building, and the year 1763; and his MAJESTY having ſignified his pleaſure to honour the deſign with his patronage, ſeveral drawings were prepared, and engraven, ſome of which were executed by the late celebrated Mr. EDWARD ROOKER: but by the time matters were brought into this train, I found myſelf ſo exceedingly preſſed with buſineſs in my profeſſion of a *civil Engineer*; and this being ſhortly after ſucceeded by an appointment, to be one of the receivers of the *Derwentwater Eſtate* for *Greenwich Hoſpital* †; that, together with the hurry naturally attending the commencement of ſuch an appointment, obliged me to ſuſpend at that time, the further proſecution of the ſubject; and the conſequent ſucceſſion of engagements, not only in this, but at the ſame time in ſome of the principal undertakings in this kingdom, in my line of profeſſion, which called me forth *almoſt* againſt my will ‡, put a total ſtop to any further proceeding upon the deſcription of the *Edyſtone Lighthouſe*, till the year 1783; when a ſevere attack upon my health rendered it adviſeable, for the *preſervation of life*, to deſiſt from entering upon any *freſh* undertakings; by which means at the end of that year, I had ſo far got myſelf cleared of the preſſure of former engagements, and was ſo far recovered in point of health, as ſeriouſly to begin to think once more of re-commencing my deſign.

I ſhall now proceed to give an account of the *Edyſtone Rocks*, and circumſtances relative thereto, principally from my own obſervations on the ſpot, during the time of erecting the *preſent* Lighthouſe; and of *former Buildings thereon*, ſo far as at this time I am able to collect the particulars.

† This aroſe from the patronage of the Earl of EGMONT, then firſt Lord of the *Admiralty*, to whom I had not the honour of being perſonally known; and the good offices of my much honoured friend the preſent Lord HOWE, then one of the Lords, and now *firſt* Lord of the *Admiralty*.

‡ In the ſpring of the year 1767 the *Speaker's Warrant* was ſerved upon me to *oblige* me to attend the Houſe of Commons, upon the propoſition of the *Firth and Clyde Canal*, then propoſed to be made from ſea to ſea in the ſouth of *Scotland*.

BOOK I. CHAPTER I.

CONTAINING

A General Account of the EDYSTONE ROCKS.

1. THE ſubject I have before me, will I conceive be rendered more perſpicuous, by beginning with a general deſcription of the *Edyſtone Rocks*, as they exiſt in nature, independently of any building; as this will at once explain the ſource and reaſon of thoſe difficulties, that muſt neceſſarily ariſe in the conſtruction of an edifice upon them.

Name.

2. THE *Edyſtone Rocks* are ſuppoſed to have got this appellation from the great variety of contrary *Sets* of the tide or current amongſt and in the vicinity thereof; both upon the tide of *Flood*, and the tide of *Ebb:* and this uncertainty of the current, would be ſtill further increaſed, from the following circumſtances, to thoſe who might not formerly be fully acquainted with the general *Set* of the *Channel-Tide* in theſe parts.

3. THE turn of the tide to the eaſtward from the weſt, and the contrary; that is to ſay, *up* channel and *down*, not happening at the time of high and low water, as is commonly the caſe in tide rivers; but the change of direction or time of *Still Water*, being when the water has flowed to half its height from low water, and when it has fallen from high water to half its ebb, it is ſaid to change its direction at *Half Tide*; and the technical term for this diſpoſition of the tides is, that they are ſaid to run *Tide and Half Tide:* and it would be ſo in this diſtrict of the channel, whether there were any rocks here to interpoſe and diſturb the regular *Set* of the tide, or not: which compounded with the particular Sets, occaſioned by the interpoſition of this *Congeries* of irregular rocks, makes the currents in reality ſo irregular, that there is much need of a knowledge of the local ſituation, to ſhun the danger of coming near them; and therefore they may very properly be termed (as they are) the *Edyſtone* Rocks.

Situation.

4. THE Edyſtone Rocks are ſituated nearly S. S. W. from the middle of *Plymouth Sound*, according to the *true* meridian; which I always mean when not otherwiſe particularly expreſſed; that is, allowing two points of variation (as in the preſent times) of the north end of the magnetic needle to the weſtward; this will make their bearing by the compaſs, from the middle of the Sound, now, at or about S. W. and the diſtance, as nearly as I can collect it from obſervations, is 12½ miles; and from the ſame point in the Sound to the Jetty Head called the *Barbican* in the port of Plymouth is 1½ mile more, which makes the diſtance of the Edyſtone from the port of Plymouth to be nearly 14 miles. See Map of the Coaſts, N° 2.

The promontory called *Ram-Head* is the neareſt point of land to the Edyſtone, which bears from thence ſouth, ſcarcely one point weſt, diſtant about 10 miles; and conſequently by the compaſs is nearly S. W. b. S.——Thoſe rocks are nearly in a line, but ſomewhat within that line, which joins the *Start*, and the *Lizard* points: and as they lie nearly in the direction of veſſels coaſting down and up the channel, they muſt, before a lighthouſe was eſtabliſhed thereon, have been very dangerous, and often fatal to ſhips under ſuch circumſtances; and many rich ſhips and other veſſels, have in former times been actually lost upon those rocks, particularly such as were homeward bound from foreign Ports: it being even now, a common thing in foggy and thick hazy weather, for homeward-bound ships, from long foreign voyages, to make the *Edystone Lighthouse*, as the first point of land of *Great Britain*; so that in the night, and nearly at high water, when the whole ranges of these rocks are covered, the most careful mariner might run his ship upon them, if nothing was placed there by way of warning.

5. I WILL by this time suppose my reader to have also laid before him the chart N° 1, of the *Seas surrounding* the Edystone lighthouse; from which he will see, that a line drawn from the *Lizard* point, to the nearest point of land upon the coast of *France* towards *Ushant*, will form the openings of the headlands of the *British Channel*, into the *Bay* of *Biscay* and the *Atlantic* Ocean; these headlands being distant from each other about 31 leagues. It is further observable, that the lighthouse lies, not so much as one half of that opening, in a north-east direction, within, or *up Channel* of the said line; and that the *Bay* of *Biscay* and *Atlantic* Ocean lie open to the *Edystone*, from the S. b. W. point to the W. b. S.; and in consequence, that it lies open to the *swells* of the *Bay* and *Ocean*, from all the south western points of the compass; which swells are generally allowed by mariners to be very great and heavy in those seas, and particularly in the *Bay* of *Biscay*. It is to be observed, that the soundings of the sea from the south westward towards the Edystone, are from 80 fathoms to 40, and every where till you come near the Edystone, the sea is full 30 fathoms in depth; so that all the heavy seas from the south-west, come uncontrouled upon the *Edystone Rocks*, and break thereon with the utmost fury.

6. A CIRCUMSTANCE that greatly tends to augment the force and height of the seas so breaking upon those rocks, is their particular form and position, as will in part be understood from the *general Plan* of the Edystone rocks N° 3, by which it will be seen, that they not only stretch across the channel in a north and south direction to the length of above 100 fathoms; but that they lie in a sloping manner toward the south-west quarter: and the sloping (or *sliving* of the rocks as it is technically called) does not cease at low water, but still goes on progressively, so that at 50 fathoms westward, there is 12 fathoms water; nor do they terminate altogether, at the distance of a mile; but at two miles distance there is doubtless *clean Ground*, being a white sand, as common to this part of the channel.——From this configuration it happens, that the seas coming uncontrouled from the deep water, and rather suddenly at *last*, though gradually meeting the slope of the rocky bottom, they are swelled to that degree in storms and hard gales of wind, as to break upon the rocks, with the most dreadful violence; as may in some degree (and in some degree only) be comprehended from the *Tablet* in the *Title page*. Nor is the effect of this slope less sensible, in proportion, in moderate weather; and it is frequently very troublesome even in calm weather; for the libration of the water, caused in the *Bay* of *Biscay*, in hard gales at S. W. continues in those deep waters for many days, though succeeded by a calm; insomuch, that when the sea is to all appearance smooth, and even, and its surface unruffled by the slightest breeze, yet those librations still continuing, which are called the *Ground Swell*, and meeting the slope of these rocks, the sea breaks upon them in a frightful manner, so as not only to obstruct any work being done upon the rock, but even the landing upon it, when, figuratively speaking, you might go to sea in a *Walnut-shell*.

7. A STILL further circumstance, that even yet increases the difficulty of working upon the rock in moderate weather, will be apprehended from considering the particular plan and elevation N° 7 of what is now called the *House Rock*; every building having been made upon it, as the largest and highest; where, in the plan, upon the line A B, there is a sudden drop of the surface of the rocks, forming a step, of about 4½ or 5 feet high; this face or front exhibited in the upright view, also by the letters A B, somewhat overhangs the perpendicular towards the west; so that the seas which in moderate weather come swelling towards this step, meet so sudden a *check* thereby, that they frequently fly to the height of 30 and 40 feet, even when people are working upon the rock; and the broken water coming down upon the area of the House, the workmen must of necessity be thoroughly wetted, and often do their business in a very uncomfortable situation. I would not however be understood that this is the case, at *all times* in moderate weather; but only when the ground swells come home from the Bay; for when the wind is in any

any of the easterly or northerly points, that is, quite round from the south, by the E. and N. to the west point, if moderate it produces no such effect; but yet, after a ground swell has been raised by a hard gale of wind at S. W. a wind blowing only moderately from the favourable points, will not quell it in less than 4 or 5 days time; and it is to be noted, that the south-westerly are the most prevalent winds of this part of the country, in the summer months, (when alone any thing can here be attempted with success) and that when the wind blows *very fresh* at any point, all work here must cease*.

8. FROM what has already been observed, it will appear, that the turn of the current of the tide from the westward towards the east is at half flood; and that it remains in the same direction from that time forwards to high water, and afterwards till the half ebb: hence as the current of the tide, will in consequence during the whole of the time from half flood to half ebb, *aid* the ground swell from the west; and the water at this time is also high upon the rocks, it will very rarely admit of any business being done upon the rock, in the most moderate weather, during this interval; which of course at once cuts off half the time, in the period of every tide.

9. THE particular declivity of the rocks in a state of nature, will be readily judged of, by having recourse to Plate N° 6 that contains the elevation of the last Lighthouse; which is shewn by a south view at the low water of a spring tide. The high water of the same tide, supposed unagitated, would not rise to the top of the *Peak* of the rock, as it stood at the time of my taking the elevation, by three feet perpendicular; but the seas are scarcely ever so quiet here, as not to break entirely over it at high water. The sudden drop, step, or break of the house rock to the west, will be best explained by examining the Plate N° 9, containing the section of the present building; which section being upon the east and west points, distinctly shews this drop, or overhanging step, that creates so much trouble; there being, here, no other part of the rock before it, to hide it from the eye.

10. IT has been noticed, that the rocky ground at the bottom, extends considerably to the westward of the visible rocks; it does so also to the east, and to the north; in general, 14 to 20 fathoms deep at low water, at the distance of from a quarter, to half a mile; and, as I apprehend, still deeper to the southward; but of this last I have no minutes, having had no occasion to be particular there.——This rocky bottom is also another natural impediment to the working upon the rock; for every undertaker must alike experience the necessity of having a vessel of a competent size, to receive and lodge himself, his workmen and materials; and to have it *moored* in such a situation as to be sufficiently near, to effect a landing on the rock with small boats, whenever it shall appear practicable so to do; and carry to, and return from the same what materials he has occasion for. No man would however think of mooring his vessel to the south of the rocks; because, if it broke loose with a hard gale at south, he would be intercepted by the rocks in his passage home; or if moored to the west or east, if broke loose by hard gales from those quarters respectively, he would inevitably be driven upon the rocks, and the more perilous would be his situation, by being in the *drift* of the channel's tide; but on all the northern points, the land being within sight, no very heavy seas can ever come from this quarter; and therefore, if here he was to break loose from moorings, he will have every advantage in getting into port: but in this situation, though eligible for mooring, for the reasons abovementioned, the rocks are so very sharp, that a vessel lying at anchor in moderate weather, is in danger of having her *cable* or *hawser* chafed asunder, and of losing her anchor. Nothing therefore is to be done here *properly* without *chains*; and the weight thereof, that is necessary to prevent their being broke, or cut by the violent blows to which they will unavoidably be subject from those sharp rocks, is such as must render them unwieldy and troublesome in the management; especially to a vessel that for other reasons, cannot be encumbered with hands; and in reality,

* This perhaps cannot be better illustrated than by observing; that to set the workmen *forward*, at different periods of the work, when there was to be a *change* in the mode of construction; I have been obliged to continue on board our store vessel at an anchor, frequently a week, sometimes 10, 12, 14, and once 18 days together, even in the months of *July* and *August*; when though the swell was quite gentle every where else; yet was it so furious upon the rocks, as to prevent our landing, though the common artificers were to be paid 6*d*. an *hour* for their work there.

I found more difficulty and hindrance from this circumstance of a rocky bottom, than I could possibly have imagined.

The component Matter or Substance.

11. THE *congeries* of rocks called the *Edystone*, appear to me to be all of the same kind of stone, and of a kind so peculiar, that I have not seen any stone exactly like it in *Cornwall* or *Devonshire*, or indeed in any part of the kingdom; but the most similar to it that I have seen, was in *Scotland*, yet that varied in some degree from it. It is of the kind that in *Cornwall* they call a *Killas* or hard slate*; but the substance thereof appears to be the same nearly, as the *Moor-stone* or *Granite* of that county; and it is in every *respect* quite as hard. It differs from the Moor-stone in this; instead of being composed of grains or small fragments, united by a strong cement, interspersed with a shining *talky* substance, as the *Cornish* Moor-stone in general appears to be; it is composed of the like matter formed into *Laminæ* commonly from one-twentieth to one-sixth part of an inch in thickness; the shining talky particles lying between the *Laminæ*†. It coheres as strongly together as Moor-stone, if split according to the direction of the grain; but if attempted to be split across the grain, it is abundantly harder, and therefore, when worked by tools, it can by no means be brought to an *Arrist* or sharp corner; because the texture is so much stronger one way than the other, that the force which is necessary to make an impression in the harder direction, is sufficient to crumble off the *Laminæ* from each other in that where they are less united. This stone is also in a considerable degree *elastic*, as will be shewn in the sequel, especially in endeavouring to divide it *with* the grain, which lies according to the *sliving* of the rocks; and is nearly one foot *dip* to the westward, in two feet horizontal, that is, in an angle of about 26 degrees with the *horizon*. The kind of work which can the most easily be done upon this rock is in *boring* or *drilling* holes into it, crossways of the grain, as will be observed in its proper place; every thing else goes on with much labour, and difficulty, except that of splitting it in the direction of the grain.

General Directions.

12. THE time of the tides here, that is of high and low water, is nearly the same as at *Plymouth*, viz. VI at full and change of the moon. The common *Spring* tides flow from 16 to 18 feet, and the equinoctial tides from 18 to 20 feet; *neap* tides flow from 11 to 12 feet, and sometimes to 14 feet.

The proper time of sailing from Plymouth for the Edystone is at high water at *Plymouth*: because the *Ebb Tide* from Plymouth Sound, will assist in getting out of the Sound, and then meeting the *Channel's* tide running eastward, the current will naturally set you so much east, that if your wind is slack, the return of the current to the west, at half ebb at the Edystone, will bring you back thither, in course, before low water, and give you the best chance of landing. The most favourable wind, both for going out, landing, lying there and returning, is at N. W.; for that wind not only answers for the passage both ways; but being a *Land-wind*, it must blow hard before it raises any considerable sea at the rock; and the landing-place being on the east side of the house rock, that *reef*, stretching north and south, becomes a *Pier* or *Mole* for breaking off the sea, from half ebb to low water, and from thence till half flood; which interval of time, when the weather permits, is the best for landing and staying there. The most unfavourable wind for every purpose is the S. W. as will easily be conceived from what has been already described.

* Pryce's Mineral. Cornub. explanation of terms, p. 323.

† This is the account of it that I received from my ingenious friend the late Mr. WILLIAM COOKWORTHY of *Plymouth*, *Chemist*, who has been very curious in his researches upon the fossils, and particularly the *Moor-stone* of *Cornwall*; having found that to be a substance, which being acted upon by an intense fire, becomes the proper basis of *China-ware*; and a species of Moor-stone having been found by him not discoloured by the *talky* matter, a manufactory upon this principle has since been carried on at *Bristol*.

Having tried the specific gravity of *Moor-stone* and that of *Edystone*, I find the difference inconsiderable: Moor-stone being 2,625; Edystone 2,65[illegible] times that of water.

CHAP.

C H A P. II.

Concerning the Conſtruction of the Lighthouſe upon the Edyſtone built by Mr. WINSTANLEY.

13. THE many fatal accidents that were frequently happening to ſhips by running upon the Edyſtone rocks, and particularly to thoſe that were homeward-bound, we muſt ſuppoſe to have made it a thing very deſirable to have a Lighthouſe built thereon, and that for many years before any competent undertaker appeared: for, from the circumſtances which have been fully ſtated in the preceding account of the natural ſtate of theſe rocks; it would appear to thoſe then beſt acquainted with them, that the difficulties neceſſarily attending ſuch an undertaking, were likely to prove inſuperable: and perhaps in reality it may have been a peculiar advantage to every undertaker, and to the undertaking itſelf, that no one could, previous to the actual commencement of the work, be fully ſenſible of the difficulties which would inevitably attend it; and which he muſt ſurmount or fail of ſucceſs.

14. HOWEVER, formidable as it was, we learn that in the year 1696, Mr. HENRY WINSTANLEY of *Littlebury* in the county of *Eſſex*, Gent. was not only hardy enough to undertake it, but was furniſhed with the neceſſary powers to put it in execution. This it is ſuppoſed was done in virtue of the general powers lodged in the *Maſter*, *Wardens* and *Aſſiſtants* of TRINITY HOUSE at *Deptford Strond*, to erect ſea marks, &c. by a ſtatute of QUEEN ELIZABETH, whereby they are impowered "to erect and ſet up beacons, marks and ſigns for the ſea, needful for avoiding the dangers; and to renew, continue and maintain the ſame."——But whether Mr. WINSTANLEY was a proprietor or ſharer of the undertaking under the TRINITY HOUSE, or only the directing engineer, employed in the execution, does not now appear.

15. THIS gentleman had diſtinguiſhed himſelf in a certain branch of mechanics, the tendency of which is to raiſe wonder and ſurprize. He had at his houſe at *Littlebury* a ſet of contrivances ſuch as the following:——Being taken into one particular room of his houſe, and there obſerving an old ſlipper careleſsly lying on the middle of the floor; if, as was natural, you gave it a kick with your foot, up ſtarted a *Ghoſt* before you: if you ſat down in a certain chair, a couple of arms would immediately claſp you in, ſo as to render it impoſſible to diſentangle yourſelf till your attendant ſet you at liberty: and if you ſat down in a certain arbour by the ſide of a canal, you was forthwith ſent out *afloat* to the middle of the canal, from whence it was impoſſible for you to eſcape, till the manager returned you to your former place.——Whether thoſe things were ſhewn to ſtrangers at his houſe for money, or were done by way of amuſement, to thoſe that came to viſit the place, is uncertain, as Mr. WINSTANLEY is ſaid to have been a man of ſome property: but it is at leaſt certain, that he eſtabliſhed a place of public exhibition at *Hyde Park Corner*, called WINSTANLEY's *Waterworks*, which were ſhewn at ſtated times, at one ſhilling each perſon: the particulars of thoſe waterworks are not now known; but, according to the taſte of the times, we muſt naturally ſuppoſe a great variety of *jets d'eau*, &c.*

Thoſe particulars relative to Mr. WINSTANLEY are indeed of little importance at preſent, either to the public or to the deſign of this publication, otherwiſe than as they may ſerve to give a ſketch of the talents and turn of mind of this original undertaker; and to account for the whimſical kind of buildings that he erected upon the Edyſtone, for the purpoſe of a Lighthouſe; as it would ſeem, from the deſign

* It appears that the exhibition of theſe waterworks continued ſome years after the death of Mr. WINSTANLEY, as they were exiſting in the month of September 1709, being mentioned in the *Tatler* of that date.

thereof, that it was not sufficient for his enterprizing genius, to erect a building upon a spot, where of all others it was the least likely to stand unhurt; but that he would also give it an elevation, that in appearance should be the most liable to subject it to damage from the violence of wind and seas.

16. THE following comprehends an account of two different buildings that he erected there, and is chiefly extracted from what was written upon the large copper plate print addressed to Prince GEORGE of *Denmark*, then Lord *High Admiral* of *England*, containing a perspective elevation of his finished Lighthouse; which, drawn orthographically and reduced to the same scale as the subsequent buildings are adjusted to, is shewn in *Plate* N° 5 of the present work. The account I refer to, is intituled by Mr. WINSTANLEY,

" *A Narrative of the Building.*

17. " THIS Lighthouse was begun to be built in the year 1696, and was more than four years in building: not for the greatness of the work, but for the difficultie and danger in getting backwards and forwards to the place; nothing being or could be left safe there for the first two years, but what was most thoroughly affixed to the rock, or the work at a very extraordinary charge: and though nothing could be attempted to be done but in the summer season, yet the weather then at times would prove so bad, that for ten or fourteen days together, the sea would be so raging about these rocks, caused by out-winds, and the running of the ground-seas coming from the main ocean; that although the weather should seem, and be most calm in other places, yet here it would mount, and fly more than 200 feet, as has been so found, since there was lodgment upon the place: and therefore all our works were constantly buried at those times, and exposed to the mercy of the seas*; and no power was able to come near, to make good or help any thing, as I have often experienced with my workmen in a boat in great danger; only having the satisfaction to see my work imperfectly at times, as the seas fell from it, and at a mile or two distance; and this at the prime of the year, and no wind or appearance of bad weather: yet trusting in *God*'s assistance for a blessing on this undertaking; being for a general good, and receiving most inexpressible deliverances, I proceeded as follows.

18. " THE *first* summer was spent in making 12 holes in the rock, and fastening 12 great irons† to hold the work that was to be done afterwards; the rock being so hard, and the time so short to stay by reason of the tide or weather, and the distance from the shore, and the many journeys lost that there could be no landing at all; and many times glad to land at our return at places, that, if the weather permitted, would take up the next day to get to Plymouth again‡.

19. " THE *next* summer was spent in making a solid body, or round pillar twelve feet high, and fourteen feet diameter; and then we had more time to work at the place; and a little better landing, having some small shelter from the work, and something to hold by; but we had great trouble to carry off and land so many materials, and be forced to secure all things as aforesaid every night § and time we left work, or return them again into the boats.

20. " THE *third* year the aforesaid pillar or work was made good at the foundation from the rock to 16 feet diameter, and all the work was raised, which to the vane was eighty feet. Being all finished, with the lantern, and all the rooms that were in it, we ventured to lodge there soon after Midsummer, for the greater dispatch of this work. But the first night the weather came bad, and so

* See the tablet in the title page.

† One of the irons about 3½ inches diameter octagon, was cut out in the operations of 1756.

‡ From this description it appears that they had not any store vessel to lie at moorings by way of constant retreat; but performed the work by single journeys.

§ Hence it appears they did not work in the night.

continued,

continued, that it was eleven days before any boats could come near us again; and not being acquainted with *the height of the ſeas riſing*, we were almoſt all the time drowned with wet, and our proviſions in as bad a condition, though we worked night and day, as much as poſſible to make ſhelter for ourſelves. In this ſtorm we loſt ſome of our materials, although we did what we could to ſave them; but the boat then returning, we all left the houſe to be refreſhed on ſhore; and as ſoon as the weather did permit, we returned again and finiſhed all, and put up the light on the 14th of November 1698; which being ſo late in the year, it was three days before Chriſtmas before we had relief to get on ſhore again, and were almoſt at the laſt extremity for want of proviſions; but by good Providence, then two boats came with proviſions, and the family that was to take care of the light, and ſo ended this year's work *.

21. "THE *fourth* year, finding in the winter the effects the ſea had upon the houſe, and *burying* the lantern at times, although more than ſixty feet high; early in the ſpring, I encompaſſed the aforeſaid building with a new work of four feet thickneſs from the foundation, making all ſolid near twenty feet high; and taking down the upper part of the firſt building, and enlarging every part in its proportion, I raiſed it 40 feet higher than it was at firſt, and made it as it now appears; and yet the ſea, in time of ſtorms, flies in appearance, *one hundred feet above the vane*; and at times doth cover half the ſide of the houſe and the lantern, as if it were under water †."

22. BESIDES the above narrative, this print of Mr. WINSTANLEY's contains the following information.

"This Lighthouſe bears from *Plymouth* (or the entrance of the *Sound*) S. by W. and from the *Ram Head*, S. half a point eaſtwardly; and is diſtant from the anchoring in the foreſaid Sound 4 leagues, and from Ram Head about 3 leagues and an half; which is the neareſt ſhore from the ſaid houſe: and the Iſle of *Mayſtone* bears from the Lighthouſe about N. E. by N. and is alſo four leagues diſtant; ſo that the ſhips coming from the Eaſt or Weſt, have much the ſame advantage of the light, that are bound for Plymouth. All the rocks near this houſe are on the eaſtward ſide, but ſtretching north, and moſt ſouthwardly: all are covered at high water; but on the weſt ſide, any ſhip may ſail cloſe by the houſe, there being 12 or 13 fathoms water, and no hidden rock; but towards the E. by N. about a

* Though Mr. WINSTANLEY has not himſelf left any particular repreſentation of the building, deſcribed as the produce of theſe three years work; yet I am enabled to preſent the curious reader with the elevation thereof in plate N° 4. This is drawn orthographically to the ſame ſcale as the reſt; from a perſpective print ſaid to be drawn at the rock by JAABIELL JOHNSTON, *painter*. I never ſaw but the ſingle copy in my poſſeſſion, and therefore at this time I muſt ſuppoſe it extremely ſcarce.

From the appearance of the baſement, it would ſeem to be of ſtone; and though Mr. WINSTANLEY does not ſay in his deſcription of the 2d year's work, which was that of making a *ſolid body*, or kind of round pillar, that it actually was of *ſtone*; yet from the manner of the expreſſion one would infer that to be the caſe; and which will appear more probable if we may ſuppoſe Mr. WINSTANLEY and his workmen ignorant at that time, of the proper manner of compoſing a cement capable of becoming hard under the utmoſt violence of the ſea; and in want thereof, he would doubtleſs after a winter's expoſure, find the joints of his ſolid pillar to be much waſhed, and the work itſelf looking ragged: it was therefore a natural expedient to ſurround the former pillar as deſcribed in the 3d year's work, with a caſe of ſtone of a foot thick; and not only to make the joints with all imaginable care, but to ſurround every joint with a *band* or *girdle* of iron or copper plate, of ſome inches in breadth, to hold in and ſecure the mortar from the waſh of the ſea; which mode of ſecurity is inferred from the repreſentation.

The height of the ſtone pillar here repreſented is 12 feet above the rock upon the upper ſide, and 17 feet on the lower ſide; it muſt therefore be ſuppoſed, in ſpeaking of 12 feet high, Mr. WINSTANLEY means above the rock on the higher ſide; or, as the print from whence this is taken, appears to be made from an *Eye Draught*, it may be an inaccuracy in the draughtſman.

The elevation appears to be taken from the ſouth at half tide, or when the ſea is overflowing the landing place; which of courſe occaſions the rock to make a ſmaller appearance in this draught, than in any of the reſt.

A is the eye-bolt and ring upon the landing-place. B the ſloping ſurface of the rock. C the ſtone baſement. D the ſtore room. E the ſtate room. F the open gallery. G the kitchen. And H the lantern for the lights.

† See the tablet in the title page; which yet is ſhort of the height deſcribed by Mr. WINSTANLEY by 50 feet.

quarter

quarter of a mile diſtant from the houſe, lies an hidden rock that never appears, but at low ſpring tides, and therefore, not ſo well known, is the more dangerous.

23. "THE ſea ebbs and flows at this rock on ſpring tides 19 feet, and at high water all the rocks are covered, though a ſmooth ſea; and it is high water at the ſame time as at Plymouth; but it runs *tide and half tide*, ſo that it runs Eaſt 3 hours after it is high water, and yet the ſea falls lower; and it runs Weſt 3 hours after it is low water, and yet the ſea riſeth. At low tides, eſpecially ſpring tides, three great ranges of rocks appear very high, and lie almoſt parallel, ſtretching towards the S. E. and N. W. the houſe ſtanding the moſt Weſt of all. The forementioned hidden rock is a full cable's length from *all* theſe rocks, and lies as aforeſaid*."

24. THE plate N° 5 I have already had occaſion to remark is drawn orthographically from Mr. WINSTANLEY's perſpective elevation, from whence the above narrative is taken, and wherein

A repreſents the rock at low water.——B the landing place, covered at half tide, and all the time the current runs Eaſt.——C the entry door.——DE the baſement, which in the fourth year he deſcribes to have been added to the original one of 16 feet, ſo as to make an addition of four feet in thickneſs on every ſide; from hence it ſeems, that on the weſt ſide at D, it has been a work of ſtone; the joints appearing to have been covered with hoop plates, as before deſcribed of the original baſe; whereas the eaſt ſide E has the ſame appearance of having been wood; and to have been bound together with iron ſtraps, as the whole of the ſuperſtructure evidently was.——F is the ſtore-room with a projecting cabin to the ſouth-eaſt.——G the ſtate-room.——H the kitchen.——I the open gallery or platform.——K the lodging-room.——L the attending, or look-out room.——M the lantern for the lights, ſurrounded by a gallery or balcony.

N. B. The baſe is ſuppoſed completely to contain the original ſtone baſe of 16 feet diameter, which with the addition of four feet all round, makes the baſe of this ſecond ſtructure to be 24 feet diameter; and it appears to be partly round, and in part a *polygon*: but the works above the baſe are evidently upon a *dodecagonal* plan, or polygon of 12 ſides, till they riſe to the baſe of the look-out room, where, with all above, the building aſſumes an *octagonal* figure.

25. IT is very unneceſſary for me to enter into a further criticiſm upon either of thoſe ſtructures, as, with the information that I have collected, my reader will abundantly do that for himſelf; it is ſufficient to ſay, that it was no ſmall degree of heroic merit in Mr. WINSTANLEY to undertake a piece of work, that before had been deemed *impracticable*; and by the ſucceſs which attended his endeavours to ſhew mankind, that the erection of a building upon the *Edyſtone* was not in itſelf a thing of *that* kind: and it will be a further confirmation of the exceeding violence of the ſeas upon thoſe rocks; and of the augmented ſhock by the interpoſition of a building, when I mention, that on my firſt going to Plymouth in the year 1756, I was informed by an old gentleman who remembered both Mr. WINSTANLEY and his lighthouſe, that after it was finiſhed, it was commonly ſaid, that in time of hard weather, ſuch was the height of the ſeas, that it was very poſſible for a *ſix-oared* boat to be lifted up upon a wave, and driven through the open gallery of the lighthouſe.

26. EXCEPT the above, I have met with no occurrences concerning this building till the month of November 1703, when the fabric needing ſome repairs, Mr. WINSTANLEY went down to Plymouth to ſuperintend the performance thereof: and we muſt not wonder, if from the preceding accounts of

* For a more perfect account of the general ſhape and ſituation of the Edyſtone rocks, ſee the general plan thereof Plate N° 3; relative to which it is to be noted, that at the beginning of this century, the variation of the compaſs by Mr. FLAMSTEED was N. 7° ½ weſterly; whereas it is now become nearly 2 points of the compaſs to the W. of N.; which, with the common inaccuracy of reputed bearings, ſufficiently accounts for the difference of thoſe given by Mr. WINSTANLEY, from theſe ſet down in this plan.

the

the violence of the feas, and the ftructure of the Lighthoufe, the common fenfe of the public led them to fuppofe, this building would not be of long duration; and the following is an anecdote which I received, to the fame effect from fo many perfons, that I can have no doubt of the truth of it.

Mr. WINSTANLEY being amongft his friends previous to going off with his workmen, on account of thofe reparations; the danger being intimated to him, and that one day or other the Lighthoufe would certainly be overfet; he replied, "He was fo very well affured of the ftrength of his building, "he fhould only wifh to be there in the greateft ftorm that ever blew under the face of the heavens, "that he might fee what effect it would have upon the ftructure."

It happened that Mr. WINSTANLEY was but too amply gratified in this wifh; for while he was there with his workmen and light keepers, that dreadful ftorm began, which raged the moft violently upon the 26th November 1703 in the night; and of all the accounts of the kind, which hiftory furnifhes us with, we have none that has exceeded this in *Great Britain*, or was more injurious or extenfive in its devaftation.

The next morning, November 27th, when the violence of the ftorm was fo much abated, that it could be feen whether the Lighthoufe had fuffered by it, nothing appeared ftanding, but, upon a nearer infpection, fome of the large irons, whereby the work was fixed upon the rock; nor were any of the people, or any of the materials of the building, ever found afterwards; fave only part of an iron chain, which had got fo faft jambed into a chink of the rock, that it could never afterwards be difengaged, till it was cut out in the year 1756.

27. THE above accounts are what I have received from old people at Plymouth; the following anecdotes are extracted from a book, publifhed foon after the melancholy accident to Mr. WINSTANLEY and thofe with him, entituled The STORM, printed *London* 1704.

"The lofs of the Lighthoufe called the *Edyftone* at *Plymouth*, is another article, of which we never heard any particulars, other than this; that at night it was ftanding, and in the morning all the *upper part of the gallery* was blown down, and all the people in it perifhed; and by a particular misfortune, Mr. WINSTANLEY the contriver of it; a perfon whofe lofs is very much regretted by fuch as knew him, as a very ufeful man to his country. The lofs of that Lighthoufe is alfo a confiderable damage; as 'tis very doubtful whether it will ever be attempted again; and as it was a great fecuritie to the failors; many a good *fhip having been loft there in former times*.

"It was very remarkable, that, as we are informed, at the fame time the Lighthoufe aforefaid was blown down, the model of it in Mr. WINSTANLEY's houfe at *Littlebury* in *Effex*, above 200 miles from the Lighthoufe, fell down and was broke to pieces*." Page 223.

"At *Plymouth* they felt a full proportion of the ftorm in its utmoft fury; the Edyftone has been mentioned already; but it was a double lofs; in that the Lighthoufe had not been long down, when the *Winchelfea*, an homeward-bound *Virginia* man, was fplit upon the rock where that building ftood, and moft of her men drowned." P. 212.

* This however may not appear extraordinary, if we confider that the fame general wind that blew down the Lighthoufe near *Plymouth*, might blow down the model at *Littlebury*.

CHAP. III.

Account of the second Lighthouse built upon the Edystone by Mr. RUDYERD.

28. THE great utility that the Lighthouse of Mr. WINSTANLEY had proved itself to be of, during its continuance, would of course prompt mankind to wish for another in its place; and the loss of the *Winchelsea* Virginia man just mentioned, with others that may naturally be supposed to have shared the same fate, would doubtless prove powerful incentives to awaken the attention of those most nearly concerned, to attempt a work, that with whatever difficulties it might in reality be attended, yet Mr. WINSTANLEY's building had demonstrated to be a thing, not in its own nature *impossible* or *impracticable*.

It was not however begun afresh quite so soon as it might naturally have been expected; for Mr. WINSTANLEY's Lighthouse having been destroyed the 26th November 1703, it was not till the spring of the year 1706, that an act of parliament of the 4th of QUEEN ANN was passed for the better enabling the *Master, Wardens* and *Assistants* of TRINITY HOUSE at *Deptford Strond*, to rebuild the same; so that in the steps necessary for this, we must suppose some obstruction; but the work itself was begun in the July following*.

29. BY this act of parliament, the duties payable by shipping, passing the Lighthouse, were vested in the corporation of TRINITY HOUSE at *Deptford Strond*, and it included powers to them to grant a lease thereof to an undertaker or undertakers, such as they should approve. In consequence of these powers they agreed with a *Captain* LOVEL or LOVET for a term of 99 years, commencing from the day that a light should be exhibited, and continuing so long as that exhibition should last during the said term.

* Extract from the preamble to this act 4th of ANN, chap. 20th.

"And whereas there now is, and time out of mind has been, *a very dangerous rock* called the *Edystone* lying off of *Plymouth* in the county of Devon, upon which divers ships and vessels have been cast away and destroyed: and whereas upon application some time since made to the said *Masters, Wardens* and *Assistants* by great numbers of masters and owners of shipping to have a *Lighthouse* erected upon the said rock, offering and agreeing in consideration of the great *charge, difficulty* and *hazard* of such an undertaking, to pay the said Master, &c. one penny per ton outwards, and the like inwards, for all ships and vessels which should pass such Lighthouse (coasters excepted, which should pay twelvepence only for each voyage) they the said Master, &c. having a due regard to the safety and preservation of the shipping and navigation of this kingdom, did in the year 1696 cause a Lighthouse to be begun to be erected on the said rock, and in three years time a light was placed therein; and the said Lighthouse in the term of five years was, with much hazard and difficulty, and at a very great expence, fully built and completed to the great satisfaction of the flag officers and commanders of the fleet and ships of war, and of all others concerned in trade and navigation: the same being not only useful for *avoiding the dangerous rock upon* [illegible] *built*, but also a *guide and direction to ships passing through the channel* from and to all parts of the world. And whereas the said Lighthouse was preserved and kept up for several years notwithstanding the *great force and violence* of the *wind* and *sea* (to which it was [illegible]) [illegible] the late dreadful storm in November 1703, when the same was blown down and destroyed: and whereas it was found by experience that the said Lighthouse (during the standing thereof) was of public use and benefit to this kingdom, a means to preserve her Majesty's ships of war, and the shipping, lives and estates of her subjects.——And forasmuch as the speedy rebuilding the said Lighthouse is [illegible] *necessary* for avoiding the dangers attending the trade and navigation of this kingdom; and in regard the same work [illegible] *charge, hazard and expence*, and all due and proper *encouragement ought to be given thereunto*; to the end therefore that the said Master, &c. may be encouraged to new-erect and build, or cause to be new-erected and built the said Lighthouse with all convenient speed, and [illegible] keep and maintain the same for the benefit of the navigation and trade of this kingdom, be it enacted, &c." It [illegible] the payment of the duties above mentioned, and double on foreign vessels "from and after the *kindling* or placing [illegible] in the said Lighthouse."

30. UPON

30. UPON this foundation Captain LOVET engaged Mr. JOHN RUDYERD to be his engineer or architect and furveyor: and the event has fhewn that he made a very proper choice; though it does not appear that Mr. RUDYERD was bred to any mechanical bufinefs, or fcientifical profeffion, being at that time a *Silk Mercer* who kept a fhop upon *Ludgate Hill, London*; nor do we find that in any other inftance he had diftinguifhed himfelf by any mechanical performance before or after: yet this is no proof but that he might have made thefe kind of fubjects his private amufements; and it is indeed true, that a natural genius with very flender experience, will go much further in *Defign*, than experience alone is capable of; but when genius and a competent experience are united in the fame perfon, it is to be looked upon as a happy combination; and their productions likely to be the moft complete and perfect. However, Mr. RUDYERD's want of perfonal experience, was in a degree affifted by Mr. SMITH and Mr. NORCUTT, both fhipwrights from the king's yard at *Woolwich*; who worked with him the whole time he was building the lighthoufe.

It is not very material now in what way this gentleman became qualified for the execution of this work; it is fufficient that he directed the performance thereof in a mafterly manner, and fo as perfectly to anfwer the end for which it was intended *. He faw the errors in the former building and avoided them; inftead of a polygon he chofe a circle for the outline of his building, and carried up the elevation in that form. His principal aim appears to have been *ufe* and *fimplicity*; and indeed, in a building fo fituated, the former could hardly be acquired in its full extent, without the latter. He feems to have adopted ideas the very reverfe of his predeceffor; for all the unwieldy ornaments at top, the open gallery, the projecting cranes, and other contrivances, more for ornament and pleafure, than ufe, Mr. RUDYERD laid totally afide; he faw, that how beautiful foever ornaments might be in themfelves, yet when they are improperly applied and out of *place*; by affecting to fhew a tafte, they betray ignorance of its firft principle, *Judgment*: for whatever deviates from propriety is erroneous, and at beft infipid.

31. IN like manner as Mr. WINSTANLEY; Mr. RUDYERD alfo, after the completion of his work, publifhed a print entituled *a Profpect and Section of the* LIGHTHOUSE *on the* EDYSTONE ROCK *off of* PLYMOUTH; and he dedicated it to *Thomas Earl of* PEMBROKE, then *Lord High Admiral of Great Britain and Ireland*; with this motto, *Furit natura coercet ars.* The drawing by B. LENS, the engraving by I. STURT, both eminent artifts of their time. This print I fuppofe to be very fcarce, not having feen any other but the fingle copy I have in my own poffeffion.

* Since writing the above, on perufal of the MSS. by my valuable and learned friend the Rev. Mr. MICHELL, he has communicated to me an anecdote concerning Mr. RUDYERD, when I leaft expected it: and as it is in itfelf curious, and comes fo well authenticated, I will give it a place here; and perhaps it will come in better by way of note, than by being interwoven in the context:

The following particulars Mr. MICHELL had often heard his father repeat in his life-time, of this Mr. RUDYERD. They were both born in *Cornwall*; and his father being 18 years old when Mr. RUDYERD's Lighthoufe was begun, was at a time of life when he was likely to pick up the current ftories of the times; as well as fufficiently in the way to hear them, from his fituation in the neighbourhood. ——According to the late Mr. MICHELL's account, Mr. RUDYERD's father and mother were of the loweft rank of day-labourers, with a large family of children; and in as low repute in all other refpects, as in point of rank; being looked upon as a worthlefs fet of ragged beggars, whom almoft nobody would employ, on account of the badnefs of their characters. *Our* Mr. RUDYERD, however, was from a child of a very different difpofition from the reft; born with a good head, and an honeft and a good heart, in fhort the very reverfe of the reft of the family, fo that he was confidered by them as a fullen boy, as he would not affociate with them in going out upon their pilfering fchemes; and probably on that account, as hath been fuppofed, he ran away from them; and by good luck, and from fomething promifing in his afpect, got into the fervice of a gentleman, fuppofed at *Plymouth*; and in this ftation he appeared to fo much advantage to his mafter, and became fo great a favourite with him, that he gave him the opportunity of reading, writing, accounts and mathematics; in all which he made a very ready and great progrefs; and afterwards his mafter affifted him very greatly in life, by procuring him fome employment that raifed him above the rank of a fervant, and laid the foundation of his future fuccefs in the world. ——The above account ftrongly evinces that though education and example may do much; yet that there is fomething in natural difpofition, that is not totally to be eradicated by education. Had Mr. RUDYERD's parents been of the moft amiable character, if one of their children had turned out the reverfe, who would have wondered? We fhould readily have explained it, that it arofe from ill impreffions from without: but the wonder in this cafe is, that in fpite of all the force of evil example, here is a mind capable of emancipating itfelf, by the moft violent of all remedies, that young people generally take, that of feparation from parents and houfhold by *flight*.

32. THE

32. THE Plate N° 6 is an orthographic elevation and section of Mr. RUDYERD's Lighthouse. The *manner* of it, is herein copied, on account of the compendium thereby suggested; which shews part of the outside and part of the inside, so as to be at once, both an elevation and a section; this seems worthy of imitation, as it avoids a greater multiplicity of designs than the subject necessarily requires: but the proportions of the several parts of the structure, are designed and drawn from fresh materials.

33. WHETHER it was owing to a kind of indolence, that some ingenious men are subject to, or to want of health, that we hear nothing more of Mr. RUDYERD after the publication of this print, does not now appear: I am rather inclined to suppose the latter; for had he continued in health and vigour, even if he had some slight *turn* of the former kind, yet the eminent abilities he shewed in this building, after finishing it with *eclat*, must have called him forth to the public service on some other subject. I therefore must conclude, that even when the design for this print was prepared for the engraver, Mr. RUDYERD's application must have been slackened by want of health; and that the drawing must have been compiled from some sketch or sketches of the building made *antecedent* to its execution: because in many particulars, it deviates from the proportions the building actually had; as fully appeared when there was occasion to examine it, by after surveyors: and that, in some particulars, which could not afterwards be changed, nor in reality were they. Yet as what is written upon the face of Mr. RUDYERD's print, is the only piece of writing of *his* that has been preserved, it will be proper to insert a transcript of it, pointing out by notes the principal inaccuracies thereof.

34. "THIS *Edystone Rock* lyeth 3 leagues S. E. and N. W. of *Ram Head* *, and four leagues from *Plymouth*. The building was begun in July 1706; a light put up thereon and made useful the 28th July 1708, and compleatly finished in 1709. The rock *slives* from E. to W. 10 feet 11 inches in 24 feet, which is the diameter of the foundation †: 25 feet 6 inches is the largest circle that can be drawn upon the rock ‡. The face of the rock is divided into seven equal ascents. There are 36 holes cut into the rock, from 20 to 30 inches deep; 6 inches square at top, narrowing to 5 inches at 6 inches deep, from thence spreading and flatting to 9 by 3 at the bottom. They are all cut smooth within, and with great dispatch (though the stone was harder than any marble or stone thereabouts) with engines for that purpose. Every cramp or bolt was forged exactly to the bigness of the hole it was designed for; they weighing from 2 cwt to 5 cwt each, according to their different lengths and substances §. These bolts served to tye the solid to the rock."

He mentions further in the literal references, that the outside timbers (since called the *uprights*) were seventy-*two* in number; and so indeed they might have been *intended*, but the real number was seventy-*one*.

35. AS nothing would stand upon the sloping surface of the rock without artificial means to stay it; Mr. RUDYERD judiciously concluded, that if the rock was reduced to level bearings, the heavy bodies to be placed upon it, would then have no tendency to slide; and this would be the case, even though but

* It is supposed that by some error in the transcriber or engraver, these bearings should have been S. b. E. and N. b. W.; for then they will agree tolerably with Mr. WINSTANLEY's account, and with the variation of the compass at that time. The distances are doubtless according to vulgar reckoning.

† The diameter of this Lighthouse upon its base could not exceed 23 feet 4 inches, as I have fixed it; which I conclude from the extent of the work upon the surface of the rock, by which it was reduced into steps or level bearings.

‡ The diameter of the base of the present Lighthouse is 26 feet, nor does its circumference any where come nearer the border than one foot, so that a circle of 28 feet, which is 2 feet and 6 inches larger than Mr. RUDYERD describes, may in reality be drawn upon the rock: but the base was somewhat enlarged by cutting off the top of the rock in 1756.

§ Several of the bolts, or, as since called, *branches*, here described, were cut out of the rock in the year 1756; and found to be very different in shape, size, and weight from what is here described; which seems rather what was intended before the work was begun, than what really was [illegible]. See the detached figure of one of them in Plate N° 7. The *ascents* were in reality very *unequal*.

imperfectly

imperfectly executed; for the sliding tendency being taken away from these parts that were reduced to a level, the whole would be much more securely retained by the iron bolts or branches, than if for the retention of the whole, they had depended entirely upon the iron-work; as manifestly appears to have been the case with the building of Mr. WINSTANLEY.——According to Mr. RUDYERD's print, the inclined surface of the rock was intended to have been reduced to a set of regular steps, which would have been attended with the same good effect, as if the whole could have been reduced to one level; but in reality, from the hardness of the rock, the shortness and uncertainty of the intervals in which this part of the work must have been performed; and the great tendency of the *Laminæ* whereof the rock is composed, to rise in *spawls*, according to the inclined surface when worked upon by tools, urged with sufficient force to make an impression; this part of the work, that is, the *stepping* of the rock, has been but imperfectly performed, though in a degree that sufficed.

36. THE holes made to receive the iron branches, appear to have been drilled into the rock by *Jumpers**, making holes of about 2½ inches diameter; the extremities of the two holes forming the breadth for the branch, at the surface of the rock, were about 7½ inches; and these holes were directed so that at their bottoms they should be separated somewhat better than an inch more, that is, so as to be full 8½ inches. In the intermediate space, a third hole was bored between the two former; and then if the three holes were broke into one, by square-faced *Pummels*, this would make the holes sufficiently smooth and regular†. By this means he obtained holes of a dovetail shape, being 2½ inches wide, 7½ broad at top, 8½ at bottom, and 15 and 16 inches deep; and, as these could not be made all alike, every branch was forged to fit its respective hole. The main pieces of each branch were about 4½ inches broad at the surface of the rock, and 6½ at the bottom; and this being first put down into the hole, the space left for a key would be 3 inches at top, and two inches at bottom, which would admit it to be driven in so as to render the whole firm, and the main branch fixed like a dovetail or *Lewis*.——I shall now proceed to describe the manner of filling the interstices with lead, so as to make all solid, and exclude the water.

37. THE holes being each finished, and fitted with their respective branches, and cleared of water, a considerable quantity of melted tallow was poured into each hole: the branch and key being then heated to about a *blue* heat, and being put down into the tallow, and the key firmly driven, by these means, all the space unfilled by the iron, would become full of tallow, and the overplus made to run over: when this was done, all remaining hot, a quantity of coarse pewter, being made red hot in a ladle, and run into the chinks, as being the heaviest body, would drive out the superfluous melted tallow: And so effectually had this operation succeeded, that in those branches which were cut out in 1756, and had remained fast, the whole cavity had continued so thoroughly full, that not only the pewter, but even in general, the tallow remained apparently fresh: and when the pewter was melted from the irons, the scale appeared upon the iron, as it had come from the smith's forge, without the least rust upon it.——I have been the more minute in this description, because it shewed the perfection of this method of fixing iron-work into stone, even in the case, where the salts of sea water are ever in readiness to penetrate, could they have found the least admission.

38. ALL the iron branches which are shewn, as I found them, in Plate N° 7, having been fixed in the manner abovementioned; they next proceeded to lay a course of squared oak balks, lengthwise upon the lowest step, and of a size to reach up to the level of the step above.——Then a set of short balks were laid crossways of the former, and upon the next step compoundedly, so as to make good up to the surface of the third step.——The third *stratum* was therefore again laid lengthwise, and the fourth crossways, &c. till a basement of solid wood was raised, two complete courses higher than the highest part

* The instruments so called are well-known tools for boring holes in the harder kind of stone.

† In this way I tried the making dovetail holes, and found the method very practicable: and in this way afterwards, in the course of the work we made various temporary affixtures to the rock; and made the *Lewis* holes in the Moor-stones.

 of

of the rock; the whole being fitted together, and to the rock as clofe as poffible, and the balks, in all their interfections with each other, trenailed together. They were alfo fitted to the iron branches where they happened to fall in; for the branches do not feem to have been placed with any complete regularity or order, but rather where the ftrength and firmnefs of the rock pointed out the propereft places for fixing them: they were however to appearance difpofed, fo as to form a double circle, one about a foot within the circumference of the bafement, and the other about three feet within the former; befides which, there were two large branches fixed near the center, for taking hold of the two fides of a large upright piece of timber, which was called the *Maft*; by which two branches, it was ftrongly fixed down; and being fet perpendicular, it ferved as a center for guiding all the reft of the fucceeding work.

The branches were perforated, in their refpective upper parts, fome with three, and fome with four holes; fo that, in every pair (collectively called a branch) there would be at a medium feven holes; and as there were at leaft 36 original branches, there would be 252 holes, which were about ⅞ of an inch in diameter; and, confequently, were capable of receiving as many large-bearded fpikes or *Jag-bolts*, which being driven through the branches into the folid timber, would undoubtedly hold the whole mafs firmly down; and the great multiplicity of trenails in the interfections, would confine all the *ftrata* clofely and compactly together.

39. I CANNOT omit here to remark, that though the inftrument we now call the *Lewis*, is of an old date; yet, fo far as appears, this particular application of that idea, which Mr. RUDYERD employed in fixing his iron branches firmly to the rock, was made ufe of for the firft time in this work: for though Mr. WINSTANLEY mentions his having made 12 holes, and fixed 12 great irons in the rock, in his firft year's work; yet he gives no intimation of any particular mode of fixing them, but the common way with lead: and the ftump of one of the great irons of Mr. WINSTANLEY's, that was cut out in the courfe of the work of the fummer 1756, was fixed in that manner; but we remarked, that the low end of this bar or ftanchion was a little *club-ended*, and that the hole was fomewhat *under-cut*; fo that, when the lead was poured in, the whole together would make a fort of dovetail engraftment: however, when thefe irons, by great agitations became loofe, and the lead yielded in a certain degree, they would be liable to be drawn out; as the orifice by which they entered, muft have been large enough to receive the iron club. ——Mr. RUDYERD's method, therefore, of *keying* and fecuring, muft be confidered as a material acceffion to the practical part of *Enginecry*; as it furnifhes us with a fecure method of fixing *ring*-bolts and *eye*-bolts, ftanchions, &c. not only into rocks of any known hardnefs; but into piers, moles, &c. that have already been conftructed, for the fafe mooring of fhips; or fixing additional works, whether of ftone or wood.

40. IN this way, by building *ftratum fuper ftratum*, of folid fquared oak timber, which was of the beft quality*, Mr. RUDYERD was enabled to make a folid bafement of what height he thought proper: but in addition to the above methods, he judicioufly laid hold of the great principle of Engineery, that WEIGHT *is the moft naturally and effectually refifted by* WEIGHT. He confidered, that all his joints being pervious to water, and that though a great part of the ground joint of the whole mafs, was in contact with the rock, yet many parts of it could not be accurately fo; and therefore, that whatever parts of the ground joint were not in perfect contact, fo as to exclude the water therefrom, though the feparation was only by the thicknefs of a piece of poft-paper, yet if capable of receiving water in a fluid ftate †, the action of a wave upon it edgewife, would upon the principles of *Hydroftatics*, produce an equal effect towards lifting it upwards, as if it acted immediately upon fo much *area* of the bottom, as was not in clofe contact.

* It is faid that the timber ufed in this building was *winter felled*.

† When water is received into the pores of wood or ftone and other folid bodies, I do not confider it as in a ftate of fluidity.

41. THE

41. THE more effectually therefore to counteract every tendency of the seas to move the building, in any direction, he determined to interpose *strata* of *Cornish Moor-stone* between those of wood; and accordingly having raised his foundation solid, two courses above the top of the rock, he then put on five courses, of one foot thick each, of the Moor-stone*. These courses were as well jointed as the workmen of the country could do it; to introduce as much weight as possible, into the space to contain them: they were however laid without any cement; but it appears that iron cramps were used to retain the stones of each course together, and also upright ones to confine down the outside stones; for though Mr. RUDYERD makes no mention of the cramps, I learnt this circumstance by conversing with a person actually employed in the preparation of the stone, as will be more fully stated hereafter.

42. WHEN five feet of Moor-stone were laid on, which according to the dimensions would weigh 120 tons; he then interposed a couple of courses of solid timber as before; the use of which was plainly for the more effectual and ready fastening of the outside uprights to the solid, by means of *Jag*-bolts†, or screw-bolts; and that these bolts might the more effectually hold in the wood, in every part of the circle (which could not be the case with timbers lying parallel to each other, because in two points of the circle opposite to each other, the timbers would present their ends towards the bolt) he encompassed those two courses with circular, or what is technically called *compass* timbers, properly *scarphed* together, and *breaking joint* one course upon the other. We must not however suppose, that these courses were composed wholly of circular timbers to the center, but that the circles of compass timbers on the outside, were filled up with parallel pieces within; and that the compass timbers were, in the most favourable points, jag-bolted to the interior parallel pieces.

The two uppermost courses, after clearing the rock, and before the five Moor-stone courses came on, were furnished with compass timbers, as well as some others below, which are also distinguished in Plate N° 6, exhibiting the orthographical elevation and section beforementioned of Mr. RUDYERD's Lighthouse, as it stood antecedent to its demolition by fire in the year 1755.

The two courses of wood above the Moor-stone courses beforementioned, terminated the *entire solid* of the basement; for a *Well Hole* was begun to be left upon these courses for stairs in the center, of six feet 9 inches in the square; and hereupon was fixed the entry door, or rather, one course lower, making a step up, just within the door; in consequence of this, the entire solid terminated about nine feet above the higher side of the base, and 19 feet above the lower side thereof‡.

The detached sketch Fig. 2, Plate N° 6 gives the plan of the five Moor-stone courses included in the entire solid, compiled from old working draughts, that appear to have been given out by Mr. RUDYERD during the course of the work, for forming and fixing these courses: the continued lines represent the joints of course N° 1; and the dotted lines, those of course N° 2, which shew how they broke joint upon one another: and the courses being alternately of these different figures, they would mutually break joint in the same manner.——In the original drawings, they were represented by black lines and red lines. ——From hence it appears, that though no cramps are represented, yet besides the mast in the center, there are ten holes of about two inches diameter each; eight of them forming an octagon round the center, and two more in two of the opposite stones that abut upon the mast: and I have no doubt, but that the use of those holes was for the passage of iron bars or bolts, which firmly laying hold of the two compass

* In Mr. RUDYERD's print six courses of Moor-stone are exhibited in this place; but in reality there were but five, as many occasions of repair have afterwards evinced; which is a further argument, that the print was compiled from a design or sketches made *before* the building was erected.

† *Jag* or *bearded* bolts or spikes, are such as with a chissel have a beard raised upon their angles, somewhat like that of a fish-hook, so that when driven forcibly into the wood, those beards, by laying hold, oppose their being drawn out again.

‡ The difference in the declivity of the base from that mentioned § 34 is to be attributed to the difference betwixt the original design and the execution.

courses

courses under the Moor-stone, then passing through the five Moor-stone courses, and lastly through the two compass courses above the Moor-stone, would, besides the upright cramps, be a further means of tying all these nine courses firmly together as one solid; that solid being firmly tied by the trenails to the courses below, and those ultimately to the branches. This mode of binding appears still the more probable, as in Mr. Rudyerd's copper-plate representation, there is the appearance of iron bars proceeding through all the courses of stone, and to the termination of the solid at the store-room floor; but of these I find no traces either in the said drawings, or the building above the entire solid, further than has been already described.

43. IN Mr. Winstanley's house, the entry was from the rock into an internal staircase, formed in the casing mentioned in the work of the 4th year, upon the S. E. side; he therefore needed only a few external steps, as shewn in Plate N° 5. But Mr. Rudyerd's entry door, being full eight feet above the highest part of the rock, he would consequently need a ladder. This he made of iron of great strength; and being open, whenever the seas broke upon this side of the house, they readily found their passage through, without making any very violent agitation upon it.

44. THE two compass courses terminating the entire solid, having been established, as already mentioned, he again proceeded with five Moor-stone courses; of which Fig. 3 is the plan, Plate N° 6, nearly the same as the former; allowing for the necessary difference, resulting from there now being a central well hole for the stairs, and a passage from the entry door, as described, to the well hole: this passage was 2 feet 11 inches wide, and, as it appears, took up the whole height of the five courses. The weight of these five courses, according to the dimensions, amounted to 86 tons.

He then again proceeded with two compass courses, covering the door head and passage, so as now to leave no other vacuity, than the well hole; and upon these he laid four Moor-stone courses*, the weight of which amounted to 67 tons. He then proceeded with two compass courses, and after that, with beds of timber cross and cross, and compass courses interposing; and last of all, with one compass course, upon which he laid a floor over all, of oak plank of three inches thick, which made the floor of the store-room.

45. THE height of this floor above the bottom of the well, was near 18 feet; above the foot of the mast 33 feet; above the rock on the higher side 27 feet; and above the foot of the building on the lower side 37 feet. In all this height, no cavity of any kind was intended for any purpose of depositing stores, &c.——From the rock to the bottom of the well, all was solid, as we have shewn; but as the building increased in height, and consequently was more out of the heavy stroke of the sea, a less degree of strength and solidity would be equivalent to the former, and therefore admit of the convenience of a staircase *within* the building, with a passage into it: which last, being made upon the east side, would be withdrawn from the heavy shock of the seas from the south-west quarter, and the rock being there highest, the ascent by the iron stair upon the outside, would be the least; the whole therefore to the height of the store-room floor, as abovementioned, having been made with all possible solidity, was denominated *the solid*.

46. THE height of Mr. Rudyerd's store-room floor, was fixed as high as the floor of Mr. Winstanley's *state*-room, which was over his store-room†; and as many were doubtless still living who had seen and examined Mr. Winstanley's Lighthouse, during the four years that it stood in a finished state; and as in that time there would be an opportunity of knowing from experience, to what height the unbroken water of the waves mounted in bad weather; we may very well suppose, that Mr. Rudyerd regulated the height of his solid from that information.

* Mr. Rudyerd's design shews five courses; but this is clearly a mistake, as might be seen at any time, by counting them in the staircase.

† See § 24 and Plate N° 5.

47. WE

41. WE have already ſeen, that the two compaſs courſes of wood, which capped the firſt bed of moorſtone, and terminated the entire ſolid, were forcibly ſcrewed down by ten large iron bars or bolts to the beds of timber below the moorſtone, and theſe by the trenails and branches to the rock. We muſt ſuppoſe this precaution to have been taken, to prevent any derangement from the heavy ſtrokes of the ſea in ſtorms and hard gales, which were liable to happen in the very fineſt part of the ſeaſon, before there was any proper opportunity of connecting the upper part of the work with the lower, by means of the upright timbers, that were to form the outſide caſe; becauſe, till the work was brought to that height, there could be no proper means of beginning to fix them: and as we do not find any traces or mention of binding the upper courſes with the lower, after the ſtaircaſe was ſet forward; we muſt ſuppoſe that the outſide caſing had been then begun from the rock, and carried on progreſſively, ſo as to become a *bond* of the upright kind: for, all ſuch timbers as were high enough, having been ſcrewed faſt to the compaſs courſes, would be thereby ſecured to the lower courſes; otherwiſe, from what I have myſelf experienced of the ſituation, I ſhould have expected, that whenever the two courſes of compaſs timber were put upon the ſecond bed of moorſtone, if a hard gale ſhould have come on at South-Weſt, it would not only have lifted up and carried away the timber beds, but poſſibly would have deranged the moorſtone courſes; notwithſtanding the upright cramps to the outſide ſtones.

42. THE ſolid being in this manner completed, the upper part of the building comprehending four rooms, one above another, was chiefly formed by the outſide upright timbers; having one *Kirb* or circle of compaſs timber at each floor, to which the upright timbers were ſcrewed and connected; and upon which the floor timbers were reſted. The uprights were alſo jag-bolted and trenailed to one another, and in this manner, the work was carried on to the height of 34 feet above the ſtore-room floor; and there terminated by a planking of three inches thick, which compoſed the roof of the main column, as well as ſerved for the floor of the lantern, and of the balcony round it.

43. THUS the main column of this building conſiſted of one ſimple figure, being an elegant *Fruſtum* of a cone, unbroken by any projecting ornament, or any thing whereon the violence of the ſtorms could lay hold; being, excluſive of its ſloping foundation, 22 feet 8 inches upon its largeſt circular baſe; 61 feet high above that circular baſe; and 14 feet 3 inches in diameter at the top: ſo that the circular baſe was ſomewhat greater than one-third of the total height, and the diameter at top was ſomewhat leſs than two thirds of the baſe at the greateſt circle.

44. THE junction of the upright timbers upon each other, was by means of *Scarfs*, as they are technically called in ſhip-building and carpentry; that is, the joining of timbers end to end by overlapping The timbers were of different lengths from 10 to 20 feet, and ſo ſuited, that no two joinings or ſcarfs of the uprights might fall together. The number of uprights compoſing the circle was the ſame from top to bottom; and their number being 71, their breadth at the bottom would be one foot nearly; their thickneſs there was 9 inches; and as they diminiſhed in breadth towards the top, they alſo diminiſhed in thickneſs. The whole of the outſide ſeams was well caulked with *Oakum*, in the ſame manner as in ſhips; and the whole *payed* over with pitch, conſequently upon a near view, the ſeams running ſtraight from top to bottom, in ſome meaſure reſembled the *fluting* of columns; which in ſo ſimple a figure, could not fail to catch the attention of the beholder, and prove an agreeable engagement of the eye.

The whole of the building was indeed a piece of *Shipwrightry*: for it is plain from the preceding account, that the interpoſed beds of moorſtone had nothing to do with the frame of the building, it being entire and complete excluſive thereof: the beds of moorſtone could therefore only be conſidered in the nature of ballaſt, and amounted, from what has been before ſtated in the whole, to the weight of above 270 Tons.

45. ALL the windows, ſhutters and doors were compoſed of double plank, croſs and croſs, and *clinked* together; which falling into a *rabbet*, when ſhut, their outſide formed a part of the general

 ſurface,

surface, like the port-holes in a ship's side; without making any unevenness or projection in the surface. ——There were however, two projecting parts terminating this *Frustum*; one at the top, and the other at the joining with the rock; the utility of which seems to render them indispensable. They were each of them a projection of about 9 inches. The top projection, which is in the nature of a cornice, consisted of a simple *bevil*, and the use of it was very great; for in time of storms and hard gales of wind, when, according to the accounts of Mr. WINSTANLEY's building, the broken sea rises to a far greater height than the whole structure, it would be likely to break the windows of the lantern, unless there was something to throw it off, as *their* use does not admit of any defence by shutters. Therefore Mr. RUDYERD applied this simple cornice, judging it sufficient to have the effect of throwing off the sea in time of storms; and yet not of so much projection, as that the sea at the height of 71 feet above the foot of the building could have power enough to derange it.

The bottom projection, which has been called the *Kant*, and which fills up the angle formed between the uprights and the sloping surface of the rock, so as to guard the foot of the uprights from that violence of action which the waves naturally exert when driven into a corner, was certainly a very useful application: but whether it was originally constructed by Mr. RUDYERD himself, or was applied some time after, upon finding a want thereof, is at present uncertain.——I am rather inclined to think the latter, and that for two reasons: First, there is nothing of the kant shewn in Mr. RUDYERD's print of the building; the feet of the uprights being shewn as applied to the naked steps, both in section and elevation, without any thing of the kant; but as there were in reality many other deviations, I am more strongly inclined to think it was not there, upon the first completion, for the second reason; that is, because the iron stanchions or branches, that were let into the rock by way of confining the kant in its place, were not fixed into the rock in the method of *Key* and *Dovetail*, as Mr. RUDYERD had done all his principal and original branches; but were fixed in with club ends, in the way of Mr. WINSTANLEY's irons: whereas a workman versed in Mr. RUDYERD's method, would not only find it much more firm, but even more easy in the execution, than the old method.

46. UPON the flat roof of the main column, as a platform, Mr. RUDYERD fixed his lantern, which was an octagon of 10 feet 6 inches diameter externally. The mean height of the window frames of the lantern above the balcony floor, was nearly nine feet, so that the elevation of the center of the light above the highest side of the base was 70 feet; that is, lower than the center of Mr. WINSTANLEY's second lantern by seven feet; but higher than that of his first by 24 feet.——The width of Mr. RUDYERD's lantern was however nearly the same as that of Mr. WINSTANLEY's second: but instead of the towering ornaments of iron work, and a vane that rose above the top of the cupola no less than 21 feet, Mr. RUDYERD judiciously contented himself with finishing his building with a round ball, of 2 feet 3 inches diameter, which terminated at three feet above the top of his cupola. The whole height of Mr. RUDYERD's lantern, including the ball, was no more than 21 feet above his balcony floor; whereas that of Mr. WINSTANLEY, including the iron ornaments, was above forty.

The whole height then of Mr. RUDYERD's Lighthouse, from the lowest side to the top of the ball, was 92 feet, upon a base of 23 feet 4 inches, taken at a medium between the highest and lowest part of the rock that it covered.

47. IN the elevation of this building, contained in plate N° 6, the rock is represented at the low water, as seen from the South, in the manner I found it in the year 1756; to which, the present plate of the elevation of his Lighthouse is adapted, from the best documents concerning it that have come into my hands.

A shews the rock.——B the landing place.

a a the steps or flats to which the rock was reduced.——b b the branches.——c c, &c. floors of wood laid lengthwise of the steps.——d d floors laid crossways of the same.——e e courses of compass timber.

——D live

——D five courses of moorstone, which with two courses of compass timber marked E completed the entire solid, to the top of which led

F the iron ladder to G the entry door, and through G H the entry or passage into——H I the well-hole for the stair case.——K L the mast.——M five courses of moorstone, the height of which composed the entry or passage.

N two beds of compass timber, making good the passage to the stairs.

O four beds of moorstone, capped with two beds of compass timber, after which succeeded courses of timber alternately *cross* and *cross*, with compass courses interposed as shewn in the section.

P Q shew the upright timbers, as they appeared externally, being 71 in number.

p q the same in the upright section.

I the store-room floor, and R the door of the store-room; which was so much further to the North than the entry, that when casks and stores were drawn up perpendicularly by a tackle, suspended from above, they would clear the iron ladder.

S the state-room.——T the bed chamber.——V the kitchen.——W the balcony——X the lantern.——Y the lantern door into the balcony; and—Z the cupola and ball.

f f four curved pipes for venting the smoke from the candles in the lantern.

g the top of the copper funnel, which passed through the lantern, from the kitchen fireplace which was of brick.

h the upper bevil, or projection by way of cornice for throwing off the sea, to prevent it from breaking the lantern windows in time of storms; which was necessary, though the panes were of *ground Glass*, on account of strength.

i knees to strengthen the junction of the uprights with the balcony floor, and also in part to support the weight of the lantern.

k k k the original kirbs of compass timbers to form the uprights to a circle, and support the weight of the floors.

m m m *Kirbs* applied of late years for strengthening the frame of the building.

n n the kant at the foot of the uprights, and o o one of the stanchions by which the kants were fastened down.

48. SUCH a platform as the balcony round the lantern was absolutely necessary, on account of cleaning the outside of the windows; which gather a saline incrustation upon them, every storm and hard gale of wind; and the rails not only served the purpose of preventing persons from tumbling over, but were of use in hoisting the flag, as a signal to the shore, that something was wanted. This is sufficiently explained by Plate N° 5: but the flag-staff was not always in one fixed place, as there represented; as it could occasionally be *lashed* to the most proper part of the rails for its exhibition to the shore; and to suit the wind, so as that the flag might fly clear of the building.

Also instead of any cranes as shewn by Mr. WINSTANLEY, a pair of *tackle* blocks were occasionally, when wanted, hooked to the hand-rail of the balcony, and taken in when done with; for there was little chance of getting any thing into the house, except when a boat could lie in the Gut, and then it might be landed directly into the store-room.

The chink at p is the place where a part of a chain, apparently one of Mr. WINSTANLEY's crane chains, was jammed in so fast on the destruction of that Lighthouse, that it remained so during the whole continuance of Mr. RUDYERD's Lighthouse, and was shewn as one of the curiosities of the place.

49. I HAVE endeavoured to describe this building with all possible minuteness, because it affords a great, and a very useful lesson to future Engineers. We are sure that a building such as Mr. WINSTANLEY's, was not capable of resisting the utmost fury of the sea; because, in four years after its completion, it was totally demolished thereby: but Mr. RUDYERD's building having sustained the repeated attacks of that element in all its fury, for upwards of 46 years after its completion; and then being

being destroyed, not by water, but by fire; we must conclude, it was of a construction capable of withstanding the greatest violence of the sea in *that* situation. And by withstanding it *there*, this Lighthouse proves the practicability of a similar erection in any like exposure in the known world: for, having attentively read and considered what is contained in the respective voyages of ANSON, BYRON, COOK, and PHIPPS, the most scientific navigators that modern times have produced, I do not find in all their accounts, such an exposure to the sea's uttermost violence, as at the *Edystone Rocks*.

50. Mr. RUDYERD informs us, as abovementioned, that a light was put up in this building the 28th *July* 1708, and that it was completely finished in 1709*. The means of exhibiting this light, would have been not only curious, but useful, had it been handed down to us. The best information that I have been enabled to procure upon this point is, " that a light was exhibited from the house in a lantern, that was raised upon eight fir *Balks*, which butted upon the solid, and were weather-boarded with deal." ——At this time we must suppose that the solid was completed; and, in a great part, its exterior casing also; but that this casing was not got much above the solid: if therefore those eight pillars were raised, so as to be capable of hoisting a light above the floor of the third room; then, in the course of that summer, they might very well perfect the two low rooms, for lodging the lightkeepers, during the ensuing winter; and finish the two remaining rooms and principal lantern, the next season of 1709, as Mr. RUDYERD relates; that being the fourth and last summer of the progress of that work.

51. THE following anecdote has been related to me by such a variety of persons, that I cannot doubt of its having some foundation in truth, though no mention has been made thereof by Mr. RUDYERD. The relation will therefore I trust be acceptable to my readers, as it at once shews the great estimation in which this building has been held by foreigners, even such as were, at the very time, enemies of this country.

LEWIS *the* XIV. being at war with England, during the proceeding with this building, a French privateer took the men at work upon the Edystone rock, together with their tools, and carried them to France; and the captain was in expectation of a reward for the achievement. While the captives lay in prison, the transaction reached the ears of that monarch: He immediately ordered them to be released, and the captors to be put in their place; declaring, that though he was at war with England, he was not at war with mankind; he therefore directed the men to be sent back to their work with presents; observing that the Edystone Lighthouse was so situated, as to be of equal service to all nations having occasion to navigate the channel that divides France from England †.

52. I HAVE seen a paper in the hands of one of the present proprietors, upon which were put down the quantities of materials said to have been expended in the construction of this building: *viz.* 500 tons of stone; 1200 tons of timber; 80 tons of iron, and 35 tons of lead; and of trenails, screws, and rack-bolts 2500 each ‡.

* This is further ascertained by the following extract from the preamble of an act of the 8th of ANNE, chap. 17.

" And whereas the said *Master, Wardens*, and *Assistants* (of TRINITY HOUSE) having a due regard to the safety and preservation of the shipping and navigation of this kingdom, did soon after the passing of the said act, (4th of ANNE, chap. 20.) cause the said Lighthouse to be begun, and to be rebuilt; and by the great care and diligence of the persons employed therein, the said work was carried on with such expedition, that a light *useful for shipping* was placed therein on the 28th July 1708; and the said Lighthouse hath since, with much hazard and difficulty, and at a very great expence been fully built and completed, to the great satisfaction of the flag officers and commanders of her majesty's fleet and ships of war, and of all others concerned in trade and navigation."

† Mr. RUDYERD's remarks upon the face of his print, that " to expedite the work and to protect the workmen, these four men of war, at sundry times, were appointed to this station, *viz.* 1st, The *Roebuck* of 42 guns.——2d, The *Charles Galley* of 36.——3d, The [illegible] *Prize* of 3[illegible].——4th, The *Albrew* of 24." Which appointment was probably in consequence of the accident above related.

‡ This must be supposed the account of rough materials, otherwise the stone and timber must greatly exceed the real quantity.

CHAP.

CHAP. IV.

Containing Subſequent Tranſactions and Occurrences from the Finiſhing Mr. RUDYERD's *Lighthouſe, to the total Demolition thereof.*

53. FROM the time of finiſhing the Lighthouſe in 1709, we have no further particulars till about the year 1715, when Captain LOVET, the proprietor of the leaſe, under the Corporation of the *Trinity Houſe*, beforementioned, being deceaſed, his property was ſold at public biddings by a Maſter in Chancery, in conſequence of a decree and directions from that court: when it was purchaſed by three perſons, *viz.* ROBERT WESTON, Eſq; RICHARD NOYES, Eſq; of *Grays Inn*; and ——— CHEETHAM, Eſq; an Alderman of *Dublin*. The agreement of the purchaſers was to divide the leaſehold property thus acquired into eight ſhares, of which Mr. WESTON had three, Mr. NOYES two, and Mr. CHEETHAM three.

54. THIS houſe, we are told, ſtood in no need of any material repairs for ſome years; but in or about the year 1723, defects were diſcovered, which required great attention: for now it was firſt obſerved, that ſome parts of the uprights were decayed at the but ends, by means of a ſmall worm, which had eaten ſome inches into them, eſpecially thoſe on the loweſt ſide of the houſe. Hereupon the gentlemen proprietors appointed Mr. JOHN HOLLAND, then a foreman ſhipwright in his Majeſty's dock-yard at *Plymouth*, to ſurvey and direct the repairs; which he very judiciouſly did, from time to time, till he was advanced to the office of aſſiſtant builder in *Woolwich Yard*: on which occaſion, the overſeeing and conducting of the repairs was transferred to a creditable ſhipwright at Plymouth dock; upon whoſe reports of the ſtate of the building, from time to time, Mr. HOLLAND gave directions in what manner to proceed: but this not being ſo ſatisfactory to the proprietors, as when under the immediate inſpection and direction of Mr. HOLLAND; and ſome conſiderable repairs being neceſſary in the year 1734, Mr. HOLLAND, by leave of the Lords Commiſſioners of the ADMIRALTY, was ſent down to Plymouth to conduct the ſame.

This is the period when the ſtructure of that edifice, and the defects it was liable to, became better underſtood; for one of the gentlemen principally intereſted, followed Mr. HOLLAND to *Plymouth*, and reſiding there a conſiderable time, made many obſervations in his viſits to the building; and ſeeing how the works were carried on, formed ſuch a plan for the future conducting of this ſtructure, as might probably have preſerved it for a number of years, againſt the attacks of thoſe elements to which from its critical ſituation it was the moſt obviouſly expoſed †.

55. IN this place it may be proper to take notice of an experiment which was tried in 1734, to prevent the ill effects that might happen from the worm: and that was by covering the outſides of 15 pieces of the uprights, at the bottom of the houſe, with *copper*, and their inſides with lead; and two pieces were covered entirely with copper, as high as the worm deſtroyed: but I am informed, this did

† In this year Mr. HOLLAND made a very curious draught of the Lighthouſe, in which every one of the outſide upright timbers was diſtinctly repreſented; ſo that every one of them could numerically be referred to; and the places and nature of the ſcarfing or joinings diſtinguiſhed. This was done by ſuppoſing the whole of the uprights to be ſeparated at one particular joint, from top to bottom; and then all the reſt opened till they were brought into one plane: the figure thus formed would become a kind of *Evolute* of the ſurface of the whole building; and was peculiarly adapted to illuſtrate the experiments, reports and repairs that were then carrying on, and might from time to time thereafter be wanted or recommended: this draught diſtinctly repreſents the *kant* at the bottom; and hereby it was firſt known, that the real number of uprights was 71; and not 72 as had been before imagined.

not thoroughly anſwer expectation; for in 1744, one of thoſe pieces that was entirely coppered, was taken out, and found to be worm-eaten *.

56. THE latter end of 1744 after all the neceſſary repairs were finiſhed, there happened a dreadful ſtorm on the 26th September, which being from the Eaſt, tore away no leſs than 30 pieces of the uprights all together †; which in part made an opening into the ſtore-room: this diſaſter however, by great exertion, was entirely repaired by the 14th December following, under the inſpection and direction of Mr. JOSIAS JESSOP, then (and indeed until his death no more than) that ſpecies of foreman ſhipwright, called a *Quarter-man* in Plymouth dock. This perſon, whoſe modeſty and ingenuity cauſed him to be deſervedly reſpected by many, Mr. HOLLAND recommended to the proprietors to be their overſeer, which they ſtill rank among the eminent ſervices he did them ‡.

Mr. HOLLAND, who had been promoted to be King's *Builder* at Deptford Yard, continued his good offices to the time of his death, which happened not till the year 1752; and then the execution of the important office of repairing this building, was ſolely intruſted to Mr. JESSOP, who diſcharged his duty herein, with the greateſt integrity, diligence and accuracy, till the calamity happened, which totally deſtroyed the building, and which could neither be foreſeen nor avoided.

57. IT ſeems that for many years after the eſtabliſhment of this Lighthouſe, it was attended by two men only; and indeed the duty required no more; as the principal part of that, beſides keeping the windows of the lantern clean (and in general the rooms) was the alternately watching *four hours*, and *four hours*, to ſnuff and renew the candles; each at the concluſion of his watch taking care to call the other and to ſee him on duty before he himſelf retired: but it happened, that one of the men was taken ill and died; and notwithſtanding the Edyſtone *Flag* was hoiſted, yet the weather was ſuch for ſome time, as to prevent any boat from getting ſo near the rocks as to ſpeak to them §.——In this dilemma, the living man found himſelf in an awkward ſituation; being apprehenſive that if he tumbled the dead body into the ſea, which was the only way in his power to diſpoſe of it, he might be charged with murder; this induced him for ſome time to let the dead corpſe lie, in hopes that the boat might be able to land and relieve him from the diſtreſs he was in.——By degrees the body became ſo offenſive, that it was not in his power to get quit of it without help; for it was near a month before the attending boat could effect a landing; and then it was not without the greateſt difficulty that it could be done when they did land. To ſuch a degree was the whole building filled with the ſtench of the corpſe, that it was all they could do

* It will now ſeem that this experiment of plate copper (which I have from the beſt authority) that did not ſucceed in preventing and deſtroying the worm, is not eaſily to be reconciled with the preſent practice of ſheathing ſhips bottoms therewith, which is held to be an effectual remedy, as being a poiſon to the worm: this we may however infer, that this, as well as many other good propoſitions, have been given up too haſtily: for though here was a trial of 10 years, yet the practice was condemned as *ineffectual* upon a *ſingle inſtance*.——On conſulting my ſcientifical friends reſpecting this fact, ingenious reaſons have been ſuggeſted, why the conſtant ſtate of immerſion that takes place in a ſhip's bottom, may more effectually convey the poiſon into the wood, than where it is forſaken by the ſea every tide; and even that the ſtrokes of the ſea may at the Edyſtone be ſo great as to waſh the poiſon out again from the wood, that in a ſituation of leſs violence could gradually and ſlowly inſinuate itſelf; and probably ſomething of this kind may have been the caſe: but on lately converſing with a very intelligent *builder* of one of his *Majeſty's yards*, I am informed, that it is not uncommon for the timber of ſhips to be eat by the worm under the copper ſheathing, where the joints have not been carefully cloſed; ſo that in fact it is not ſo much its being a *poiſon*, as the means of the [illegible] *evaſion*, by a coating that they cannot penetrate, that prevents their deſtroying the wood: we may therefore, rather impute the want of ſucceſs in the year 1734, to their not being ſkilful to cloſe the joints of the copper plates ſufficiently compact.

† It was in this ſtorm that Admiral BALCHEN was loſt in the *Victory*.

‡ After the appointment of Mr. JESSOP, and in conſquence of the numbers of uprights torn away in the ſtorm of 1744, which enabled [illegible] into the conſtruction of the ſolid than had been known before; he made a ſtill more accurate *Evolute*, and alſo a model of the *Lighthouſe*, and it is principally from the meaſures of this Evolute, that I have compiled the preſent draught, Plate N° 6.

§ The ſign, when any thing was wanted by the Lightkeepers, was to hoiſt a large flag upon a flag-ſtaff from the balcony rails (as has been obſerved in the references to the Plates N° 5 and 6) on the leeward ſide, ſo as to be fully extended by the wind, clear of the building: [illegible] moderate weather from the heights about *Ram-Head*: and that it might never be hung out in vain, it was a [illegible] at the perſon [illegible] firſt notice to the agent at Plymouth, received from him half a guinea; the agent immediately on this [illegible] a boat, to land, if poſſible, and at leaſt to know what was wanted.

ſo

to get the dead body diſpoſed of, and thrown into the ſea; and it was ſome time after that, before the rooms could be got freed from the noiſome ſtench that was left. This induced the proprietors to employ a *third* man; ſo that in caſe of a future accident of the ſame nature, or the ſickneſs of either, there might be conſtantly one to ſupply the place.

This regulation alſo afforded a ſeaſonable relief to the Lightkeepers; for ever ſince there were three, it has been an eſtabliſhed rule, that in the ſummer, in their turns, they are permitted each to go on ſhore, and ſpend a month among their friends and acquaintance.

58. WHETHER the abovementioned two men, of which one died, were the two to which the following account that I found very current in the country, referred; or it was a couple preceding them, is now uncertain: but a boat landing there with viſitants of curioſity (as not unfrequently happens in the ſummer ſeaſon) after examining the place and ſtructure; they obſerved to one of the men, how very comfortably they might there live in a ſtate of retirement. "Yes," ſays the man, "very *comfortably*, if we could have the uſe of our *tongues*; but it is now a full month ſince my partner and I have ſpoke to each other." The appointment of *three* has moſt likely put a ſtop to this piece of unſeaſonable taciturnity; for though we have ſeen it is poſſible to find two, yet it is ſcarcely probable there ſhould be found *three together* of this mind *.

Being now upon the chapter of anecdotes, I will proceed to give one, that ſhews how very different the ideas of mankind are concerning the nature of *confinement*. It happened in ſome one of the laſt years of the continuance of the late building; and I was told the ſtory by the very *ſkipper* who bore a part in the converſation. Says the ſkipper to a ſhoemaker in his boat, who he was carrying out to be a lightkeeper; How happens it, friend *Jacob*, that you ſhould chuſe to go out to be a lightkeeper, when you can on ſhore, as I am told, earn your half crown and three ſhillings a day in making leathern hoſe †; whereas the lightkeeper's ſalary is but £. 25 a year, which is ſcarce ten ſhillings a week? Says the ſhoemaker, I go to be a lightkeeper becauſe I don't like *confinement!* After this anſwer had produced its ſhare of merriment; he at laſt explained himſelf, by ſaying, that he did not like to be *confined to work*.

59. WE now come to the laſt awful ſcene, containing the fatal *cataſtrophe* of this celebrated building.

On the 22d of Auguſt 1755 the workmen returned on ſhore, having finiſhed all neceſſary repairs of that ſeaſon: between which time and the 2d of December following, the attending boat had been off ſeveral times to the Edyſtone, and particularly on the 1ſt of December, and had landed ſome ſtores, when the lightkeepers made no manner of complaint; and ſaid all was right, except that one or two of the bricks in the kitchen fire-place, had been looſened by a late ſtorm ‡.

60. WHAT in reality might occaſion the building's firſt catching fire, it has never been poſſible fully to inveſtigate; but from the moſt diſtinct account, it appears to have commenced in the very top of the lantern, that is, in the *cupola*.

If I might hazard conjectures, I would ſuppoſe, that the whole building being of wood, and the heat of the candles in the lantern conſiderable §, and this repeated every night for between 40 and 50

* It is very poſſible I might have paſſed over this anecdote in ſilence, had it not been alluded to in one of the ſpeeches of Lord NORTH, in the time of the late war, where he gives this as an inſtance how the *public ſervice* is liable to be obſtructed by *private diſſentions*; however juſt this remark, yet as it may be a ſatisfaction to the maritime part of the public to know it; I beg leave to ſay, I never heard that *this line* of the *public* ſervice was ever intermitted or obſtructed by this or any diſſentions among the parties themſelves.

† Leathern pipes ſo called.

‡ This is another proof of the violent agitation this building was put into by ſtorms and hard gales of wind.

§ *Viz.* 24 candles burning at once, five whereof weighed two pounds, and it was uſual to go into the lantern to ſnuff them every half hour.

years together, we may well ſuppoſe the wood above them, and particularly the lining of thin boards that ſupported the uppermoſt cover of ſheet lead, to be brought into a perfect ſtate of dryneſs and inflammability; and this of courſe being covered with a thick cruſt of ſoot, collected by receiving the ſmoke of the candles, the whole together would become in reality a maſs of *tinder* and *matches*. Now if we can ſuppoſe it poſſible for a ſingle ſpark to fly from one of the candles, and lodge itſelf in this maſs of combuſtible matter, the conſequence is obvious: or, if we ſuppoſe, that in length of time, the copper funnel in paſſing the cupola, had been corroded by the ſalts of the ſea falling into it in ſtorms, and alſo by the pit-coal ſoot from the kitchen fire, ſo as to open a hole into the upper part in the cupola, by which, a ſpark might iſſue from the fire below, the conſequence would be the ſame *. But whether either of theſe may be eſteemed a probable account of the origin of the fire, or not, it is certain, that when the lightkeeper then upon the watch (about two o'clock in the morning of the 2d of December) went into the lantern as uſual to ſnuff the candles, he found the whole in a ſmoke; and upon opening the door of the lantern into the balcony, a flame inſtantly burſt from the inſide of the cupola: he immediately endeavoured to alarm his companions; but they being in bed and aſleep, were not ſo ready in coming to his aſſiſtance as the occaſion required.——As there were always ſome leathern buckets kept in the houſe, and a tub of water in the lantern; he attempted as ſpeedily as poſſible to extinguiſh the fire in the cupola, by throwing water from the balcony with a leather bucket, upon the outſide cover of lead: by this time, his comrades approaching, he encouraged them to fetch up water with the leather buckets from the ſea; but as the height would be at a medium full 70 feet, this, added to the natural conſternation that muſt attend ſuch a ſudden and totally unexpected event, would occaſion this buſineſs of bringing up water, at the beſt to go on but ſlowly. Meanwhile, the flames gathering ſtrength every moment, and the poor man, though making uſe of every exertion, having the water to throw full four yards higher than his own head, to be of any ſervice; we muſt by no means be ſurpriſed, that under all theſe difficulties, the fire, inſtead of being ſoon extinguiſhed, would increaſe; and what put a ſudden ſtop to further exertions, was the following moſt remarkable circumſtance.

As he was looking upward with the utmoſt attention, to ſee the direction and ſucceſs of the water thrown; on which occaſion, as *phyſiognomiſts* tell us, the mouth is naturally a little open; a quantity of lead, diſſolved by the heat of the flames, ſuddenly ruſhed like a torrent from the roof, and fell, not only upon the man's head, face and ſhoulders, but over his cloaths; and a part of it made its way through his ſhirt collar, and very much burnt his neck and ſhoulders: from this moment he had a violent internal ſenſation, and imagined that a quantity of this lead had paſſed his throat, and got into his body. Under this violence of pain and anxiety, as every attempt had proved ineffectual, and the rage of the flames was increaſing, it is not to be wondered that the terror and diſmay of the three men increaſed in proportion; ſo that they all found themſelves intimidated, and glad to make their retreat from that immediate ſcene of horror, into one of the rooms below: where they would find themſelves precluded from doing *any thing*; for had they thrown down ever ſo much water there, it could not have extinguiſhed what was burning above them; nor indeed, produce any other effect, than that of running down into the rooms below; and from thence finally through the ſtaircaſe, back again into the ſea: they ſeem therefore to have had no other reſource or means of retreat, than that of retiring downwards from room to room, as the fire advanced over their heads.

61. HOW ſoon the fire was ſeen from the ſhore, is not very certain; but early in the morning it was perceived by ſome of the *Cawſand* fiſhermen †, and intelligence thereof given to Mr. EDWARDS

* This ſuppoſition is not without grounds, as the lightkeepers, after the accident, declared, that the fire broke out from the chimney or funnel into the cupola, but were not believed *then*, as the whole of it that paſſed through the lantern was of *copper*.

† *Cawſand Bay* is a capacious bay within the confines of Plymouth Sound; it lies juſt within the Sound, on the weſt ſide; the ſouthermoſt point of this bay is Point *Penlee*, which is alſo the extreme point of Plymouth Sound on the weſt ſide; and the two fiſhing towns of *Kingſton* and *Cawſand* are ſituated at the bottom of the bay. See the Map, N° 2.

of

of *Rame* in that neighbourhood, a gentleman of some fortune, and more humanity. This prompted him immediately to send out a fishing-boat and men, to the relief of the people he supposed in distress upon the Edystone *.

The boat and men got thither about ten o'clock, after the fire had been burning full eight hours; and in this time, the three lightkeepers were not only driven from all the rooms, and the stair-case, but to avoid the falling of the timber, and red-hot bolts, &c. upon them, they were found sitting in the hole or cave on the East side of the rock (See Plate N° 6 Letter q, also Plate N° 14 Letter X) under the iron ladder, almost in a state of stupefaction; it being then low water.

62. AT this time the wind was eastwardly, and did not blow very fresh; but just hard enough to make a landing upon the rock, at the proper landing-place (which is on the East side) quite impracticable, or attended with the utmost hazard. It therefore became a difficulty, how the men were to be taken off; for the ground swell upon the West side produced so great a surf upon the sloping surface, that no boat could attempt to land there. They however fell upon the following expedient: having a small boat with them, they moored their principal boat by a *grapling* to the westward; but as near the rock as they durst; and then launching their small boat, they rowed it towards the rock, veering out a rope, which they had fastened to the large boat, till they got near enough to throw a coil of small rope upon the rock; which having been laid hold of by the men, they one by one fastened it round their waists, and jumping into the sea, they were towed into the small boat; and from thence delivered into the large one: and as they found that it was out of their power to do any further service, this boat hastened to Plymouth to get the men relieved. No sooner however were they set on shore, than one of them made off, and has never since been heard of: which would on the first blush induce one to suppose, there was something culpable in this man; and if it had been a house on shore one would have been tempted to suspect he had been guilty of some foul play: but the circumstance of its being a Lighthouse, situated so as to afford no retreat in the power of its inhabitants, seems to preclude the possibility of its being done wilfully; as he must know, he must perish, or be in extreme danger of so doing at least, along with the rest. I would therefore rather impute his sudden flight, to that kind of *panic*, which sometimes, on important occasions, seizes weak minds; making them act without reason, and in so doing commit actions the very reverse in tendency of what they mean them to have; and of which they have afterwards occasion to repent: but the man already described to have suffered so much by the melted lead, was sent to his own house at *Stonehouse*, a village near the place where they landed.

63. IT was not long after the alarm was made at Cawsand, that the dreadful news reached Plymouth; and as from the composition of the structure, it was thought that a considerable part of it might be saved, at least of the foundation, endeavours were not wanting for that purpose; for Mr. Alderman TOLCHER, the agent and collector of the duties, who was a perfect enthusiast for the welfare of the Lighthouse; and his son Mr. JOSEPH TOLCHER, immediately went out to sea; both gentlemen were ever, but then more than ever, indefatigable in their endeavours for its preservation. When they came there, alas! what could they do? There was no landing, except at the imminent hazard of their lives; and if landed, they could not do any thing. They could therefore only have the supreme mortification to behold, that after the rooms and all the upper works were totally destroyed, the fire was rapidly communicating itself into the solid; and there being many beds of solid timber above all the stone, their connexion with those below, by means of the mast and stairs in the well-hole, and by the upright timbers on the outside, would not suffer a doubt to remain, that after such a mass of fire was generated above, it would gradually communicate itself to the beds of timber interposed between those of Moor-stone, and by that means consume the whole.

* I am informed by my esteemed friend Dr. Mudge of *Plymouth*, that the philanthropy of this worthy gentleman on this occasion, cost him his life; for his exertions gave him so violent a cold as to bring on complaints of which he shortly after died.

64. THE late worthy Admiral West, who then lay with a fleet in Plymouth Sound, on hearing of the accident, immediately sent out a sloop properly manned, with a boat and an engine therein, which also carried out Mr. Jessop the surveyor; this vessel also arrived early in the day on which the fire happened. In endeavouring to make a landing of the engine, on the West side, it being then about low water, the boat, men and engine were at once tossed upon the rock by a wave, which on its retreat left them thereon; and before the engine was got out of the boat, another wave came, set them afloat, and swept them back again to their former situation: *British Tars* are not dismayed with small matters; however, *this* accident sufficiently taught them to be thankful for an escape with their lives; and to make no further attempt to land: yet they notwithstanding tried to play the engine from the boat; but the agitation of the sea near the rock was such, that they very soon broke the engine pipe; and so ended this well meant expedition, in a total disappointment.

65. THE only hopes that then remained, were from a great addition to the wind, which then blew; or a shift of wind to the S. W. quarter: for, the rocks being nearly perpendicular on the East side; and the seas being in some measure broken by the *South Reef* stretching on the East side of the *House Reef*, (See Plate N° 3.) it is only in hard gales of wind that the sea breaks in quantity, and bodily over the house reef from the East towards the West; whereas, the wind if only fresh at S. W. increases the ground swell, which is almost constant (more or less) from that quarter, to a degree that would infallibly have put out the fire: but if we are believers in *Fate*, we must suppose that this building had been destined to a total destruction: for the wind continued almost invariably at the same quarter, and with the same degree of strength; so that there was constantly sea enough to prevent all attempts to land, and yet not enough to cause the seas to break so high, and in such quantity as to put out the fire.

In the succeeding days, it was observed that the interposed beds of timber were sufficient to heat the Moor-stone beds red hot; and that the whole mass became one great body of red hot matter. Nor was it till the 7th of the same month, that the joint action of the wind, the fire and the seas totally completed the catastrophe so fatally begun; and then left no other evidence of the destruction they had made, than that the greatest number of the iron cramps and branches were left standing upright upon the rock.

66. WE will now return to the poor unfortunate man, who had received so peculiar an injury by the melted lead. His name was Henry Hall of *Stonehouse* near Plymouth, and though aged 94 years, being of a good constitution, he was remarkably active considering his time of life: he had invariably told the surgeon who attended him (Mr. Spry, now Dr. Spry of Plymouth, who constantly administered the proper remedies to such burns and hurts as could be perceived) that if he would do any thing effectual to his recovery, he must relieve his stomach from the lead, which he was sure was within him: and this he not only told Dr. Spry, but those about him, though in a very hoarse voice; and he also said the same thing to Mr. Jessop, who went to see him several times during his illness, and who gave me this information. The reality of the assertion seemed however then incredible to Dr. Spry, who could scarcely suppose it possible, that any human being could exist, after receiving melted lead into the stomach; much less that he should afterwards be able to bear towing through the sea from the rock; and also the fatigue and inconvenience from the length of time he was in getting on shore, before any remedies could be applied. The man did not shew any symptoms however of being either much worse, or of amendment, till the sixth day after the accident, when he was thought to be better: he constantly took his medicines, and swallowed many things both liquid and solid till the tenth or eleventh day; after which he suddenly grew worse; and the twelfth day being seized with cold sweats and spasms, he soon afterwards expired.

Mr. Jessop was desired by Dr. Spry to attend the opening of the body; but being averse to sights of that kind, he excused himself from seeing the operation; as did also the daughter of the deceased, and another woman who was in the house. On opening the stomach Dr. Spry found therein, a solid piece of lead of a flat oval form, which weighed *Seven Ounces* and five drachms, and this he immediately shewed

to

to the two women, and afterwards to Mr. Jessop. I have also seen the piece of lead since in the hands of Mr. Tolcher, and it appeared to me, as if a part of the coat of the stomach firmly adhered to the convex side thereof.

67. BY a letter of the 19th December, Dr. Spry transmitted an account of this very singular case to the *Royal Society*, inclosing the exact weight and figure of the lead; but that learned body thinking the circumstance very unlikely and extraordinary, and doubting the truth of it, the reading of the paper was deferred till a further elucidation was received.

As Dr. Spry had on this occasion been deprived of the benefit of eye-witnesses; and supposing his character called upon, not only as a professional man, but as a man of veracity; he endeavoured to support himself by experiments of the same kind upon different animals.——He therefore tried what would happen by pouring melted lead down the throats of dogs and fowls, to the amount of, from six drachms to six ounces; and found that those animals survived the operation, till they were killed to extract the lead: and Dr. Spry says, he kept one dog with lead in his stomach, with intent to try how long he might survive.

The account of these experiments is contained in a letter of the 30th January 1756, from Dr. Spry, addressed to Lord Macclesfield, then *President* of the Royal Society; and it was further corroborated by a letter from the late Dr. Huxham of Plymouth, F. R. S. to the late Sir William Watson, F. R. S. who speaks not only to the ingenuity and veracity of Dr. Spry, but of his being himself eye-witness to the extraction of a lump of lead of near three ounces weight, from the crop of a cock, that previous to being killed, though he seemed dull, yet readily pecked and swallowed several barley-corns that were thrown to him *.

Though the authenticity of this wonderful (and till this instance unheard of) capacity of animal bodies was thus investigated †; yet Dr. Spry was still so unfortunate as to fall under a censure of a different kind; that of cruelty towards the animals, in trying the experiments mentioned.

For my own part I cannot but think that Dr. Spry was somewhat hardly used: he attempted no experiments upon other animals, till he found his account disbelieved by the most eminent of his profession; his character therefore and future prospects in life were endangered, he being then a young gentleman of some expectations. What therefore was the comparison between the lives of a few dogs and poultry, to the loss of character of a man bred to a profession, upon his success in which, as depending upon the good opinion of others, must depend likewise that benefit and utility which he might be of to his fellow-subjects? Such however was Dr. Spry's lot, that in establishing his abilities in his profession, he was then by some stigmatized with the imputation of inhumanity.

68. IT has been thought by many, that if the poor lightkeepers, when in the midst of their distress, had been possessed of reflection enough to have thrown out their combustible stores, such as chests of *Candles*, *Coals*, &c. there might have been a probability of saving the whole, or some part of the *solid* of the Lighthouse; in which case, the repair would have been ready and easy; and the following summer might have been sufficient for its reinstatement: but in my own opinion, the doing of this could not have retarded the progress of the fire a single hour; for, in the three upper rooms there was little more to burn than in the store-room, had it been emptied of stores; and the same communication by the uprights,

* Those that are further curious on this subject, will find a full account thereof in the 49th vol. of the *Philosophical Transactions* page 477, wherein Dr. Spry fully describes the complaints and method of treatment of his patient; and in the succeeding articles are other particulars above referred to.

† Though there is at present no doubt of the fact of the lead being taken out of the man's stomach after he had survived it 12 days; yet these experiments by no means prove, that it would not be instant death to the human species, in by far the *greatest number* of cases.

would

would have taken place here, as above; and the ſtore-room floor, being itſelf, and every thing underneath it, of wood, for a depth or thickneſs of between ſix and ſeven feet; and this open in the center by a ſquare of above ſix feet, in which were included the ſtairs and the maſt, there could be no want of communication for the fire, from the rooms to the ſolid, even excluſive of all the ſtores: nor can I conceive any thing within the reach of human art could have ſaved the building, even if the rock had been acceſſible; unleſs there had been time enough for ſhipwrights or carpenters to have been ſent out with proper tools, before the fire had got ſo low as the ſtore-room: then indeed it would have been very practicable to have cut the uprights quite round the building, where they were only a ſingle thickneſs, as was the caſe above the ſtore-room floor; and by ſupporting the *Saw-gate* with wedges, the whole of the ſuperſtructure, together with the maſt, might have been expeditiouſly ſevered from the ſolid: but even after this, under the circumſtances beforementioned, it would have been very problematical, whether a battery of chain ſhot from a ſhip of war, carrying heavy metal, could have ſo ſpeedily and effectually diſperſed the ſuperſtructure ſo ſevered, as to have prevented its fragments from ſetting fire to the ſolid below: and to ſuch a maſs of combuſtibles, had the ſolid caught fire, a ſingle fire-engine, or even two, which would be rather more than could have been worked upon the rock, with any degree of convenience, would have proved very inadequate.

Nothing therefore, as it ſeems, but a ſtorm, or hard gale of wind at South-weſt, as already hinted, could have effectually put out the fire, ſo as to have ſaved any material part of the building, which, after a duration of forty-nine years from its commencement, was doomed to inevitable deſtruction, by an element, not ſo much as thought of as an *Enemy*; or guarded againſt, as ſuch, in its erection.

BOOK II.

An Account of preparatory matters towards building the present Lighthouse *upon the* EDYSTONE ROCK *with* STONE.

CHAP. I.

Containing the Proceedings from the destruction of Mr. RUDYERD's *Lighthouse in December* 1755, *to* Mr. SMEATON's *departure from* LONDON *to* PLYMOUTH *in March* 1756.

69. THE Lighthouse happily effected by Mr. RUDYERD, having been totally consumed by fire in December 1755, as before related; and the Proprietors, having the remainder of a term therein of above half a century, they immediately applied themselves in the most strenuous manner towards the erecting of another Lighthouse in the place of that which had been, both for themselves and the public, so unfortunately destroyed. In this however there arose some difficulties; for a space of 30 years having elapsed, since the purchases of shares by the three families which I have mentioned, § 53, in this interval a number of changes (as might reasonably be expected) had happened in the property. Some shares of the Lighthouse having been devised by will to be divided amongst children, and settlements on marriage having taken place with respect to other shares thereof; the claimants therefore were now become numerous. The whole interest of the third person mentioned, Mr. CHEETHAM, being three shares, was however at this time vested in a Mrs. HOFSLEGGER, they having been settled upon her in marriage; and on this account, the principal impediment occurred; for without the expenditure of a considerable sum of money, such as it might be supposed three-eighths of the erection would cost, the whole of her shares could not be valued at any thing; no duties being payable while no light was exhibited*: and as her estate in the Lighthouse was only for life, it was not to be expected that she should advance a sum of money, from the expenditure of which the greatest benefit might probably devolve upon her successors. In consequence of this circumstance, an early application to *Parliament* took place, and an act was obtained enabling Mrs. HOFSLEGGER to sell so much of her property and interest in the Lighthouse, as would pay for that share of the building she was to retain.

On the other hand it may be reckoned among the fortunate circumstances attending this *Catastrophe*, that the three-eighths purchased by the WESTON's, not only remained in that family, but continued so far united, that, though separately taken they were in different branches, yet the executive part for the whole of these shares was in one person: and as at this time the claimants under the NOYES's family were more than a dozen in number, it still more fortunately happened, that ROBERT WESTON, Esq; from his having for years past taken a most discreet part, respecting the management of this property, and having so considerable a share in his own person, had the utmost trust and confidence reposed in him by the whole body of the proprietors: but it may be reckoned among the most fortunate of all the circumstances for the future undertaking, that this gentleman was not more remarkable for his strict integrity, than for his discernment and universal *Philanthropy*.

* An early piece of justice, which indeed has always marked the Proprietors, appeared by their advertisement in the *Gazette*, and other newspapers, in the first fortnight after the accident happened, importing that the duties had ceased till a fresh exhibition of a light; and that the money which had been, or should be paid by ships, after the demolition, would be returned by the agents who received it.

He conſidered that this was not a work proper to be advertiſed; or put into the hands of a general undertaker in the building way; and that it would not be better for the ornaments to be derived from the *five Orders*: that it was a work of a very peculiar kind; and that to reinſtate it, would not ſo much require a perſon who had merely been bred, or had even rendered himſelf eminent, in this, or that given profeſſion; but rather one who from natural genius had a turn for contrivance in the mechanical branches of ſcience; and that ſuch a one would be the moſt likely perſon to take into conſideration the peculiarities, the advantages, and diſadvantages of the ſituation, as well as other circumſtances: in ſhort, that it required a perſon who would not ſtand in need of being led by the actual execution of a ſimilar performance; but who ſolely from the nature of the thing, would be likely to find out the proper methods of executing a building of the like kind with that, which had approved itſelf upon an experience of near 50 years; ſuch a perſon being the moſt likely to diſcern how far the late building was defective, how far theſe defects were capable of a remedy; and what improvements could be made upon the former conſtruction.

60. IN this view Mr. WESTON laid aſide thoſe prejudices of the ignorant, who conſider the *Royal Society* as a body of *theoretic Men* only, having nothing amongſt them practical, or applicable to the real buſineſs of human life; he well knew that though in a multitude there might be many of that denomination; yet that there were alſo many real artiſts in this body: and that ſince its inſtitution by *King* CHARLES *the Second*, the moſt important inventions, applicable to the greateſt purpoſes of human life, had originally ſprung from the joint labours of ingenious men, either actually members, or connected by correſpondence with thoſe who were ſo: and this without a view to any particular emolument or reward.

Under theſe circumſtances, Mr. WESTON applied to the late Earl of MACCLESFIELD, the then *Preſident of the Royal Society*; a nobleman ſcarce known to him, but by public character. On communicating the object of his viſit, Lord MACCLESFIELD told him, that there was one of their Body whom he could venture to recommend to the buſineſs; yet that the moſt material part of what he knew of him was, his having within the compaſs of the laſt ſeven years, recommended himſelf to the ſociety by the communication of ſeveral mechanical inventions and improvements; and though he had at firſt made it his buſineſs to execute things in the inſtrument way (without having ever been bred to the trade) yet on account of the merit of his performances, he had been choſen a member of the ſociety*: and that for about three years paſt, having found the buſineſs of a *Philoſophical Inſtrument Maker* not likely to afford an adequate recompence; he had wholly applied himſelf to ſuch branches of mechanics, as he (Mr. WESTON) appeared to want; that he was then ſomewhere in *Scotland*, or in the north of *England*, doing buſineſs in that line: that what he had to ſay further of him was, his never having known him undertake any thing, but what he completed to the ſatisfaction of thoſe who employed him; and that Mr. WESTON might rely upon it, when the buſineſs was ſtated to him, he would not undertake it, unleſs he clearly ſaw himſelf capable of performing it.

This kind of character which the noble Earl was pleaſed to honour me with, proved fully ſatisfactory to Mr. WESTON, and as his Lordſhip did not know how to direct to me, he learnt from him, that as I was well acquainted with Mr. B. WILSON an eminent painter in *Great Queen-ſtreet*, he would probably get a direction to me from that gentleman.

Upon this, he immediately applied to Mr. WILSON, who undertook to write to me (being then in *Northumberland*) which he did very laconically, ſignifying that I was made choice of as a proper perſon to rebuild the *Edyſtone Lighthouſe*: this was early in the month of January 1756.——I had at that time, but barely heard that the Edyſtone Lighthouſe was deſtroyed by *Fire*; and having ſeen a popular print of it, I underſtood that it was a building very critically placed out at ſea, upon a ſingle rock: but as I had no doubt that its foundation part at leaſt, was built with *Stone*, though its upper works had the appearance of timber, I could not readily conceive how it could be *totally* deſtroyed. I concluded therefore, that the object was to *repair* or reſtore the *Upper Works*: and therefore I received the call without joy,

* Mr. SMEATON was choſen Fellow of the *Royal Society* 15 March 1753.

or

or indeed much emotion of any kind; concluding, as moſt public works of conſequence were undertaken upon advertiſements, the meaning was, that I ſhould return to London to give in my propoſals along with other candidates.

I therefore returned my friend for anſwer, that I ſuppoſed it was meant I ſhould go back to town in order to form a ſcheme, which if it had the good luck to be thought preferable to that of others, I was to be employed in the *Repair* of the building: if this was the caſe, I had engagements and proſpects before me, that I could not leave upon any uncertainty; but that if I was abſolutely choſen to this buſineſs, I ſhould think it ſo great an honour done me, that in one month I would diveſt myſelf of all other engagements, and attend the gentlemen in town. To this I received an anſwer from my friend, even more laconic than before. That it was a *total* demolition, and that as NATHAN ſaid unto DAVID "*Thou art the Man.*"

61. HAVING acquitted myſelf of the buſineſs in which I had been engaged in the North, I arrived in London the 23d February 1756; and the next day, agreeable to a meſſage I had received for that purpoſe, waited on ROBERT WESTON, Eſq; till then totally unknown to me. The hours ſpent in this interview, were taken up in my attention to a relation of the nature of the ſtructure of the former Lighthouſes of Mr. WINSTANLEY and Mr. RUDYERD; and in examining ſeveral plans, models and drawings in Mr. WESTON's poſſeſſion, that referred thereto.——I was till then, I may ſay, almoſt a total ſtranger to thoſe ſtructures and their ſituation (which indeed by the deſcription now given of them appeared very formidable) as I never happened to have been in thoſe parts; and a mechanical deſcription of them never fell in my way: but from the information now given me, I thought a little time and ſtudy would make me ſufficiently maſter of the ſubject, to enable me to give my opinion in general, what plan it would be beſt to purſue.

It is true I found myſelf at firſt under ſome little reſtraint, from that freedom I would ever wiſh to exert; by diſcovering in the courſe of this day's converſation, a ſtrong propenſity in this gentleman for purſuing the former deſign; I mean that of Mr. RUDYERD: but when what has been already ſaid upon that ſtructure is conſidered, I muſt own that Mr. WESTON's attachment was very reaſonably founded. There were other circumſtances too, which might have been a ſtill greater clog and impediment to the ſcope of my thoughts, had the gentlemen Proprietors ſuffered themſelves to have been biaſſed thereby; I mean a *partial View* to their own *immediate Intereſt*. But I was ſoon releaſed from every ſuppoſition of this kind; for on putting the query, that if any improvement could be made in the ſtability or durability of the ſtructure, whether the Proprietors would wiſh to adopt it; though it ſhould incur a greater expence than a mere re-erection of the laſt building? He replied, with an emphaſis which gave me no doubt of his ſincerity; that if there was a poſſibility of rebuilding the Lighthouſe in any better or more durable manner than it had been, though almoſt half of the original leaſe from the Corporation of TRINITY-HOUSE was then expired, yet the matter being now in their hands, they ſhould think themſelves bound, for the ſake of poſterity, to do every thing that lay in their power to render the new building not only effectual for their own time, but as *permanent* as poſſible.——And, on coming away, Mr. WESTON ſaid, I was not to think myſelf at all indebted to him, or any of the Proprietors for the undertaking I was likely to be engaged in; ſince if either he or they could have heard of any perſon more capable of deſigning and executing ſuch a work, he ſhould not have ſeen me at his houſe that day: which valediction, though in the groſs ſenſe, it might be ſaid to contain little of *Obligation*; yet as it at once ſhewed me that I was likely to be received with that degree of truſt and confidence which is ſo eſſential to the ſucceſs of an arduous undertaking; it thereby became a pleaſing earneſt of that diſpoſition in the Proprietors, which muſt ever be ſatisfactory to an artiſt; that of wiſhing to have his work, whatever it might be, performed in the *beſt* manner; and therefore could not in this ſenſe, fail to be more highly agreeable than any other kind of compliment.

62. THE models and drawings having been ſent to me, I endeavoured by a full conſideration of them, to inveſtigate the particular plan of the reſpective architects; but could not trace out that of either

either of them to my perfect satisfaction. They afforded me just so much light as to enable me to discern the want of more information: and I found upon further enquiry, that neither the models, drawings or prints were coeval with the structures they were intended to represent, except the print of Mr. WINSTANLEY's Lighthouse published by himself in the year 1699, before referred to; for as to the models, &c. relative to Mr. RUDYERD's, save a few original drawings, that shewed how some of the courses of stone were laid, as I have already mentioned, they were all of a late date, chiefly since the year 1734; and rather useful for *repairing* than *rebuilding* the house; exhibiting no more of the inside work, than what was discovered by the openings that were made at the time such repairs were carried on; so that at best those could afford but very defective information, as to the particular original design; though they had been necessary for conducting the repairs of that building.

From similar observations, the models had also been framed; but to render these more complete, to appearance, imagination was taken in to supply what never could have been obtained by real inspection: for, as no models, draughts or sections, that had been made at the time the house was built (except as before mentioned) were handed down to posterity; conclusions were drawn, from the things that were apparent, with respect to the inward structure; so that when any part of the case, or outside timbers that covered them, were taken off to be repaired, the models and drawings that were in consequence made by such kind of piecemeal discoveries, were in reality the best evidences I have seen of the nature of the structure, and therefore could not give me a full information.

This being the case, after all I could glean from the drawings and models, as well as every insight into the nature of the work, that Mr. WESTON from several interviews could give me; I was naturally led to consider what could be done by an erection *entirely of Stone*; as along with greater natural permanency of materials than wood, it would not be liable to destruction by fire; against which no absolute defence (as it appeared to me) could be applied, if rebuilt with timber. In fact, on first hearing of the late Lighthouse having been destroyed, I had conceived that the interiour part of the foundation, and indeed for a considerable height, must have been a solid body of stone, though the outside might have been covered with wood, (as it appeared from the only figure of it I had ever seen); and which I supposed might have been thought necessary by the builder, to prevent that wash of the joints, that a very exposed situation might subject it to, in case the cement was not of the very best kind possible for water-works: and such having been my thoughts, my imagination was in consequence carried to suppose how such a building might have been put together in the most effectual manner. Coming therefore to town with these ideas, and finding how very short the best account of the real structure fell of answering my conceptions; I was encouraged, from the declaration of the only Proprietor I had seen, as being the sense of the rest, as well as from the apparent utility to the public, and possibly in the end to the Proprietors themselves, to turn my thoughts towards the practicability of a stone building: which proposition appearing in a light more favourable, in proportion as I thought more upon it; in a very few days I became so satisfied, that I desired an interview with the body of Proprietors upon a *primary* and *leading Question*.

63. AT this meeting I stated the great advantages that would arise from a *Stone Building*, which indeed were quite obvious to all; but the difficulty was, how such a building could be carried into execution; for though the Proprietors unanimously declared, that they would make no objection to any reasonable expence in procuring that durability and safety, which would be the evident result, if a building with stone could be effectually established; yet they very properly observed, that as the late building had fully answered the end, for almost *half a Century*; were any thing to fail, in case they altered the mode of the structure, for *any Reason whatever*, however laudable, they should be condemned by the public, for having attempted an alteration, though even for the service of the public; and the loss must fall upon themselves as individuals, if, on any account whatever, they should not succeed.——They likewise observed, that it had been generally thought by the best judges, that the safety and continuance of the late building, had in a great measure depended on the elasticity of the materials of which it was chiefly composed; which enabled it to give way to the violent shocks of the sea, to which it was exposed: and that

that it was faid, by thofe beft acquainted with it, that its motion in violent ftorms was fo great, that frequently the *Trenchers* were thereby thrown from the fhelves in the upper rooms: and that moft undoubtedly, in thefe great agitations, *fomething muft give way*, which a ftone building could not be expected to do, unlefs in the cafe of a total overthrow.

In anfwer to this I obferved, that the great agitation which the late building was fubject to, arofe from its want of *Weight*, as well as want of *Strength*; that what I propofed would be both much heavier and much ftronger; and therefore if the building would not *give way to the Sea*, the *Sea muft give way* to the building. I further obferved, that I had not met them at fo early a time to debate the mode of conftruction of a ftone building, or its properties; but to afk them a fimple queftion: and that was, if I could convince their *own* underftandings, that a building could be made with ftone, not only fo as to be more durable, but even more fafe from every accident that could be forefeen, and not likely to be attended with a charge enormoufly more large, whether they would *prefer fuch a Building to the laft*, which they had experienced could be confumed by fire? becaufe, if not, it was to no purpofe to fpend time in afcertaining the mode of doing a thing that muft ultimately be rejected; but rather apply that time as early as poffible, towards inveftigating the beft method of compofing a ftructure upon fimilar principles with the former: I fay *fimilar Principles*, becaufe, as already fhewn, there did not at that time appear to exift, any precife defign of the former building: but that, if under the provifo mentioned, they would prefer a ftone building; the *onus probandi* fhould be upon me; and if upon trial I could not fatisfy *their* minds, as well as my *own*, of the practicability of my propofition, I would then quietly give it up, and as ftrenuoufly apply myfelf to what fhould upon the whole appear the moft *eligible*: and as it would not take up much time to produce fomething in a *rough* way; as I underftood it was too early in the feafon for any operations upon the place, no very material time could be loft. On this they unanimoufly agreed, that I fhould make the attempt to convince them, and if convinced, they would act accordingly; unlefs controuled by fome fuperiour power.

64. IN reflecting upon the late ftructure, with a wifh to retain as much of it as poffible, confiftent with the different nature of the material I had then in view, it appeared that the general form and fize of the building, and diftribution of the rooms of the houfe, were very proper and judicious. It appeared alfo moft evidently, that had it not been for the moorftone courfes, *inlaid* into the frame of the building, and acting therein like the ballaft of a fhip, it had long ago been overfet, notwithftanding all the branches and iron-work contrived to retain it: and that in reality the violent agitation, *rocking* or vibration which the late building was defcribed to be fubject to, muft have been owing to the narrownefs of the bafe on which it refted; and which, the quantity of vibration it had been conftantly fubject to had rendered, in regard to its feat, in fome degree rounding, like the *Rockers* of a cradle. It feemed therefore a primary point of improvement, to procure, if poffible, an enlargement of the bafe, which from the models before me appeared to be practicable. It alfo feemed equally defirable, not to increafe the fize of the prefent building in its *Waift*; by which I mean that part of the building between the top of the rock, and the top of the folid; and the Plate N° 6. (which has already been fully defcribed) being fuppofed in my Reader's view, I muft imagine him quite as well informed as I could have been at the time I am now defcribing. If therefore I ftill kept ftrictly to the *conical* form, a neceffary confequence would be, that the diameter of every part being proportionably increafed by an enlargement of the bafe, the action of the fea upon the building would be greater in the fame proportion; but as the ftrength increafes in proportion to the increafed weight of the materials, the total abfolute ftrength to refift that action of the fea, would be greater by a proportional enlargement of every part, but would require a greater quantity of materials: on the other hand, if we could enlarge the bafe, and at the fame time rather diminifh than increafe the fize of the waift and upper works; as great a ftrength and ftiffnefs would arife from a larger bafe, accompanied with a lefs refiftance to the acting power, though confifting of a *lefs Quantity of Materials*, as if a fimilar conical figure had been preferved.

65. ON this occasion, the natural figure of the waist or bole of a large spreading *Oak*, presented itself to my imagination. Let us for a moment consider this tree: suppose at twelve or fifteen feet above its base, it branches out in every direction, and forms a large bushy top, as we often observe. This top, when full of leaves, is subject to a very great impulse from the agitation of violent winds; yet partly by its elasticity, and partly by the natural strength arising from its figure, it resists them all, even for ages, till the gradual decay of the material diminishes the coherence of the parts, and they suffer piecemeal by the violence; but it is very rare that we hear of such a tree being torn up by the roots. Let us now consider its particular figure.——Connected with its roots, which lie hid below ground, it rises from the surface thereof with a large swelling base, which at the height of one diameter is generally reduced by an elegant curve, concave to the eye, to a diameter less by at least one-third, and sometimes to half of its original base. From thence its taper diminishing more slow, its sides by degrees come into a perpendicular, and for some height form a cylinder. After that a preparation of more circumference becomes necessary, for the strong insertion and establishment of the principal boughs, which produces a swelling of its diameter.——Now we can hardly doubt but that every section of the tree is nearly of an equal strength in proportion to what it has to resist: and were we to lop off its principal boughs, and expose it in that state to a rapid current of water, we should find it as much capable of resisting the action of the heavier fluid, when divested of the greatest part of its cloathing, as it was that of the lighter when all its spreading ornaments were exposed to the fury of the wind: and hence we may derive an idea of what the proper shape of a column of the *greatest Stability* ought to be, to resist the action of external violence, when the *Quantity of Matter is given* whereof it is to be composed.

In Plate N° 13. Fig. 1. is a sketch representing the idea I formed of this subject. It is farther observable, in the insertions of the boughs of trees into the bole, or of the branches into the boughs, (which is generally at an oblique angle) that those insertions are made by a swelling curve, of the same nature as that wherewith the tree rises out of the ground; and that the greatest *Rake* or *Sweep* of this curve, is that which fills up the obtuse angle; while the acute angle is filled up with a much quicker curve, or sweep of a less *Radius*: and Fig. 2. of the same plate represents my conception of this matter. ——In this view of the subject, I immediately rough-turned a piece of wood, with a small degree of tapering above; and leaving matter enough below, I fitted it to the oblique surface of a block of wood, somewhat resembling the sloping surface of the Edystone Rock; and soon found, that by *reconciling Curves*, I could adapt every part of the base upon the rock to the regularly turned tapering body, and so as to make a figure not ungraceful; and at the same time carrying the idea of great firmness and solidity.

66. THE next thing was to consider how the blocks of stone could be *bonded* to the rock, and to one another, in so firm a manner, as that, not only the whole together, but every individual piece, when connected with what preceded, should be proof against the greatest violence of the sea: for, I plainly saw, from the relations I had got, that as every part of the work, even in the most favourable seasons, was liable to be attacked by violent storms; if any thing was left to the mercy of the sea and good fortune, the building of the Edystone Lighthouse with stone would be tantamount to the rolling of the stone of SISYPHUS.

On this head I considered the nature of *Cramping*; which, as generally performed, amounts to no more than a *Bond* upon the upper surface of a course of stone, without having any direct power to hold a stone down, in case of its being lifted upward by an action greater than its own weight; as might be expected frequently to happen at the Edystone, whenever the mortar of the ground bed it was set upon was washed out of the joint, when attacked by the sea before it had time to harden; and though upright cramps to confine the stones down to the course below, might in some degree answer this end; yet as this must be done to each individual stone, the quantity of iron, and the great trouble and loss of time that would necessarily attend this method, would in reality render it impracticable; for it appeared, that Mr. WINSTANLEY had found the fixing 12 great irons, and Mr. RUDYERD 35, attended with such a consumption of time (which arose in great measure from the difficulty of getting and keeping the holes dry,

dry, ſo as to admit of the pouring in of melted lead) that any method which required ſtill much more, in putting the work together upon the rock, would in conſequence inevitably, and to a very great degree, procraſtinate the completion of the building. It therefore ſeemed of the utmoſt conſequence to avoid this, even by any quantity of time and moderate expence, that might be neceſſary for its performance on ſhore; provided it prevented hindrance of buſineſs upon the rock: becauſe of time upon the rock, there was likely to be a great ſcarcity; but on the ſhore a very ſufficient plenty.

This made me turn my thoughts to what could be done in the way of *dove-tailing*.——In ſpeaking however of this as a term of art, I muſt obſerve that it had been principally applied to works of *Carpentry*. its application in the maſonry way had been but very ſlight and ſparing; for in regard to the ſmall pieces of ſtone that had been let in with a double dovetail, acroſs the joint of larger pieces, and generally to ſave iron, it was a kind of work even more objectionable than cramping; for though it would not require melted lead, yet being only a ſuperficial bond, and conſiſting of far more brittle materials than iron, it was not likely to anſwer our end at all.——Somewhat more to my purpoſe I had occaſionally obſerved in many places in the *Streets of London*, that in fixing the *Kirbs* of the walking paths, the long pieces or *Stretchers* were retained between two *Headers* or bond pieces; whoſe heads being cut dovetail-wiſe, adapted themſelves to and confined in the ſtretchers: which expedient, though chiefly intended to ſave iron and lead, nevertheleſs appeared to me capable of more firmneſs than any ſuperficial faſtening could be; as the *tye* was as good at the bottom as at the top, which was the very thing I wanted; and therefore if the tail of the header was made to have an adequate bond with the interior parts, the work would in itſelf be perfect.

What I mean will be rendered obvious by the inſpection of Fig. 3. in Plate N° 13.——Something of this kind I alſo remembered to have ſeen in BELIDOR's deſcription of the ſtone floor of the great ſluice at *Cherbourgh*, where the tails of the upright headers are cut into dovetails, for their inſertion into the maſs of rough maſonry below, and Fig. 4. of the ſame Plate is taken from BELIDOR's Plate *.

From theſe beginnings I was readily led to think, that if the blocks themſelves were, both inſide and out, all formed into large *dovetails*, they might be managed ſo as mutually to lock one another together; being primarily engrafted into the rock: and in the round or entire courſes, above the top of the rock, they might all proceed from and be locked to one large center-ſtone.——After ſome trials in the rough, I produced a complete deſign, of which Fig. 5. Plate 13. is the exact copy; the dotted lines repreſenting the courſe next above or below, which in the original was drawn from the ſame center, on the other ſide of the paper; ſo that looking on each ſide ſeparately, each courſe was ſeen diſtinctly; or looking through the paper, the *Relation* of the two courſes, ſhewing how they mutually broke joint upon one another, was clearly pointed out: and this method of repreſentation was purſued throughout; but not being practicable in copper-plate work, I am under the neceſſity of introducing the method by dotted lines, though attended with ſome degree of confuſion of the main deſign.

67. IN like manner, upon the ideas aſſumed, concerning the particular figure of the outſide of the building, with the draughts and models of Mr. RUDYERD's Lighthouſe before me; it was not long before I made out a fair ſection of a ſtone building, ſuch as to me appeared practicable on the principles before mentioned. Figure 6. in the ſame Plate, is a reduction of it to half the ſize of the original; which, with the copy of the firſt fair plan, ſhewing how all the ſtones compoſing the ſame courſe were to be mutually locked together, by a new method of dovetailing, I am the more inclined to inſert, as a part of this work; becauſe I eſteem theſe *Prototypes* more perfect in themſelves, as a *general* ſcheme, than what was on further conſideration actually adopted and executed; becauſe many things were obliged to be varied, in order to render the whole more ſuitable to the ſituation, which would not have been varied had it not been on account of particular conſiderations: and thoſe variations, together with the reaſons for the ſame, will be pointed out in the detail of the parts, in the progreſs of the work.

It is obvious that in this method of dovetailing, while the ſlope of the rock was making good; by cutting the ſteps (formed by Mr. RUDYERD) alſo into dovetails, it might be ſaid, that the foundation ſtones

* Architecture Hydraulique, Part II. Tom. I. Plate 26. Fig. 4. Page 272.

of every courſe were *engrafted* into, or rather *rooted* in the rock; which would not only keep all the ſtones in one courſe together; but prevent the courſes themſelves (as one ſtone) from moving or *ſliding* upon each other.——But after loſing hold of the rock, by getting above it; then, though every ſtone in the ſame courſe would be bonded in the ſtrongeſt manner with every other, and might be conſidered as conſiſting of a ſingle ſtone, which would weigh a conſiderable number of tons, and would be further retained to the floor below by the cement, ſo that when completed, the ſea would have no action upon it but edgeways; yet as a force, if ſufficiently great might move it, notwithſtanding its weight, and the ſmall hold of the ſea upon it; and break the cement before time had given it that hardneſs which it might be expected to acquire afterwards; I had formed more expedients than one, for fixing the courſes to one another, ſo as abſolutely to prevent their ſhifting; but deferred the choice of theſe expedients till a ſtone building had been approved and reſolved upon.——I alſo foreſaw that though the cement in the bed of each courſe, while remaining entire, by excluding the water, would in reality take away the whole tendency of the ſea to *lift* it; yet while a courſe was unfiniſhed, and the mortar not ſufficiently *ſet* or hardened, the violent action of the ſea upon the cement in that ſtate, might entirely waſh it out; and then the ſea would act in the ſame manner in lifting, as if there had never been any cement put in: I therefore formed a variety of temporary expedients to prevent this, while the courſe was *unfiniſhed*; for after a courſe was once finiſhed and the cement was hardened, there could be no danger of ſuch a thing happening: but I ſhall not trouble my reader with a recital of thoſe expedients at preſent, as they will more properly come in along with the reaſons of my choice, in the detail of the actual proceedings.

68. WHILE I was digeſting and ſettling my mind upon theſe matters, I had frequent conferences with Mr. WESTON, who had actually, two or three times, been upon the rock; and as from him I learnt that if I was then at Plymouth, a probability of landing upon the rock ſo early in the ſeaſon was not to be expected; I took ſo much time as maturely to arrange my thoughts, previouſly to a full explanation of my general ſcheme, and yet to leave time for the neceſſary preparatory ſteps, in caſe what I had then in contemplation ſhould not be approved of.——I therefore, as early as was conſiſtent with theſe circumſtances, deſired another interview with the body of Proprietors; when by the help of the two drawings above referred to in Plate N° 13. *Fig.* 5. and 6. I fully explained my deſign above ſtated; with which after mature conſideration, they declared their perfect ſatisfaction: and that the ſcheme, was not only in itſelf practicable; but, as appeared to them, the only means of doing the buſineſs *effectually* for the general good of the public.——They however obſerved, that though they themſelves were unanimous in this opinion; and though the condition of their receiving the *light* duties* was that of *maintaining* a light upon the *Edyſtone Rock*; and that though neither the form, nor materials of the building for that purpoſe were preſcribed to them; yet they thought it right, not to reſt the determination of theſe matters with themſelves only, but to have the concurrence of the Board of ADMIRALTY, and of other ſuperior opinions; which being taken, it ſeemed to them (on ſuppoſition of *their* approbation) that I ſhould not then have any thing to do, but to go down to Plymouth and prepare for the execution.

To this I obſerved, that we were not yet ripe for taking thoſe opinions; for at preſent the ſcheme was ſo much in *Embryo*, that it exiſted merely as a work of imigination, formed from the repreſentations and informations, I had *then* received: but that when I came to ſee the Edyſtone Rock, with my own eyes, and obſerved its nature and ſituation; it was a poſſible caſe, that I might *myſelf* be of a different opinion; and ultimately recommend a ſtructure as near alike, as we could tell how to make it, to the laſt. ——That the neceſſary ſteps ſeemed to be, that ſince the new ſcheme, had in its outlines been honoured with their approbation; it was now, or, as ſoon as the ſeaſon ſhould become likely to obtain a landing, would be proper for me to go to *Plymouth*, and make my own obſervations; and take ſuch exact dimenſions of the rock itſelf, as would be neceſſary to enable me to erect a ſtructure upon it of either kind: as alſo to examine into the nature and diſtance of ſuch materials, as ſhould appear to be neceſſary; by

* [illegible] Penny per ton upon all Britiſh ſhips, outward or homeward-bound, that paſs the Edyſtone; on, or from foreign voyages. [illegible] coaſters; and double theſe duties on foreign ſhips when they come into Britiſh ports. The King's ſhips being [illegible]

which

which means, on my return, I ſhould not only be able to adviſe as to the ſort of building; but to make an exact model of the rock, and of the fabric I ſhould ultimately propoſe upon it; all which, if approved by the Proprietors themſelves, it would be then time to ſubmit it to the opinion of the ſuperior *Boards*: for, we ſhould cut but a ſmall figure indeed, if after having received their approbation, we ſhould find ourſelves under the neceſſity of telling them, that what we had propoſed was premature, and would *not do*; and that we were obliged to recur to the former conſtruction.

This propoſition being approved of by the Proprietors, it was determined that the Lighthouſe ſhould have the ſame *general Form* and *Conveniencies*, as the laſt; but as to the matter, whether of wood or of ſtone, or what kind of ſtone, ſhould be referred to my further enquiry and report.

It being yet rather too early in the ſeaſon, for my journey to Plymouth to be of any probable uſe, I employed the reſidue of my time in preparing ſuch inſtruments and neceſſary matters in London, as I foreſaw might be uſeful; however, to loſe no material time, it was concluded I ſhould ſet out for *Plymouth* on the 22d of March 1756, where I arrived on the 27th.

C H A P. II.

Containing an Account of the Proceedings and Occurrences on Mr. SMEATON's *firſt Journey to* PLYMOUTH *in the Spring of the Year* 1756.

69. IN my journey to Plymouth, I had nothing to regret but the loſs of time that I ſuffered, which was occaſioned chiefly by the badneſs of the roads.——Notice having been given of my coming, I had an early viſit from the perſons who expected me; and in particular from Mr. Josias Jessop, with whoſe general character, as given to me, I have already made my reader acquainted. To him I was principally referred for what information and aſſiſtance I might ſtand in need of; and had the ſatisfaction to find him perfectly to anſwer the character that had been given me of him: who beſides being an approved workman in his branch as a ſhipwright, I found a competent draughtſman and an excellent modeller, in which laſt he was accurate to a great degree; he therefore appeared to be a very fit perſon to overlook the exact execution of a deſign given.

To him I ſoon hinted the probability of building the houſe with ſtone, at which he ſeemed much ſurprized, and aſked me, how I meant to faſten the *outſide Timbers*: I told him, that if it was built with ſtone, I meant to uſe no timber at all about it; at which he was aſtoniſhed, and ſaid, it would be impracticable in that ſituation; or if it could be done, it *would not ſtand*: but on endeavouring to come at his reaſons for thinking ſo, I found it was no other than the idea of ſecurity, which had been generally conceived to have ariſen, from the rocking of the late wooden houſe.——After ſhewing him the ſketches of my deſign, and explaining the ſame to him, as I had done to the Proprietors, he ſeemed to be tolerably ſatisfied; and ſaid, that as I propoſed to do without cramps or iron, in binding the lower part of the works together, it would certainly be a great ſaving, both of expence, and, what in this caſe was more valuable, of *Time*.

He alſo obſerved to me, that the worms had brought on ſo general a decay in the foundation part of the late Lighthouſe, not only of the outſide timbers, which could eaſily be *ſhifted**, but alſo of the interior ground timbers, that ſeveral of them had in his time been obliged to be ſhifted; and that this generally proved an operation, not only tedious and difficult, but even in itſelf imperfect; as the new timbers put in, could ſcarcely be brought to an equal bearing with the others: and that in conſequence (the greateſt number ſhifted having been on the S. W. quarter) the whole building had got a conſiderable *Liſt* or leaning to the S. W. where the rock was loweſt; and that from this cauſe of decay,

* The term *ſhifting* a timber in *Shipwrightry* ſignifies in general the ſubſtitution of a piece of new timber in the place of a piece of old.

as well as the neceſſity of repairs, every year growing more and more preſſing, it muſt have become in a courſe of years, not only exceeding difficult, but very expenſive to have kept ſtanding; even if any adequate remedy ſhould have been found out againſt the worms attacking the new timbers, as many of the old ones were in a very decayed and porous ſtate at the time of the deſtruction of the late building.

70. I WAS impatient to go off to the rock; but though the wind was fair at N. W. which was the favourable quarter; yet it had blown ſo hard, that Mr. JESSOP aſſured me we could not effect a landing upon it for a day or two longer at the ſooneſt; I therefore turned my thoughts to other matters. ——I waited upon FREDERICK ROGERS, *Eſq*; *Commiſſioner* at *Plymouth Dock*, who with great civility and politeneſs aſſured me, that no aſſiſtance to my undertaking, which he could give, ſhould be wanting. I alſo went to ſome of the artificers recommended by Mr. JESSOP to give directions for tools, to make trial of the manner, and with what expedition we might be able to work the rock; and alſo inſtruments and utenſils to enable us to take a plan thereof.

71. THE 2d of April being the firſt day there was any probability of landing on the rock, we ſet ſail; it being at that time near the height of the ſpring tides, the wind eaſterly and moderate. We got within a ſtone's caſt of the rock, but could not attempt to land, as the ſea broke upon the landing-place. ——Though we could not land, yet as the tide was at its low ebb, I had a good view of the rock, and an early opportunity of correcting many errors that I had been led into by the incorrectneſs of the ſeveral models and draughts which had come to my hands; and indeed I never ſhould have had an adequate idea of this very turbulent place without ſeeing it.

72. ON the 5th of April we made our ſecond voyage, the wind at N. W. and very moderate, ſo that though we went out of *Sutton Pool* at Plymouth before the water began to ebb, yet we did not arrive at the Edyſtone till it was nearly low water; and then I was rejoiced with ſetting my foot, for the firſt time, upon the *Edyſtone*. We ſtaid there 2½ hours; that is, till the ſea began to break from the weſt ſide over the rock at the landing-place; which my experienced guides pointed out as the laſt warning for our departure. Having employed myſelf while upon the rock in taking a *general View of the whole*, I could not perceive any remains of the houſe, either upon it, or about it; except the greateſt part of the iron branches which had been fixed by Mr. RUDYERD; and ſome of the moorſtones, which might be diſcerned lying in the bottom of the *Gut*: we ſounded 12 feet water then upon them, which compared with former obſervations of Mr. JESSOP, ſhews that the Gut was filled up full two feet perpendicular, by their having tumbled into it, and there meeting with a place of repoſe.

I then obſerved ſuch traces of the ſituations of the irons fixed by Mr. WINSTANLEY, as that it would not be difficult to make out his plan and the poſition of the edifice; from whence it appeared very probable, that Mr. WINSTANLEY's building was overſet all together; and that it had torn up a portion of the rock itſelf along with it, as far as the irons had been faſtened in it.

On this view I ſoon perceived that Mr. RUDYERD's iron *Branches*, as then called, were much ſmaller and ſhorter than he had deſcribed them to be at the bottom of his print; that many of them were looſe, and ſome broken and bent: and I remarked that in regard to the ſteps, deſcribed to be cut upon the rock, there were only five of them, of which the traces were remaining: ſo that there was but one *flat or tread* of a ſtep above the center of the houſe; and the upper part of the ſurface of the rock above that, was a ſloping plain as it had been at firſt. Three ſteps, of the five now remaining, ſeemed to have been but faintly cut, and the uppermoſt but one was ſo imperfect, that I ſuppoſed a large *ſpawl* or ſplinter had come from it; and this appeared the more probable, as the uppermoſt ſtep was ſo ſhaken, that another large ſpawl might have been eaſily raiſed from it, by a ſlight action of a wedge. Above the uppermoſt ſtep the rock ſeemed to be of a ſofter nature, was cracked in many places, and probably had received ſome damage from the fire. None of the ſteps appeared to have been cut with much regularity, either as to level or ſquare; but to have all the marks of hurry upon them.——In the center of the houſe a ſlight footing was cut for the maſt, ſuitable to a ſquare of 18 inches, with large iron branches anſwerable

able to two of its ſides; and a ſmall hole bored in the center of about 1½ inch diameter, being ſix inches deep. By conſulting Plate N° 7. many of the above matters will be made apparent to the eye.

I then proceeded to try the degree in which the rock was *workable*, and found that from a flat ſurface indifferently taken, I could with a pick ſink a hollow at the rate of five cubic inches per minute; and could cut or drill a hole with a jumper of 1½ inch diameter, at the rate of one inch deep in five minutes. I alſo tried a method of forcing two holes into one by a ſquare flat-faced bruiſer, or *Pummel*; ſo that, if there ſhould be occaſion, I might be able to make a continued groove; or let in an iron branch, in the manner of Mr. RUDYERD, and I had the ſatisfaction to find that the whole ſucceeded to my wiſhes.

73. IN conſidering what had occurred, there was not any thing that put on the appearance of *Impracticability* in the fixing a ſtone building; but I was forcibly ſtruck with the idea that nothing would more immediately tend to expedite our work, than the ſecuring a more ſafe and certain landing; as by that means we might frequently be enabled to work upon the rock, when otherwiſe we could not land thereon, or get off again when landed. I therefore loſt no time in turning my thoughts to this ſubject, as a matter of great importance: for as I ſaw it muſt frequently happen, when the veſſels cannot get in, and muſt in ſuch caſe lie off the rock, waiting for a favourable time to enter the Gut; that in the interim, tides might change, ground ſwells come on, winds ſhift, and ſtorms ariſe, which would of courſe make it adviſeable to return to Plymouth, if poſſible, though the purpoſe of the voyage was unperformed: it ſeemed therefore of the greater conſequence that no practicable opportunity ſhould be loſt, for want of proper expedients.

At this time my knowledge of theſe ſources of uncertainty, in a great meaſure depended on the relation of others; but my own after-experience, in the courſe of the performance of this work, has moſt fully and amply verified them: and I may add, that when veſſels had got with ſome facility into the Gut, they frequently could not get out again without extreme danger: for as the larger ſort had not room to turn in it, they were in reality obliged to go out ſtern forward, in caſe they came in the right way: the *Sugar-Loaf* Rock (See Plate N° 3.) being ſo critically placed, and ſhallow water on both ſides of it, that it prohibits a thorough paſſage. Indeed I was told, that by the ſkill and expertneſs of thoſe ſeamen who had frequently attended the ſervice of the Edyſtone, not only row-boats, but the attendant veſſels, after having delivered their cargoes, had been carried quite through at the top of an high tide, with a fair wind and ſmooth water*; but this neither is, nor ought to be, attempted in common.

The two voyages I had made, were in a ſmall ſailing veſſel of about ten or twelve tons burthen, built on purpoſe for attending upon the late houſe by Mr. TOLCHER the agent, and was called the *Edyſtone Boat.* ——By the experience of theſe two voyages, it occurred to me, that while the Lighthouſe was ſtanding, if the boat ſhould have happened to be ſtaved upon the rocks, while lying in the Gut, there was a poſſibility of the men being ſaved by getting into the houſe, as the lightkeepers would have been ready to throw out a rope and aſſiſt them: but if any accident of the kind was to happen now that the houſe was down, and no ſhelter or protection to be had, there was but a chance of their being ſaved; and theſe conſiderations being likely to caſt a damp upon every exertion to land, I determined to go out no more without another ſailing-boat to *attend*, and accordingly hired a fiſhing veſſel of an equal ſize with the Edyſtone boat.

74. THE 9th of April the wind and weather having become favourable for another attempt, we ſet forward at midnight between the 9th and 10th, the wind being then at N. W. and ſo moderate, that to expedite our paſſage we uſed our oars: but by the time we got a-breaſt of the Ram Head, it had veered to S. W. and began to blow ſo hard, that in three hours, finding we had made little progreſs towards the Edyſtone, we returned and re-landed at Plymouth at ſix in the morning†.

* The *Sugar-Loaf* is overflowed at half tide in ſtill water.

† The mention of this voyage might very well have been ſpared; but the brief recital of it, and of ſuch other fruitleſs attempts as occurred upon *this* viſit to Plymouth, will ſerve as a ſample, and (better than any form of general words) make my reader ſenſible of the great difficulty and uncertainty that naturally attends the landing upon the Edyſtone Rocks.

It

It was not till the 14th that we had any prospect of success at sea; the intervals between these attempts were therefore filled up in looking out a place proper for a work-yard; which to answer the purposes of a stone building, I considered should have the following properties: 1st, That it should be accessible not only to the boats or craft immediately employed in the service, but to such larger sloops and vessels as were to be employed in bringing stone from the respective quarries: for this purpose, it was necessary, that there should be a wharf or quay, or the capacity of erecting one; against which there might be nine feet, or at least eight feet depth of water at the high water of *Neap* tides. 2dly, That this should be in a harbour, interior to that of *Plymouth Sound*, where vessels might lie sheltered and in safety from all winds. 3dly, That it should be readily accessible to vessels coming in with their cargoes from the sea. 4thly, That the navigation outward for our own craft to the Edystone, should be attended with as little intricacy, difficulty and uncertainty, as possible; in short, that there should be no material obstruction to their getting out at high water into Plymouth Sound. 5th, and lastly, That there should be a level area to the amount of about 50 yards square, or a capacity of making such a one.

With this view I searched all the likely places I could hear of in and about Plymouth, to the amount of eight or ten in number; but found them all to be wanting in some of the requisites; or previously occupied in such a manner as to make it too expensive for us to acquire an establishment in them. It is unnecessary to mention the particulars and the reasons for rejection, except what relates to one of the situations, that had been the work-yard of my predecessor, and on that account may deserve a more particular notice.

This place, which is called *Emparcombe*, tradition has pointed out to be the spot where Mr. RUDYERD framed and fitted up his works ready for the sea. It is situated upon the east side of an interior bay that proceeds from the *Hamoaze** behind *Mount Edgecombe*†. The principal trace that remained of his works, was a row of cottage-houses, said to have been originally erected for the lodgment of himself and his workmen‡.——From the discretion that Mr. RUDYERD had shewn in his general proceedings, I could not doubt but that this place which he had pitched upon, must fully have answered his purpose: but as, in case of a stone building, the tonnage of the materials to carry off, was likely to be considerably more than double of Mr. RUDYERD's, I found it very indifferently suited to mine; for it seemed wanting in every requisite except the second; and was peculiarly defective in the first: and I could scarcely imagine he had made choice of it for any other reason, than that of his workmen being retired from the bustle that attends the town of Plymouth in time of war, and that it did not in the least interfere with the King's works.

Indeed I found no procurable place, completely made to my hands; but that which seemed the most nearly to contain all the requisites, or the capacity of making them, was in a field adjacent to *Mill Bay*, about a mile west from Plymouth. This bay, and particularly the west side of it, was well screened from all winds, for all kind of vessels that we could want. Its entry was sufficiently wide, but yet not too much so; the water deep and the headlands bold: and though the mouth is well protected from the surge of the *Sound*, by the island of *St. Nicholas*, now more generally called DRAKE's island; yet the passage out to the Sound, as well as the coming in, is very easy and safe. The greatest objection was, a want of depth of water towards the west shore; especially where, in other respects, the ground lay the most commodious for a work-yard: but it appeared that this inconvenience (amounting to about three feet want of depth in the shallowest part) might be remedied by first clearing a passage through the mud, and then sinking the natural bottom, which appeared to be a strong hard clay, so as to form a channel of sufficient width for the passage of vessels: and thus the business as to the obtaining of a work-yard was brought to a point ready for application to the proprietor of the field. See Plates N° 2. and 17.

75. THE weather still continuing unsavourable, my next excursion was to visit the nearest place to Plymouth where *Moorstone* which in reality is the true *Granite*, was found and worked; and that was

* The *Hamoaze* is that part of the harbour opposite the *King's Docks* near Plymouth; being the broad outfall of the river *Tamar* into the Sound.

† See the Plan N° 2 of Plymouth Sound, and of the interjacent sea including the Edystone.

‡ In the year 17[illegible], I found at this place more respectable buildings.

about

about fifteen miles from Plymouth, up the river *Tamar*, near *Calſtock*, to which place I underſtood that river was navigable. The moorſtone is found upon *Hingſtone Downs*; and here I was firſt ſhewn the method of working it: which was by ſplitting it with a great number of wedges applied to holes or notches, cut (or, as they term it, *pooled)* in the ſurface of the ſtone, at the diſtance of about four inches, more or leſs, according to the ſize and ſuppoſed ſtrength of the ſtone. Theſe pool-holes are ſunk with the point of a pick, much in the way that is done for the ſplitting of hard quarry-ſtones in general.——Here I was informed, that the harder the quality of the moorſtone, the more exactly in general it could be ſplit to the ſize or *ſcantling* required; and on the contrary, that the more ſoft and capable of being worked with the pick or other tool, the leſs regularly it would ſplit: ſo that to bring this kind of ſtone to a true ſquare, would require in the whole, near the ſame quantity of labour, whether of the harder or the ſofter ſpecies.——The moorſtone of this place ſeemed to be of the harder ſpecies; but of the quantity remaining, the ſtones were not of ſo large a ſize as I expected to have met with.

In enquiring as to the prices of the work, I foreſaw it would be to no purpoſe to aſk the expence of ſhaping ſtones to the particular figure I wanted; becauſe the workmen being totally unuſed to any work of that ſort, the queſtion would only have puzzled them, and the anſwers of courſe would at beſt have been indiſtinct, if not tending to miſlead: I therefore founded my enquiries upon the price at which they could produce *Aſhler* *, by the foot ſuperficial, when brought to a true ſquare; and what was their price per gallon in forming ſtone *Troughs*, ſome of which I found they were in the practice of making. By anſwers to the firſt, I was enabled to form a judgment, at what price they could work moorſtone by the foot, to a perfect regularity, after it was ſplit into the proper ſcantlings for that purpoſe; and from the price of working out the hollows of ſtone troughs, I could judge of the expence of hollowing out the work by downright dint of labour of the pick, where no advantage could be derived from the uſe of the wedge or the hammer.

The operation of ſplitting granite is very curious; for, the apparent texture being without any particular direction, the parts ſeeming to be irregularly and coarſely huddled together, ſomewhat reſembling a *Plumb Pudding*; one would not imagine, that any degree of regularity could take place in their diviſion by ſplitting; but the caſe is ſo far otherwiſe, that gate-poſts are afforded in the rough ſquare, at a very moderate price; and I have in this country frequently ſeen poſts of *Granite* twelve feet long, and not above eight inches ſquare, uſed inſtead of wood, for the mere purpoſe of ſupporting a *Hovel*, no part of them being ſo much as an inch out of ſtraight, or flat: but it is to be conſtantly obſerved, that the ſtrength of the ſtone, on each ſide of the biſection, is ſo managed, as to be nearly equal, otherwiſe the *ſplit* will conſtantly encroach upon the weaker ſide. Indeed without this remarkable property in granite of ſplitting regularly, it would have been of little uſe in human life: for it is of ſo hard a nature, that ſteel will not *cut* it; and yet hard ſteel will *bruiſe* it; ſo that the prominent parts being gradually crumbled away by repeated blows, its ſurface can be brought to a great degree of regularity: and as the ſplitting procures plain ſurfaces nearly regular, as already obſerved, the accidental prominences can be reduced to regularity by a moderate degree of labour.

76. ON the 14th of April we went out to ſea between five and ſix in the morning, for the *fourth* time, the wind being then at Eaſt, and very moderate; but it had been at N. W. the preceding evening, which determined us to get every thing ready for the morning's tide. We had ſcarcely got out of the Sound before it became more freſh and veered to the S. E.; appearances were now againſt us, but I determined to run out to the Stone; for though it was not very likely we ſhould effect a landing, yet as the wind was fair to run to the harbour of *Fowey*, or as it is commonly called *Foy*; a port about ſix leagues to the N. W. from the Edyſtone, and a place I wanted to viſit on account of there being in that part of the county, a much more conſiderable quantity of moorſtone, as well as hands employed in working it, than I had yet ſeen, we proceeded in our voyage. As we ran further out, the wind became more freſh, and when we got out to the length of the Edyſtone, it blew hard: there was no poſſibility of

* A term uſed by maſons for ſtones prepared in the ſquare for building with regular courſes.

landing; but I caufed our boat to lie off and on, at the diftance of about one hundred fathoms, to obferve the action of the fea upon the rocks, when the wind blew from the S. E. quarter; which indeed was very violent, the feas being broken into a very large and heavy fpray. On fteering for *Fowey* we ftood before the wind, and therefore though the gale increafed, ftill our little boat and attendant behaved very well: we however had fo much fea as to make a fafe harbour very acceptable to us; and as Fowey was pointed out to me, as a place of refuge when the wind came round in fuch a manner as to prevent our return to Plymouth, it became expedient to examine its moft material properties with attention.

The entrance of this harbour is rather narrow for large fhips; but the headlands are very bold, and there is nothing to fear but what is in view. There is deep water both in the entrance and in the harbour itfelf, which is confiderably enlarged in width after paffing the headlands; in fhort, when you are in it, it is both fafe and commodious.——As the depth of the water enables merchant fhips of almoft any fize to go in or out, at any time of the tide, when the wind ferves, this harbour becomes of confequence; being critically fituated in the bottom of the extenfive bay formed between the *Ram-Head* and *Deadman's* Point; and where many good fhips, had mariners been *fufficiently* acquainted with it, might have found a fafe retreat from bad weather and fhipwreck; it is therefore to be lamented, that from erroneous accounts, formerly given in fome of the pilot-books concerning this harbour, fhips have not ventured to go into it, when they might very fafely have done fo, owing to the falfe idea entertained of it; which was that of its being a tide harbour, with a *Bar* at its mouth; than which nothing can be more contrary to the truth.

In fact, *Fowey Harbour* may be called the *Key* to the Edyftone fervice: for as from the Edyftone, Plymouth Sound and Foy Harbour lie nearly at a right angle; when it blows right a-head from Plymouth Sound, a veffel fteering to Foy will have the wind upon her beam; and as this will be a wind from the land, there never can be any great fea from that quarter, at fo moderate a diftance from the fhore; fo that any good fea-boat, may make her courfe good to Fowey: and fhould the wind be due North, a veffel may yet run under fhelter of the Deadman, and afterwards *turn into* Foy: but if the wind is to the Weftward of the North, fhe may then run under protection of the high land at the *Bolt* point to the Eaftward, and get into a fmall harbour called *Yealm*; though in the courfe of my experience, we feldom had occafion to ufe it: for it never happened when the wind was too far to the Weft to get into Fowey, but we could always fetch Plymouth Sound, by making a fingle *Tack* or two at the moft.

77. NEXT morning the 15th, the wind blew hard at S. W. we therefore fet out for *Lanlivery*, about fix miles from Foy; and here we found WALTER TRELEVEN and fon, to whom I was directed as the principal people in this diftrict for working of moorftone. WALTER aged 60 acquainted me, that he worked at the ftone-work for the late Lighthoufe under his elder brother PETER TRELEVEN, who had the contract under Mr. RUDYERD. He informed me, that none of the ftones ufed therein were above a ton weight; that they were all cramped with iron, each to its neighbour; and the outfide courfes to thofe below; but fo, that none of the cramps could be feen on the outfide; that they were all finifhed at that place, being *tried* together upon a flooring of boards, and the cramps let in, and that the cramps were made from a pattern he had from Mr. RUDYERD.——PETER TRELEVEN, aged 80, was ftill alive, but fo infirm and ill that he could not fee us: I therefore defired his brother WALTER to afk him a few queftions; and particularly whether there was any kind of mortar or cement ufed in the ftone-work; it being Mr. JESSOP's notion, from what he had obferved, that there was not, which PETER TRELEVEN confirmed: but it feems that neither he nor WALTER had ever the curiofity to go upon the Edyftone Rock.

We then went to fee the ftone, and the way by which it was to be carried down to the water fide to be fhipped. The pieces of ftone are here in general of much larger fizes than thofe we faw at *Hingftone Downs*, and are of a quality much more free to work, but will not fplit fo true, as I had before been informed. I faw one ftone apparently without crack or flaw, which curiofity prompted me to meafure, and found it to contain no lefs than 400 tons*. The diftance of the place of working the moorftone to *Parr*, the place

* The moorftone or granite of this country that is wrought for fale, not only at this place, and at Hingftone, but every where that I have

place of ſhipping it, is about three miles, through very bad roads, and by means of carriages but indifferently contrived, which in this country they call *Ploughs*: they were not then in practice of drawing above a ton and a half at a time, and to move this, they were obliged to yoke a team, conſiſting of a great many bullocks and horſes. I made ſimilar enquiries here, to thoſe I made at Hingſtone, to aſcertain the price of work, and found it upon the whole to amount nearly to the ſame as there. The ſtone here, though of a quality conſiderably ſofter, was yet very ſufficiently hard for any purpoſe of building, and equally unperiſhable by the effects of weather, with the hardeſt: and as the quality of its being more eaſily to be worked with the pick, ſeemed better adapted to produce the dovetail ſhapes I had in view, at a moderate price, and as ſtones could be got here of any ſize that could be moved from the place, the ſtone of this diſtrict ſeemed upon the whole more likely to ſuit my propoſed operations, than what I had before ſeen.

We were informed that a great part of the ſtone wherewith the walking paths of *Weſtminſter Bridge* were laid, were gotten from this place. It diſtinguiſhes itſelf, by being of a much coarſer grain, with long white ſpar-like pieces, frequently of two inches and upwards in length, and which from ſimilarity they there call *Dog's Teeth*; whereas the moorſtone of Hingſtone, was of a ſmaller and cloſer grain, and much interſperſed with the black *Mica* or *Talc* which is one of its component parts.——The morning of Saturday the 16th, the wind ſtill continuing freſh at S. W. we this day took the opportunity of returning to Plymouth by ſea from Fowey *.

ON Sunday and Monday the 17th and 18th, it blew very hard at N. W. On Tueſday morning the 19th, the weather being very fine, clear and calm, we went out the *fifth* time for the Edyſtone; but the little breeze there was being right a-head, we tacked and rowed the whole day; and at night found ourſelves about four miles from the rock. As the day was perfectly ſerene, we had the mortification of ſeeing every thing calm and quiet about the rock, without being able to get near it. Upon the turn of the tide in our diſfavour, we dropt anchor, in hopes of completing our voyage the next day's tide; but in the night it began to rain and blow ſo hard from the S. E. that we were glad to weigh anchor and come home; and in returning, the wind veering to the N. E. and blowing very hard almoſt right a-head, we had a laborious work in turning to windward and regaining Plymouth.

The event of this laſt voyage pointed out to me very ſtrongly, that the much greater tonnage of the ſtone, which muſt be neceſſary to be carried out and fixed, in caſe of a ſtone building, than was neceſſary in the compoſitions of my predeceſſors, would make the uncertainty and delay that they have deſcribed to be attendant upon their voyages, in order to fix their work, bear far heavier upon my ſcheme than upon theirs; and thereby occaſion the whole time of the performance to be lengthened; a circumſtance that would be very diſagreeable to all concerned. It therefore appeared to me, that had a veſſel been fixed within a quarter of a mile, or ſome ſuch competent diſtance from the rocks, and which ſhould be capable of lodging the workmen with all their tools, and looſe materials; the ſeveral pieces of wrought ſtone only excepted; that then the workmen might by means of ſmall row boats or *Yawls* have effected a landing both of themſelves and their materials; and have been at work upon the rock the greateſt part of that day; which we, as voyagers, loſt the whole of in fruitleſs labours and endeavours, to get to the place of action. On conſulting Mr. JESSOP upon this idea, he recommended that we ſhould build a ſtrong and very well *found* ſloop of about 50 tons burthen, with iron chains for mooring her upon the rocky ground, which, as has already been obſerved, every where prevails in the vicinity of the rocks of the Edyſtone: and that her inward lining or *cicling*, as it is termed, ſhould be *caulked* equally well with the outſide planking: ſo that the outſide planking might then ſuffer great derangement, and even be in part

I have had an opportunity of obſerving it, is not produced from quarries; but lies in pieces, generally roundiſh, upon the ſurface of the earth, ſomewhat ſunk into the ſame; and this is uſed in preference, as being the moſt eaſy to come at: but the *Miners* find, that it lies underground in very thick and ſolid *Strata*, through which they are frequently obliged to ſink *Shafts* or pits, for a great number of fathoms. It is called *Moorſtone* from its being generally found upon the high grounds of this country, which are chiefly moors.

* Doubtleſs it was this port that Mr. WINSTANLEY mentions, § 18, that he was frequently obliged to go to for ſhelter, and that it took him the greateſt part of the next day to get back to Plymouth.

destroyed

destroyed by touching upon the rocks, while the inside remaining entire and water tight, would be sufficient for the bueyancy of the vessel; and if sloop-rigged, she would lie very snug and close while at her moorings; and in case of being accidentally broken loose by a heavy storm, she would be easily manageable and got under way, so as to be able to reach *some* port; either Plymouth, or to the East or West, and be easily replaced after the gale was over. To this scheme there appeared only one objection, and that was the difficulty there might be in clearing the water from between the *Plankings*; but that it seemed, might readily be obviated by making two pumps; one to act between the plankings, and the other within the vessel. But being apprized that a vessel was then fitting out in the river *Thames*, with chain moorings, not only to enable her to lie upon the rocky ground; but to continue there all winter, as a temporary *floating Light*; in some degree to supply the want of a Lighthouse; we concluded, that in case this vessel was ordered to be moored sufficiently near the rocks, to answer the double purpose of the *Building* and of the *Light*; that, provided there was sufficient room and accommodation, the expence of the *Store-Vessel* above proposed might be saved; and therefore it was proper to postpone our putting any thing in hand relative to this object, till the determination in respect to the floating light-vessel was known: and in case that did not turn out to our purpose, the other expedient might then be adopted.

79. DURING this interval on shore, I occupied myself in various miscellaneous matters, and in procuring the best information I could of such things as it appeared necessary to have some knowledge of before the principal work was set about. In particular, on repeating my visit to *Commissioner* ROGERS, he took an opportunity of shewing me a piece of *Portland Stone*, that had been cut out from a part of the *King's Docks* there, which had been wholly lined with that material.——This specimen had been drilled with a great number of holes, something similar to the perforations made by the worms of ships; and as this had doubtless wholly happened since the stones were placed there, it was a circumstance of a kind somewhat alarming. These holes I observed had been made by a small kind of shell-fish, something like a muscle, and that they were in general much smaller at the entry on the outside, than they were within; and apparently enlarging as the shell of the fish had grown in size. I was further informed, that these holes had appeared most numerous, or at least were of the most material ill consequence, near the draw-gates of the sluices, by which the water is drained off from the docks: for by this means, those sluices had become so leaky, that it became necessary from time to time to cut out several of the injured stones, and replace them with new ones.

Afterwards in looking among the marble rocks upon the shore of *Mill Bay*, near the place I had pitched upon as proper for our work-yard, I found several detached pieces of those rocks, that had in like manner been drilled through, resembling a honeycomb; and I likewise found some, near low water mark, where the solid rock had been entered in the same manner; from which I perceived, that the Portland stone had not suffered merely on account of its want of hardness; for the marble, which is much harder, seemed to be equally penetrable; nor had the pieces thus pierced suffered any decay in the nature of a rot; because the intermediate parts, between the holes, seemed to retain their original hardness: from these circumstances it appeared probable that every kind of *calcareous* stone might be subject to the like defect; and therefore that *Portland* stone ought not to be used for the *outside* of the Edystone Lighthouse, especially of the lower works: though it might be used with great advantage for the works within, on account of the greater ease with which it might be wrought.

I was not indeed led into this opinion, by any doubt I entertained that a house built entirely with this stone, would last much longer than a wooden fabric would have done; but in contemplating the use and benefit of such a structure as this, my ideas of what its duration and continued existence ought to be, were not confined within the boundary of an *Age* or two; but extended themselves to look towards a possible *Perpetuity*: and though it did not absolutely appear from what I had seen and heard, that a Portland stone building placed upon the Edystone rock, would in fact be penetrated by this kind of shell-fish; which seemed to be in a great measure confined to, and under *low Water-mark*; yet in cases where it is not necessary, it is certainly unadviseable to run the least risque; for no one can say *what* the difference

difference of situations may effect: and though the building, if attacked by any kind of known animal, might very reasonably be expected to endure much beyond the term which I understood the Proprietors had in their present grant; yet as I knew it to be agreeable to their wishes, I concluded that to give it all possible safety and probability of permanency, it would be advisable to make use of *Moorstone* for the foundation, if not for the whole of the outside work; it being of a quality not found either liable to be impaired by the above means, or subject to any kind of decay whatever by the injury of weather or time.

The owner of the fishing-vessel that had hitherto attended us, being weary of the service, I hired a sloop of 25 tons burthen, with a commodious cabin, and decked over; but being too large to go into the Gut, it could only lie at an anchor, and be used as an attendant *Store Vessel*.

80. THE 21st of April, the wind came about to the N. W. and was moderate; I therefore determined upon another attempt, and accordingly at twelve at night, went on board and proceeded on our *Sixth* voyage. We had a light breeze from the North, which carried us out leisurely to the Edystone, without the least difficulty, where we were so happy as to effect a landing between five and six, on the morning of the 22d; it was then nearly low water, and the tide at dead of the neap. The day being perfectly serene, we staid upon the rock till twelve at noon; which was till after high water: and though the sea at half a mile's distance appeared as smooth as the *Thames* in a calm day, yet a ground swell from the S. W. frequently run up very high upon the rock; and twice, a little after high water, ran over the highest point of it, though the dead level of the surface of the sea at high water, was full nine feet below the summit. My operations being now disturbed, we retreated to our vessels till two, when we again landed, and I went on with my business till nine in the evening, having worked an hour by candle-light.

The weather continuing fine, the Edystone boat lay in the Gut all night, a thing scarcely ever before attempted: the sloop to which Mr. JESSOP and I retired, lying at half a mile's distance to the North. At five next morning the 23d, I again landed and pursued my operations till eleven, when being a second time interrupted by the ground swell, we went to the sloop for refreshment, with an expectation of recommencing the work at two o'clock, as we had done the preceding day: but about one o'clock the wind began to freshen from the S. W. and at two it blew so hard, as to render our attempt to row the yawl into the Gut ineffectual. The wind still increasing, we lay at our anchors till five, in hopes of a change for the better; and then our situation became so uneasy that we made a signal for Plymouth, where we arrived at half past seven, which, though with the wind very fresh, and in our favour, was looked on as a quick passage.——In lying off the rock with the wind somewhat fresh at S. W. I observed on the retreat of the tide, that when the seas broke against the overhanging *Breast* of the rock on the West side, see Plate N° 9. the broken sea would fly 30 or 40 feet high; whereas a much greater ground swell at high water, meeting only with the regular slope, though it mounted much higher bodily, yet scarcely broke at all.

81. IN this place, I think my reader will expect some general idea of what had employed me upon the rock for three successive tides, amounting in the whole to full nineteen hours; and this was the taking such dimensions as would enable me to make an accurate model of such part of the surface of the rock as we were likely to have any concern with in the rebuilding: and which was principally effected by the application of an instrument that I had prepared on purpose; the idea whereon it was contrived I took from LEON BAPTISTA ALBERTI's treatise of *Statues*, added to EVELYN's translation of FREART's *Parallel* of *Architecture*. Wherein placing a kind of dial upon the head of the statue, with an index or ruler, turning about on the center of the dial, and from this ruler letting fall perpendicular lines, the several parts of the instrument will shew the situation, distance from the center, and depression of any given point of a statue below the plane of the dial, that the artist is desirous of ascertaining for his guidance; which instrument he calls a *Definitor*.

With this intent, I brought with me from London, the plate and index of a large *Theodolite*; being a foot in diameter, and sufficient to shew the single minutes of the degrees of the circle. This plate I screwed firmly down upon the surface of a steady wooden three-legged stool, which when set level, would overtop every part of the rock.——Being set up, it was so adapted to the rock, that the center of the Theodolite was, as nearly as I could place it, perpendicularly over that hole in the rock, which I conſidered as having been the center of the late building; and the whole was adjuſted to marks now fixed upon the rock, ſo that it could be taken down and ſet up, as often as we might have occaſion; and ſo as preciſely to anſwer the ſame poſition of parts.——To the index of the Theodolite was ſcrewed a ruler, 16 feet in length, and divided into feet, inches and parts of inches, commencing from the center. This ruler was preſerved from bending by its own weight, in any material degree, by a *Rib* raiſed upon its upper ſide; and it could be brought juſtly horizontal by means of a pocket *Spirit-Level* being placed upon it. The figure and manner of uſing it will be ſeen in the Elevation of the rock, ſhewn in Plate N° 7. ——It is obvious that this index-ruler being carried horizontally round, along with the index of the Theodolite, would ſucceſſively paſs over every point of a circle of 32 feet in diameter: and that, a perpendicular being let fall from it, ſo as to anſwer to any point given upon the rock, within that area, the index would mark the degree and minute of the circle in which it is placed. The diſtance of that perpendicular from the center of the inſtrument would ſhew its diſtance from the aſſumed center of the former building; and the height of the perpendicular would ſhew the dip or depreſſion of the given point below the plain of the inſtrument. The two former will be ſufficient for laying down an exact *Plan* of the ſurface of the rock, as reduced to an horizontal plane; and this plan, being laid upon the plain ſurface of a proper block of wood or ſtone, and holes being drilled into the block from the reſpective points, at right angles to its plain ſurface, and to depths taken from the ſame ſcale as the plan was made by, will aſcertain the reſpective points within the block, ſufficiently for the forming a proper *Model* thereof.——The neceſſity of an exact performance of this part of the work, was proportional to the difficulty I had to get the proper meaſures taken; and indeed I was the more deſirous that every thing relative hereto ſhould be done with accuracy, as by that means many voyages and viſitations would be ſaved, in adapting the work to the rock, in the courſe of our future proceedings.

As we were liable to be expoſed to freſh gales of wind through every ſtage of our operation, there was no truſting to the perpendicularity of *Threads* and *Plumbets*: I therefore purſued the following method. ——Having made indelible marks with the point of a jumper, upon the ſurface of the rock, at all notable places, I had a wooden meaſuring rod of about twelve feet long, and 1½ inch ſquare, divided into feet, inches and parts of inches, beginning from the bottom; this was ſhod with a rounded end or ſhoe of iron, which being ſet upon the mark to be aſcertained, the rod was put into a perpendicular poſition, by means of a carpenter's ſquare, having a ſpirit-level fixed upon one of its *Limbs*, the other limb being alternately applied to two ſides of the rod, at right angles to each other. It was ſteadied in that poſition, by temporarily applying two ſlips of deal, as *Shores* to two of its ſides that were at right angles; ſo that the lower end of the ſhores *ſtepping* againſt ſome hole or prominence of the rock, the bottom of the rod, together with the lower ends of the two ſhores, would form the baſe of an oblique triangular pyramid; while the part where the ſhores were held faſt to the upright rod formed the *Apex* of the pyramid*; this rod by this means was retained very ſtiff and ſteady in a perpendicular poſition.——The upright rod being thus fixed, the index-ruler was brought round, till it ſtopped againſt the upright rod, and then was ſhoved up, or let down by a ſhorter piece of a rod, ſlided againſt the upright one, till the index-ruler was brought to be truly horizontal, by means of the ſpirit-level being laid upon it: thus the upright rod would mark upon the index-ruler the diſtance from the center; and that ruler would mark upon the upright rod, the dip of the point on which it ſtood, below the level of the inſtrument; the braſs index at the ſame time ſhewing the degree and minute.——In this way I took off 35 in number of the moſt remarkable points, within the limits above-mentioned; obſerving to have one at each end upon the plain flat part of each ſtep, and ſo placed, that a line might be ſtretched between them from the point marked at one end, to that at the other end of the ſame ſtep, without its being interrupted by the branches, or other impediments.

It might ſeem at firſt ſight, that 35 points ſo determined, within a circle of 32 feet diameter, might be ſufficient to lay down the included area, but in reality it was not ſo; for when I had taken three times as many more, I had not completed the obſervations and meaſures I wiſhed: the rock itſelf, as well as the work my predeceſſors had made thereon, being ſo very irregular.——Theſe 35 primary points having been

* The rods were here *laſhed* together by a packthread.

determined

determined as above, the reſt were obtained from them as follows. A primary point being fixed at each end of each ſtep, between which a line could be ſtretched as before noted, the iron ſtanchions and particularities of each ſtep were readily taken off upon their own level reſpectively, by means of parallels and perpendiculars: and by ſtretching a line between any other two of the primary points given, that were neareſt and moſt advantageouſly ſituated, the ſituation of any other points wanted could be determined.——On my return to Plymouth, I made ſome progreſs in laying down to a ſcale, the meaſures taken upon paper. This enabled me to turn my thoughts towards a *real* deſign, which before had been only formed from imagination, aſſiſted by ſuch circumſtances as I could lay together from former drawings, models and verbal relations.

82. THE 28th of April the weather turning out more promiſing than it had been ſince our laſt return, I determined to attempt a *Seventh* voyage; and accordingly went on board, and lay in Cawſand Bay that evening, to be ready for the firſt of the tide next morning. Our outſet was favourable enough, but we had not got above a mile ſouth of the Ram-Head before a freſh of wind from S. E. came on, and ſo ſuddenly, that our boat, which the ſeamen were heaving into the ſloop, filled with water, and narrowly eſcaped being loſt. We notwithſtanding purſued our voyage towards the Edyſtone, but the ſea breaking with violence upon the landing-place, we could not attempt to land. However having received information of another place, where moorſtone was worked, which might be got to the waterſide, not far from *Falmouth*, and the wind being now fair for that port, we *bore away* for it, and arrived there in the afternoon. The next morning, we went on horſeback to *Conſtantine*, a place about four miles from Falmouth; where I applied to Mr. MATTHEW BOX, to whom I had been directed at Falmouth, as being the principal and almoſt the only man for moorſtone in theſe parts.

The moorſtone here, appeared to be of a quality, better both to cleave and work, than any I had before ſeen; for I obſerved by a piece of it, then under the hands of Mr. Box, that it might be cut and formed with a much ſuperior degree of execution, than I had before conceived this ſort of ſtone to be capable of.——He was at this time executing a *Grave-ſtone*, of the elevated kind, of which the pedeſtal of a column gives the idea; and in which he had formed the mouldings with ſo much delicacy and propriety, that I could not help conſidering Mr. Box as a capital artiſt in that kind of material; and therefore felt a ſecret joy in meeting with ſuch a perſon.——Such however is the nature of man, that he may be great in one branch of his profeſſion, and remain ſmall in another: for on communicating the nature of my deſign to him, I quickly found, that he conſidered the forming and erecting of a well ſhaped *Tomb-ſtone* of *Granite*, as the greateſt of all human performances; and that having lived and been brought up in a retired part of the country, from whence there never had been any conſiderable demand for moorſtone, in point of quantity, he had chiefly applied himſelf to the finiſhing of ſmaller works for the gentlemen of the county within a moderate diſtance from him. He ſeemed therefore rather frightened than pleaſed, when after I had explained a little of the nature and form of the work I ſhould be likely to need, I mentioned the extenſive order that I might poſſibly give for this article; for, to the execution of it he formed numerous difficulties, and did not know what to aſk, either for his ſtone, his work, or for the carriage down to Falmouth.

On conſidering the reſult of this interview with Mr. Box, and having now examined all the places I could hear of, where moorſtone was worked, which lie tolerably convenient for water carriage to Plymouth; I became convinced of the neceſſity of making uſe of Portland, or ſome other free working ſtone for the inſide work: for the granite, though preferable to all others in point of duration; yet being at beſt of a ſtubborn nature, and the working thereof confined to few hands, I perceived there would be no poſſibility of procuring ſo great a quantity in any reaſonable time, at a moderate expence, as the whole houſe would take, eſpecially if worked in ſuch forms, and in ſo large pieces as would be required upon the principle of my firſt ſketches.——The difficulties alſo that equally occurred to them all, as to the *Land Carriage*, ſeemed to induce the neceſſity, not only of confining the moorſtone to the outſide, but to take advantage of connecting thoſe with larger and heavier ſtones *within*, that were more eaſy to procure, in order to reduce the ſize of the moorſtone pieces, as much as would be conſiſtent with the intended

ſolidity

solidity of our work; that is, to stones from half a ton to a ton and half; but none to exceed two tons: and this appeared the more proper, as even to procure a sufficient supply of those, for the outside only, it might be necessary to give orders at *all* the places I had visited, at the same time.

The next morning, the 1st of May, being very moderate and the wind in our favour for returning, we weighed and went out to sea; but found a considerable swell from the S. E. raised by the wind of the two preceding days; and before we came near the Edystone (where I proposed to make a trial for landing if the weather should suit) the wind had come to the S. W. and blew fresh, which by opposing the S. E. swell, raised it still higher: wherefore we came that night into Cawsand Bay, and lay there to take the chance of the morning's tide; and be the more ready in case the weather should be then in our favour; but it proving otherwise, we returned to Plymouth, where we landed on Sunday morning the 2d of May.

83. WHILE I was prosecuting my work at home, of laying down the measures of the rock upon paper, I was somewhat alarmed with a report which prevailed concerning a number of French prizes that had been brought into the harbour, laden with fish; which having laid there some time, were decaying and putrefying*. The report was, that by way of easily getting rid of them, it was intended to carry them out, and sink them near the Edystone: however this I could not regard otherwise than as a false rumour; supposing that an idea of disposing of them near *that place*, could never have been seriously adopted by any one in authority sufficient to give that order.——Early in the morning of the 4th of May, the weather appearing favourable, we made our *Eighth* attempt to go out to the Edystone; and as I was going aboard our sloop, advice was sent to Mr. Jessop by Mr. Joseph Tolcher of the Custom-house, that (being appointed to that service) he was going to see the covers of the *Hatches* of forty of the fish ships above referred to, nailed down; and that they were intended to be carried out and sunk at the Edystone. This in truth put me into a great consternation; but being unwilling to lose any opportunity of completing my measures upon the rock; and concluding that this purpose could not be so speedily executed as to prevent my having an opportunity of speaking with the officer deputed to carry them out, I determined to proceed in my voyage; but we had not got abreast of the Ram-Head, before a violent squall of wind and rain obliged us to return.——I immediately waited on Commissioner Rogers to learn the truth of the above-mentioned report; who so far confirmed it, that he said they were to be sunk somewhere in the *Neighbourhood* of the Edystone: whereupon I told him, that it was sufficient to undertake to make a building that should be able to withstand the utmost violence of the sea: but it was too much to aid that powerful enemy with a *thousand battering Rams*, which these ships might be expected to prove, when broken to pieces by successive storms, and driven against the works of the building. Being asked how far from the Edystone it would be necessary to carry them; I told him it would not be safe at any moderate distance East or West, lest the flux and reflux of the tide should bring the wreck upon the rock; nor nearer than three leagues to the South. With this he promised to acquaint Admiral Mostyn who then commanded at Plymouth, and to return me an answer the next day: but as consequences of this kind seemed to have a tendency so dangerous and mischievous as to render the omission of any means I could take to prevent it, inexcusable; especially as they might be more easily foreseen than remedied, if the step was actually taken; I therefore wrote the same day to one of the Proprietors, who upon the receipt of my letter, applied to the Lords of the Admiralty, to send orders for these ships to be sunk in some place at a greater distance from the rock than seemed intended: however, the day following I saw the *Admiral*, who politely assured me, that nothing should be done, that could any way obstruct the building of the Edystone Lighthouse, and that there was *no such* thing intended.

84. AS the weather continued unpromising till the 11th of May, I not only compleated my rough plan of the rock as far as my measures had gone, but put together my thoughts, upon the subject of facilitating the landing, as also upon the proper mode of carrying on the works upon the rock with *Expedition* and at the *least possible Expence*, and communicated them by letter to the Proprietors.

* It may be a necessary explanation at this time to say, that these were vessels that had been seized from the *French* before a formal declaration of war.

On

On discoursing again with Mr. Jessop upon the subject of amending the landing at the Edystone, he informed me of an expedient they had sometimes made use of; which was, that when a vessel could not get into the Gut, so as to lie along-side the house when workmen were there for repairs, but yet could get so near, as to be out of danger, the weather admitting a barrel or log of wood with a rope fastened to it to be thrown from the rock; they took this up into the vessel or boat, and fastening timbers thereto they were successively hauled through the sea, and so got upon the rock. This had frequently been done, and though it did sometimes miscarry, and always took up time, yet it was the best method they had been able to devise; and the only one they had ever practised: but this expedient would little avail me, as a stone building appeared by every day's reflection, and the experience of every voyage, more and more feasible, as well as desirable; and as my proposed materials would not swim, a safe landing became a still more important object.

Mr. Jessop was in truth the only person I had met with, who seemed to have a competent knowledge of the situation of the rocks; and though very careful and accurate in finishing what he undertook, yet he was not a man of much invention. He had however a very clear and sound judgment in whatever his practice and experience had put him into the way of knowing; and though apparent difficulties seemed to have kept his inventive faculties in awe; yet from his long experience, he generally proved an able adviser concerning the operations proposed to be performed at the Edystone.——As I looked upon a tolerably safe way to get to and from the building, and to lie there, particularly if it was to be of stone, as almost a *sine quâ non*; and had on this occasion fully communicated and explained my ideas to Mr. Jessop and received his approbation, I took the first opportunity afterwards of acquainting the Proprietors therewith by letter, in nearly the following terms.

" I shall now describe the manner in which I propose not only to facilitate the landing upon the rock, but to increase the safety of vessels lying in the Gut.——The house-reef may in its natural position be considered as a pier, break-water, or bulwark to vessels lying there; and this would have been very complete, had it not been for the following circumstances. The rock that lies next to the northwards of that upon which the house is built, approaches nearly in height to that of its neighbour; and the top of it is about fifteen feet from the house rock*; but between those two rocks is a low part, gully or hollow that is covered at about half tide, over which the sea breaks, even in fine weather, at low water, when there is any thing of a ground swell; and the waves cascade through this gap, into the Gut, as if, for the moment, an hundred mills were at work; which, when this takes place, not only endangers the filling of the boats, but raises such a surge in the Gut, as to cause the vessels to lie very unsteadily. This gap I propose to stop up, by first fixing an oak beam of at least twelve inches scantling upon a level from the house rock, to the top of the north rock, very firmly with iron bolts at each end; which beam is to serve as a *Ridge-tree*, somewhat in the manner of that for the roof of a house. Then to bolt firmly down upon the sloping surface of the rock below, two other timbers or sills, one on each side the ridge, in such manner, that three-inch planks being well spiked down upon the ridge-tree and upon the sills on each side, should form a figure like the roof of a house. The force of the sea therefore, whichever way it comes, will be broken by running up the sloping planking, and be prevented from running over in so large a quantity, whenever there is a probability of working upon the rock †.

" Moreover the east side of the house rock, though pretty nearly upright, is remarkably ragged and indented; and particularly upon its most projecting parts‡, some of which considerably overhang; if therefore there is not a constant care to keep a boat from touching when lying alongside the rock, her gunnel would be liable to be damaged by its asperities; and by its being hooked under the projections, she would be subject to be overset even in the finest weather: and this inconvenience and hazard, not only

* See Plate N° 14.

† This part of the proposition was never executed, principally for want of time at the proper season when it was possible to have done it; but being satisfied of the practicability as well as utility thereof as a temporary expedient, if done, I give it here a place as appurtenant to the subject.

‡ See the south views of the rock in Plates N° 6, 9, and 14.

arises from the unsteadiness that is occasioned by the cascading of the water through the gully before mentioned; but when there is a breeze eastwardly, though not sufficient to occasion the sea to break upon the landing-place, or prevent working; yet by the boats being driven against the rock, they would be subject to the disasters above described: and what is more material than what I have already mentioned, if the workmen should be caught with a fresh of wind at East, the boats would be liable to be staved, whilst the men were getting themselves and tools on board."——I had already found by my own experience, that such kind of disasters we were subject to, and that we should be still much more liable to them in the course of the erection: and for an evil so great, the more simple the means, the better should the contrivance be esteemed by which it might be averted. To this end "I propose to fix timbers by bolts, upon the most prominent or projecting parts of the rock, in the manner of piles against the face of a quay, and at such distances as to be nearer together than the length of our boats; by which means their gunnels and sides being made to slide up and down against the piles, instead of the rock, there would be no danger of catching; and therefore a greater degree of security would take place, as well as that less care and attention would by that means become necessary *."

85. WHATEVER advantages might ultimately result to the public, from having a durable stone building in lieu of a perishable wooden one, yet if the time that was necessary to be taken up in the erection, was likely to be greater than had been taken up by former builders, which was four summers, this would be a very sensible and striking objection to my proposition; and as the execution thereof would naturally require a greater time, in proportion to the whole additional tonnage of materials; this led me to every consideration that had a natural or artificial tendency to expedite the work.——I found that the customary payment of such artificers as had gone out upon the repairs of the late building, was five shillings per day, (or 35 shillings per week) from the time they held themselves ready to put their foot into the vessel to go out, to the time they were re-landed and discharged; without having any regard to the time employed in actual execution: what were the wages during the former buildings being *in hand*, I never could learn: but as there always had been, so long as memory reached, a house to receive and lodge the workmen, when they once got thither, the disappointments attending the difficulty of landing and fruitless voyages were, under that circumstance, of less consequence: I was therefore solicitous to form such a scheme for carrying on the works, as should make the service full as eligible to the workmen as formerly, at the same time that it should be their *interest* to exert themselves to the utmost; or at least to spend as much time upon the *Rock* as possible; and also, that they should be enabled to bear their labour chearfully during their continuance there, by not being subjected to any unreasonable degree of fatigue, by long periods of service. In consequence of all this, the work would of course be performed, not only as expeditiously as possible, but at an expence to the Proprietors, as low, in regard to the value of day labour, as could possibly be expected upon the former establishment.

It therefore seemed to me to be necessary, not only to moor a store-vessel in the neighbourhood of the rocks during the working season, but to employ *two* complete sets of hands for the outwork, to relieve each other in turns; so that whenever weather and tides would permit, the work might be pursued day and night.——That the workmen should on no occasion fall short of the common wages of the country for their support at sea, whether circumstances favoured or not; but that their making *extra Wages* should depend upon the time they actually spent upon the rock; where in general, a reasonable degree of employment could scarcely be avoided: and that it might be as much the interest of the seamen to use their best endeavours to get the workmen landed, and to encourage them to stay as long as they could, without imminent danger; their payment, as well as that of the foremen of each company, should all follow the same kind of proportion.——Upon these ideas I drew up and transmitted to the Proprietors, the following plan for carrying on the works; and which in effect, with very little variation, was afterwards carried into execution.

* T[illegible] of piles with *Trenails* through them, to answer the purpose of a ladder, are represented at P. Q. Plate N° 14.

PLAN

PLAN *for carrying on the* WORKS *and Management of the* WORKMEN.

1ſt, That the Edyſtone ſervice ſhould by all reaſonable inducements be rendered preferable to any other common employment.

2d, That therefore (as a *puniſhment)* any one failing in his duty ſhould be immediately diſcharged.

3d, That the workmen ſhould be divided into *two* companies; one company to be out at the Rock, the other to be employed in the work-yard on ſhore.

4th, That every Saturday, the weather permitting, theſe two companies to change places; but the out-company not to return home till the in-company is carried out to relieve them.

5th, Every man to have certain fixed wages weekly; and the ſame whether *out* or *in.*

6th, Every man to receive —— per hour over and above the fixed wages, for every hour he works upon the rock.

7th, Every out-man to take all opportunities of landing upon the rock to work, when the weather ſerves, whether night or day, Sundays or work-days.

8th, The in-company not to work either nights or on Sundays, except in caſe of neceſſity, and then

9th, All *extra* work on ſhore to be paid for in proportion to double the *fixed* wages for the like time.

10th, The ſeamen to be alſo at conſtant weekly wages, with an addition of a fee certain and proportionable every tide's work upon the rock.

11th, Each company to have a foreman conſtantly with them while working upon the Rock; to be paid more than the common workmen, and in the ſame proportion.

12th, The engineer and his deputy, to go off alternately week for week; and each week to go off as often, and ſtay as long as weather will permit, or the ſervice require.

13th, In caſe of ſickneſs, or neceſſary abſence of either the engineer or deputy, the whole (if poſſible) to be taken care of by the other.

14th, All perſons to victual themſelves, but a bowl of punch to be allowed each company on their return on ſhore.

15th, The foremen, workmen and ſeamen, to be paid every time the reſpective companies return on ſhore.

16th, All work tools to be provided and repaired at the charge of the Proprietors, and to have a mark put upon each of them peculiar to the Edyſtone.

17th, Every perſon hurt or maimed in the out-ſervice to receive his common wages while under the ſurgeon's hands; and the Proprietors to pay the ſurgeon. This to be allowed on the certificate of the engineer, deputy and agent.

18th, Any perſon deſirous of quitting the ſervice, to give a week's notice to the engineer or deputy.

19th, The foreman on ſhore to take an account of every thing received into, or ſent out of the work-yard; as alſo of the day's works of the company, &c, with him; under the check of the engineer or his deputy when on ſhore.

20th, All ſmith's and plumber's work to be ſeen weighed by the foreman, engineer or deputy on ſhore; and all timber or wood work to be meaſured, and other materials taken account of by the ſame on receiving them.

21ſt, The foreman *afloat* to take account of time and landings upon the rock, to be chequed by the engineer or his deputy when afloat.

22d, An account of all matters done on ſhore to be given in weekly to the agent or accountant; and of all things done afloat by the proper foreman at the time of landing.

The further conſideration of theſe and many other matters, I referred to an interview with the Proprietors, to whom I was now in hopes of ſoon returning.

86. IN the afternoon of the 11th of May, we ſet out on our *Ninth* voyage, and got to the Rock in the evening; when we found the ſea ſufficiently quiet about it, to admit our landing; but it being near

near dark, and blowing fresh at N N. W. Mr. Jessop and the seamen thought it not safe to go into the Gut that night, being of opinion that if the wind should a little increase, or get nearer to the North, we should not be able to get out again *.

On this occasion the idea first occurred to me, that there might be a possibility of the water's being sufficiently quiet for the boat to lie alongside the rock (which used to be the criterion of the men being able to work thereon) and yet that the entrance or exit from the Gut might be impracticable or dangerous: this struck me with a most sensible chagrin, insomuch that I scarcely slept that night; partly with mortification at our present disappointment, and partly in contriving means how to remedy so great an inconvenience: for the plan I had before laid down for the greater protection and security of the craft when lying in the Gut, would not have availed us in such winds and tides as were now our obstruction; and my scheme would still be imperfect, if after I had made the lying there less dangerous, I should not be able to reach it, or get out when there pressed with danger.

The blowing up of the *Sugar-Loaf* rock was undoubtedly the first thing that occurred; but this in fact would only be a partial remedy. To level the Sugar-Loaf to its base, would of itself be a serious work; as it never could be set upon except when the sea was remarkably still and quiet; and would of course take up that time which would be the most valuable towards getting the house-rock cut for the proper reception of a stone foundation; and of consequence prove a considerable hindrance to the execution of the main design: nor could this matter be expedited by an *additional* number of hands for that service; because as they could very rarely be applied, the incumbrance arising from a greater number of men afloat, than the main service naturally required, would prove a real obstruction to the general progress of the work: besides if the Sugar-Loaf was in fact levelled with its base, yet as the Gut would remain barred up within a small matter of low water, by flat rocks, which extend almost across it in that place; to get a clear passage to the South, with a sufficiency of water for the craft at low water, notwithstanding it presented itself as far from impossible, yet seemed likely to prove a greater work than that of the Light-house itself; and consequently not to be thought of at this time.

Having observed the use that was made of *Transport Buoys*, in the moving and mooring the king's ships in the *Hamoaze*; it struck me, that if a transport buoy of a size proportioned to our sort of craft and service, was moored with chains at the distance of about fifty fathoms directly North from the Gut, to which one end of a suitable cable or hawser should be *bent* (that is, fastened) and the other carried to the landing-place in the Gut; and to prevent its being fretted against the rocks, so much of it as would be liable to touch, to be a chain; this cable and chain being kept always in repair, during the working season, as there was nothing to hinder us from sailing to this buoy, when vessels could keep the sea, they might lie there till it was a proper time of tide to go into the Gut: and then by means of this communicating cable, we should be able to hawl them into and out of the Gut against wind and tide; and for facilitating of this with a few hands, I proposed a windlass of a *new Contrivance* † to be put on board each of our larger vessels that were to go into the Gut. Our buoy would also be attended with this further advantage, that in going out, the vessel having gained it, her sails might be set before she quitted it; by which means she would get under way, and shoot clear of the rocks when the wind blew northerly.

In the morning I communicated this proposition to Mr. Jessop, who thoroughly approved of it; and added, that if a couple of *eye-bolts*, at a competent distance North and South of each other, were fixed into the rocks on the *East* side of the Gut, to which ropes might be occasionally fastened, these would keep the boats from striking against the house-rock, when the wind was easterly; and such a contrivance would have been particularly useful the very last time we went out of the Gut.

87. THE 12th of *May* we landed on the rock at seven in the morning, and staid till eleven, the wind being at S. S. W. It having been moderate during the night, the boat lay very quiet; but we at

* It has already been explained, that there is no passage to the southward, through the Gut, on account of the *Sugar-Loaf* rock.

† This was by means of *Wheel and Pinion*, scarce heard of for such a purpose at that time.

last

last found it advisable to quit it, but more on account of the rain than the wind, (though that was becoming more fresh) as we were wet quite through, and what was worse our papers were wet also: however having now taken all the most material measures, this circumstance reconciled me to every thing else.—— At weighing to come home, our anchor having got foul of the rocks, we parted our cable, and afterwards in endeavouring to weigh the anchor by the buoy rope, we parted that also: so that we were obliged to leave the anchor behind us; the risque of which would have been prevented, had we now had a transport buoy, such as that proposed.

88. AS it was my wish entirely to complete my measures, if a favourable opportunity happened, without further loss of time; while I was preparing for my departure on the morning of the 15th of *May*, the weather again appeared favourable, and we proceeded on our *Tenth* voyage. We landed on the rock at half past eleven in the morning, and staid there till half past two in the afternoon. The wind being then Easterly and beginning to blow a little fresh, we found it proper to quit the place for fear of staving our vessel against the house rock, of which there would have been much less danger, as she would have been far more manageable, had the proposed *fender* piles, or Mr. JESSOP's proposition, been in use: for though we were six hands in the Edystone boat, and used our utmost endeavours to prevent it; in coming out of the Gut the boat struck against the north rock, and sprung a leak, though no considerable damage was done to her. Having now completed all the observations I was desirous of making, which I was the better enabled to do, as it was a low spring ebb, I took my leave of the rock for the present with great satisfaction, and arrived at Plymouth that afternoon.

C H A P. III.

Containing Transactions and Occurrences during my Return from PLYMOUTH *to* LONDON *in May* 1756.

89. IN my return to London, I thought it necessary to take a view of the several places that had been pointed out to me, from whence *freestone* could be shipped for *Plymouth*; not so much indeed to acquaint myself with the nature of the stone itself, of which I had seen samples before; as to learn whether I could have the quantities worked upon the spot of such weight, dimensions and forms as I concluded would be needful; and to inform myself of the charge of freightage, and other particulars that I knew would be necessary to enable me to make any kind of estimate of the cost of the building; which I must expect would be required from me by the Proprietors; or at least that I should give them all the information that I possibly could, touching such things as related to the proposed work.

90. WITH this view I first visited the quarries at *Beare*, near the S. E. corner of *Devonshire*, and near the sea-coast. I found the bed or *Stratum* of freestone worked here, was of a considerable thickness; and with so great a cover of earth upon it, that it was worked in under-ground cavities; the superincumbent *Strata* of earth, &c. being supported by pillars formed by detached parts of the *Stratum* left standing. Here the stone, which is of the calcareous kind, and in point of hardness and texture much like the Bath stone, but whiter, lies in so solid and thick a bed, that blocks might be cut out from it of any size required: and though the *Stratum* is very compact (that is, free from fissures) yet it is of so soft and workable a nature, that I found the workmen sawing out blocks from the general mass (or *posts*) with carpenter's saws, which they could do to any dimensions required; and though this stone was capable of being thus wrought, and was so free to the tool, yet I found that it hardened considerably after being exposed to the weather, as was manifest by the buildings that had been erected many

years at the village of *Beare*: the stone in the old buildings being in general covered with a kind of mossy coating; and workmen, with reason, look upon the stone so coated, as not to be in a state of waste or decay. However, though hardened by time and weather, it yet seemed of a softer nature than I would wish for the construction of a building, that in every step of its erection would be subject to the extreme violence of the sea.

91. MY next visit was to the Isle of *Portland*, at which place I had an address to Mr. ROPER; who was the principal agent, or manager at the quarries for —— TUCKER, Esq; of *Weymouth*, the principal quarry-proprietor or worker there.——I found Mr. ROPER a very plain, sensible, intelligent person; and as this isle, as it is generally called, seemed to contain many things that awakened my curiosity, I was very glad to accept of him for my conductor or guide; and as being one of the principal residents upon the isle, and particularly versed in the works peculiar to it, no person could better have fulfilled my wishes.——Upon the commencement of the works of *Westminster Bridge*, some time about the year 1739, Mr. ROPER was sent down by the contracting mason, as foreman, with a gang of masons or stone-cutters from *London*; who were, according to moulds and drawings, to hew the stones upon the *place*, to save the freightage of the waste: for, it is to be observed, that previous to this period, the stone sent from Portland had always been shipped off in the rough, or rather what is called rough *scappelled* blocks; to be sawn and fair wrought to the particular purposes, where wanted: and after the completion of that work, having engaged with Mr. TUCKER as superintendant of his quarries, he had remained there ever since.

92. THE first thing that excited my curiosity, was the very subject I came upon, that is, the quarries from whence the stone sent from Portland is produced.——The upper surface of the island I found was tolerably flat; but elevated above the sea, according to the estimation of my eye, at least 200 feet. The *Stratum* of stone that is wrought for sale, lies nearly parallel with the upper surface of the island; and with not much cover of earth or rubbish upon it. There are several beds of stone lying in contiguity, one above another, varying in thickness in general from two to four feet and upward. Those which are usually called the *merchantable Beds* (on account of the blocks for sale being produced therefrom) are universally covered with a *Stratum* called the *Cap*, which is formed entirely of a congeries of petrified sea-shells, of a great variety of kinds, but in general so distinct and separate in their forms, that to the curious naturalist, their species seem very easy to be made out*: but as they in a considerable degree retain their respective figures, (though in some places more, in some less) spaces or cavities are left between them, which consequently very much diminish the coherence of the mass; but yet the cementing principle is so strong, that the whole together is considerably harder than the merchantable beds: and indeed so hard, that to get rid of it as easily as possible, it is generally *blasted* off with *Gunpowder*.——Were it not for these cavities, the cap-stone would not readily be worked with tools; or at least it would not be worth working at a place where there is so great plenty of stone of a better quality: but as it is necessary to remove it in the course of working the better kind of stone, though by far the greatest proportion is [illegible] into fragments, yet for the buildings on the island, the cap-stone is in general use, and also for the pier and quay wall of *Weymouth Harbour*; as also in the pier for shipping stone at Portland, blocks [illegible] from the cap; and indeed upon the whole, were it not for the expence of freight (which is the same as upon those of the best quality) for various rough purposes under water, &c. the cap would make [illegible] and durable work, as the merchantable blocks.

When the merchantable beds are cleared of the cap, the quarry-men proceed to cross-cut the large [illegible], which are laid bare, with wedges, in the way I have described as to the moorstone; only the wedges are [illegible], nor does Portland stone split so evenly as the *Granite*: and frequently in the splitting, a [illegible] of this stone, oyster and other fossil-shells are discovered in the solid substance of the [illegible].——The beds being thus cut into distinct lumps, the quarry-man with a tool called a *Kevel*, which [illegible] one end a hammer, and at the other an axe, whose edge is so short or narrow

* The [illegible] kind, called *Cornua Ammonis*, some very large; and I saw one which when cleared from all sur- [illegible]

that

that it approaches towards the ſhape of a pick*, by a repetition of ſturdy blows ſoon reduces a piece of ſtone, by *his Eye*, to the largeſt ſquare figure which it will admit; and blocks are thus formed from half a ton, to ſix or eight tons weight; or upwards, if particularly beſpoke.

93. WHEN I viewed the ſimple conſtruction of their carriages, I could not but wonder upon being told, that ſuch a very plain piece of machinery, was all they had for getting the largeſt blocks down to the water-ſide; but when I ſaw the application, my wonder ceaſed.——I have already obſerved, that the plain, upon which the quarries are ſituated, is conſiderably elevated above the ſea. It is further to be obſerved, that though the greateſt part of the circumference of the iſle to ſeaward is bounded by cliffs almoſt perpendicular, yet on the North ſide towards the main land of *Dorſetſhire*, the deſcent is more moderate, though it is rather quick every where.——It did not indeed at once occur to me, that though it would require a very great power to draw large ſtones *againſt* Gravity, or *up-hill*; and even a conſiderable one to draw them upon the plain ground; yet in moving *down-hill* their gravity would aſſiſt them.——The carriages are a kind of *Carts*, conſiſting of nothing more than a pair of very ſtrong ſolid low wheels (as well as I remember) about a yard in diameter, and a very thick axle-tree, upon which is fixed a ſtout planking or platform, that terminates in a draught-tree for ſteerage and yoking the cattle to.——The wheels and platform being low, the blocks are the more eaſily loaded thereon, and a neceſſary power is employed, according to the ſize of the block, to draw it to the commencement of the deſcent. ——To this place a quantity of blocks of different ſizes have been, at leiſure times previouſly drawn; and one of theſe blocks, of a ſuitable ſize, ſuch as experience has pointed out, is by a ſtrong chain attached to the carriage, on which the other block is placed, which is then drawn forward with the block in *tow*, till they are got ſufficiently upon the ſlope of the road, to find an inclination in the loaded carriage to move the attached block; after which all the horſes and beaſts of draught are taken off, except ſuch as are abſolutely neceſſary for the guidance; and in this way (the deſcent being continual to the pier) *two* large ſtones are got down with a degree of eaſe and expedition, that would be almoſt impracticable with *one* alone, without more complicated machinery.

94. I FOUND I could have every thing here, that I could deſire in the freeſtone way; ſo far as rough ſcappelling went; and at a price ſo moderate when delivered on board, that the freight, even to Plymouth, would be a conſiderable part of the charge: but that in regard to *hewing*, after the work of *Weſtminſter Bridge* was over, the hands brought here on that occaſion were diſperſed; or the few which were left had engaged to work in the quarries: and that except for ſuch large undertakings as *Weſtminſter Bridge*, what could be ſaved in freight, would not compenſate the diſadvantage of employing ſeparate workmen at a diſtance: for, in regard to the internal works of the iſland, there was not enough of them to maintain ſtone-cutters; and though they had juſt built a new church, which I obſerved had been neatly worked, and chiefly from the cap-ſtone, yet I found that workmen had been brought into the iſland to perform it.

95. FROM the practicability of the road in the way before mentioned, and alſo from the circumſtance of there being there the quieteſt water, the pier for ſhipping the ſtones is on the north ſide, adjoining to *Weymouth Road*; ſo that the ſtone veſſels, if catched by a ſtorm while lying there for a freight, retreat into *Weymouth Harbour*.

I did not fail to viſit the Lighthouſes, built nearly on the higheſt part of the iſland; but as they are built upon the *dry Land*, and burnt coals, I found they contained nothing ſingular, or material to my preſent purpoſe.——The various *Strata*, of which this iſland appears to be compoſed, would furniſh ſpeculation to the curious naturaliſt; but which the purpoſe of my preſent viſit did not allow me time particularly to attend to: but what ſtruck me moſt with wonder and amazement was the *Portland Beach*, which, I could not enter the iſland in croſſing the ſalt-water creek from Weymouth, without remarking:

* The *Kevel* is a tool curiouſly formed for the purpoſe; the face of the hammer end not being flat, but hollowed according to the portion of the ſurface of a cylinder: this gives a keen edge to two of its oppoſite ſides, that are parallel to the handle; and by this means biting keenly upon the ſtone, brings off a *Spawl* or large ſhiver. The edge at the pick end is about half an inch in breadth.

and

and which perhaps renders it impossible to decide whether *Portland* is really and properly an *Island* or not *. This work of nature is an immense bank or mound, formed to appearance of round pebbles of promiscuous sizes, the generality not exceeding the size of a pullet's egg; which by the action of the sea in beating them one against another (being of a very hard nature) are worn so smooth and round, that a man can scarcely walk upon them without sinking to the ankles, or a horse to his knees at every step. In consequence of the matter being so loose, it forms a considerable slope, both towards the sea and to landward. It proceeds from the N. W. corner of the isle of Portland, and keeps somewhat near a N. W. direction till it approaches the shore, at (I think) scarcely a mile distance. Had it there actually joined the shore, and had the rest of the beach been heaped upon the natural coast of *Dorsetshire*, this conformation would not have been a matter altogether singular: but on ascending the summit of the *Beach*, which is several feet above high-water mark, that I might have a more distinct view of it (which I was fully enabled to do by its being low water when I first landed upon it) I found, that not only the part from the place where I stood, to its junction with the island, made a portion of a regular *curve*; but that it was continued in a *fair Sweep* as far as the eye could trace it, nearly parallel to the general range of the natural shore, but without joining it; and in this way I was told it proceeded almost to *Abbotsbury*, at the distance of 14 miles, and there united with the shore; so that a person chusing to travel upon it from *Abbotsbury*, might with much labour and patience go to *Portland* on dry land even at high water.

A work of nature so regular in its form, must necessarily have a regular cause; what this cause may be, seems not very obvious, but it certainly is well worthy the attention of the skilful naturalist.——It would seem not to have had its origin at a very remote period; for the irregularities that the sea had washed in the ancient coast were still very distinct upon the salt-water creek (which as I have already said, every where runs behind it, till its final junction with the shore,) whereas in any great length of time, they must have been so far acted upon by frost, rain and wind, as to have been obliterated; since the present beach, like an immense bulwark, defends them from the immediate action of the sea's making any further incroachments.——It would seem also, that this beach was formed somewhat suddenly; so as to be, as it were, at *once* a defence to the ancient coast: for had a quantity of pebbles been washed up from the sea, and brought to the shore *gradually*, there does not appear to be any reason why the action that brought them thus far, should drop them *short* of the shore, and not heap them upon it; in which case, no salt-water creek would have been formed; for then the little irregular bays in the shore would have been first filled up, and the whole mass brought forward in the same kind of fair curve, as we now find it: but from whence such a mass of pebbles should come, as very soon to form so great a *Barricade* as to shut out the sea, is a problem not seeming to admit of an easy solution †.

It further appears, that this beach lying in such a direction as to receive the full action of the S. W. seas, the component pebbles are of so loose a nature, that every tide makes an apparent change in the manner of its slope to seaward; which being formed into a sort of steps, or benches, answerable to the last high-water mark, these range regularly for a considerable length, and seldom remain the same for several tides together.——In time of storms, great quantities of the pebbles are driven over the summit, and as there is no power acting in a contrary direction, to bring them back again, one might at first be led to suppose the whole beach to be in a slow state of progression towards the shore, and that in time it would fill up the salt creek: but in contradiction to this idea, I was told, that four, five, or six feet beneath the surface of the pebbles, there is every where a strong mound of *blue Clay*, having the same general shape as

* If an [illegible] Dr. Johnson, [illegible] to be a *Tract of Land surrounded with Water*, then this certainly is not an island; but [illegible] to be a tract of land, whose component *Strata* are altogether detached from the main land, in this sense it may justly be [illegible] an island.

† On [illegible] Camden's *Britannia* [illegible] 8vo edit. 1590, it would seem, that in his time this Beach must have been of far less bulk than [illegible] by the action of particular winds, and its being consolidated by others: and that Portland [illegible] now annexed to the continent. His words are, speaking of this beach, "*Flexuoso hinc meatu longe se* [illegible] *arenâ aggere erecto, freto tenui interfuso per* IX. *mill. pass. obliquius prætenditur, quem auster cum* [illegible] *Hic* [illegible] PORTLAND *quondam insula, nunc continenti adnectitur.*" Camb. Brit. page 14[illegible]. The [illegible] edition of Camden was in the year 15[illegible]6.

the

the beach. This one can hardly imagine to be in a moving ſtate: and though there may be an endleſs ſucceſſion of pebbles conſtantly waſhing up from the ſea, to ſupply the place of thoſe waſhed over the ſummit; yet ſtill, why there is not a gradual incroachment upon the ſalt creek, does not readily appear. Was there any conſiderable diſcharge of land water by this creek, that would doubtleſs keep it clear, and the reflux of the ſalt water may ſomewhat tend to the ſame end; but yet its reflux ſeems far too languid to be ſufficient for the purpoſe.

96. THOUGH I found my curioſity ſtrongly excited by this ſingular and ſurpriſing work of nature, yet I had not time fully to ſatisfy myſelf as to facts; and as I have not ſince met with any adequate account of it, I am inclined to give a place to ſuch particulars as I could relate from my own obſervations; as my doing this may excite more able naturaliſts to examine minutely into the hiſtory of it, and it ſeems very well to deſerve a more particular inveſtigation.——As I was ſtruck with wonder at the conſtruction of the Portland beach, I could not be wholly inattentive to an anecdote which occurred here, reſpecting an equal ſingularity in the manners and cuſtoms of the Portland *Quarrymen*: for at that time thoſe of the *South Sea* iſlanders were entirely unknown to us; and as I do not find the ſyſtem of Portland has been touched upon by any of our travellers or *Touriſts*, my reader I truſt will not be diſpleaſed, if I give him a ſhort ſketch thereof in a note, as it occured upon the place*.

97. HAVING ſettled my buſineſs with Mr. ROPER; that the beſt way to get our ſtone rough ſcappelled, nearly to the ſhape I required, would be to ſend rough moulds, aſcertaining the figure, with the thickneſs of the courſe marked upon each mould, and each dimenſion to be one inch bigger than the true ſize previous to being fair worked, we ſhould not by this means have much extra *Weight*; as only the medium of half an inch on a ſide would be to cut off, and which would be ſufficient to form the true figure; I then took leave of him and this curious iſland: and though I had every reaſon to be ſatisfied both with the material and my correſpondent; yet nevertheleſs in my paſſage from thence to London, I determined not to leave any thing unſeen that might contribute to my information; and for that reaſon, to

* When I was looking over the quarries at Portland, and attentively conſidering the operations; obſerving how ſoon the quarrymen would cut half a ton of *Spawls* from an unformed block, and what large pieces flew off at every ſtroke, how ſpeedily their blows followed one another, and how inceſſantly they purſued this labour, with a tool of from 18 to 20 pounds weight, I was naturally led to view and conſider the figure of the *operative* Agent; and after having obſerved that by far the greateſt number of the quarrymen were of a very robuſt, hardy form, in whoſe hands the tool I have mentioned ſeemed a mere *Plaything*; I at laſt broke out with ſurprize, and enquired of my guide, Mr. ROPER, where they could poſſibly pick up ſuch a ſet of ſtout fellows to handle the *Kevel*, which in their hands ſeemed nothing: for I obſerved that in the ſpace of 15 minutes, they would knock off as much waſte matter from a maſs of ſtone, as any of that occupation I had ever ſeen before would do in an hour.——Says ROPER, we do not go to fetch thoſe men from a diſtance, they are all born upon the iſland, and many of them have never been further upon the main land than to *Weymouth*. I told him, I thought the air of that iſland muſt be very propitious, to furniſh a breed of men ſo particularly formed for the buſineſs they followed.——The air, he replied, though very ſharp, from our elevated ſituation, is certainly very healthy to working men; yet if you knew how theſe men are produced, you would wonder the leſs; for *all* our marriages here are productive of children.——On deſiring an explanation how this happened, he proceeded: "Our people here, as they are bred to hard labour, are very early in a condition to marry and provide for a family, they intermarry with one another, very rarely going to the main land to ſeek a wife; and it has been the cuſtom of the iſland from time immemorial, that they never marry till the woman is pregnant." But pray, ſays I, does not this ſubject you to a great number of baſtards? Have not your *Portlanders* the ſame kind of fickleneſs in their attachments, that *Engliſhmen* are ſubject to? And in conſequence, does not this produce many inconveniencies? None at all, replies ROPER, "for previous to my arrival here, there was but one child, on record of the pariſh regiſter, that had been born a baſtard in the compaſs of 150 years. The mode of courtſhip here is, that a young woman never admits of the ſerious addreſſes of a young man, but on ſuppoſition of a thorough probation.——When ſhe becomes with child, ſhe tells her mother; the mother tells her father; her father tells his father, and he tells his ſon, that it is then proper time to be married."——But ſuppoſe, Mr. ROPER, ſhe does *not* prove to be with child, what happens then? do they live together without marriage? or, if they ſeparate, is not this ſuch an imputation upon her, as to prevent her getting another ſuitor? The caſe is thus managed, anſwered my friend: "If the woman does not prove with child, after a competent time of courtſhip, they conclude they are not deſtined by Providence for each other; they therefore ſeparate; and as it is an eſtabliſhed maxim, which the Portland women obſerve with great ſtrictneſs, never to admit a plurality of lovers at one time, their honour is no ways tarniſhed: ſhe juſt as ſoon (after the affair is declared to be broke off) gets another ſuitor, as if ſhe had been left a widow, or that nothing had ever happened, but that ſhe had remained an immaculate virgin."——But pray, Sir, did nothing particular happen upon your men coming down from London? Yes, ſays he, our men were much ſtruck and mightily pleaſed with the facility of the Portland ladies, and it was not long before ſeveral of the women proved with child: but the men being called upon to marry them, this part of the leſſon they were uninſtructed in; and on their refuſal, the Portland women aroſe to ſtone them out of the iſland, inſomuch that thoſe few who did not chuſe to take their ſweethearts *for better, or for worſe*, after ſo fair a trial, were in reality obliged to decamp: and on this occaſion ſome few baſtards were born: but ſince then matters have gone on according to the ancient cuſtom.

take a view of the state of the quarries at *Purbeck*; from whence, for ages, *London* had been chiefly supplied with flat paving stones, and steps.

98. HAVING made my entry into the *Peninsula*, or, as it is generally called, the *Isle* of Purbeck, by the ruins of *Corf Castle*; and observing that a considerable part of the out-wall was in a remarkably leaning condition, something like the representation of the leaning tower of *Pisa*; I stopped to examine the masonry, and particularly the mortar, of a building that was capable of so great a degree of inclination without falling to pieces.——I found its solidity, as usual in ancient buildings, did not consist in having been built with large hewn stones throughout, for the interior filling of the walls was with rough *Rubble*, and fragments of the quarries; the interstices being entirely filled up with mortar, that undoubtedly had originally been fluid, and in that state poured in: and from the nature of the component matter, as well as time, the whole mass had become strongly cemented together. I found that the mortar was composed of lime (doubtless originally of a good quality) with a considerable admixture of sharp sand and *Pebbles*.

99. ON going to *Sandwich*, or, as commonly called, *Swanage*, the principal town of the quarrymen, and having procured a guide, I first went to view the quarries where the flat paving and steps were wrought. The *Strata* here are thin, some only of three inches, and seldom any single layer above twelve inches; the whole of several contiguous beds, taken together, being at that time, not much above a yard and an half in thickness. Having a good deal of cover of earth, &c. upon them, they were then chiefly wrought underground; and the whole of the merchantable stone being taken out, the incumbent matter was supported by building rough pillars with stone of an inferior quality.

From observing the nature of the thicker layers of this stone, I was at first led to imagine that this was the place from whence that peculiar kind of marble had been obtained, of which those long, slender, polished columns are formed, that are to be met with in most of the old cathedrals, even at a great distance from *Purbeck*; and which at those distant places are often taken for an artificial composition *.——I was shewn a district of ground where flat paving stone had been formerly wrought in *Strata* near the surface; so that it was then easily come at, and in great plenty; but the continual demand for the *London Market*, had in a great degree exhausted the quarries so circumstanced, and reduced the product chiefly to what they got underground in the manner I saw; so that the flat paving had already very considerably advanced in price, and was likely to advance still much higher †.

100. FROM hence I was carried to see the quarries where a species of stone was got in blocks, much of the nature and colour of Portland, which is called *Purbeck-Portland*.——These quarries are situated at, or near the point of high land, about three miles from Swanage, called St. *Alban's Head*. The strata of merchantable stone lie here in the upper part of the cliffs, as they do at Portland; but having more cover, they are in some measure worked underground. This stone is of the like nature, and puts on so much the appearance of the Portland, that it is often used in lieu of it. It is however inferior in colour, harder to work, and according to the information I then got, not in general near so durable ‡. But what seemed to me likely for ever to prohibit this field of stone from coming into competition with

* That great naturalist Dr. WOODWARD, is however, it seems, of opinion, that those slender columns extant in many of our cathedrals, are dug from the quarries of the same kind of stone at *Petworth* in *Sussex*.

† About the year 1764 the *Calder Navigation* in *Yorkshire*, having been opened, this gave water carriage to London of the immense [illegible] of the paving (there called *flags*) from the quarries of *Elland Edge* and *Cromwell Bottom*; by which means the schemes for new-paving the cities of *London* and *Westminster* were carried into effectual execution. This is not a marble or calcareous stone, like the Purbeck, [illegible] of the grit kind, yet of so close and fine a grain, as to be equally strong and durable, and, like moorstone, much less [illegible] I mean the kind really produced at the above quarries; for there is stone from other places, of the same appearance, [illegible] under the same denomination, which is much inferior in hardness and durability.

‡ The stone properly called *Purbeck ashler*, is of the same nature as the flat paving and steps, and sufficiently durable for all purposes; but a great part of these *Strata* are under twelve inches; yet some of them run to 18 and 20 inches thick, as I am *now* informed.

Portland

Portland, is; that as it cannot bear the expence of land-carriage down to *Swanage* to be shipped, the workmen are obliged to let it down with ropes from the place where it is wrought, to the surface of the sea, either into vessels lying at the foot of the cliffs where there is deep water, or where there is a dry *Strand* at low water; but there being little shelter from the winds and seas, this can only be done in very moderate weather, and particular winds; wherefore the shipping it there, must necessarily be somewhat precarious. For these reasons, though for the interior works of the Edystone the quality seemed not objectionable, and the stone could be afforded at somewhat less price than Portland; yet from the uncertainty of shipping, being somewhat further from Plymouth, and few hands, comparatively speaking, being employed here, to what were employed in the quarries of Portland *, it seemed a place much less capable of *expediting* my orders; and therefore, that Portland was to be preferred: expedition in getting the work forward being of so much greater consequence to what I had in view, than any small difference in the price.

Immediately on leaving the isle of Purbeck, I pursued my journey to London, where I arrived on Friday the 21st of May; having taken no more than five days in performing the whole, including all observations; and nothing further occurred in it which I think worthy the observation of my reader.

C H A P. IV.

Containing Transactions in LONDON *after my First Journey to* PLYMOUTH.

101. IMMEDIATELY on my return to London, I attended the Proprietors at a general meeting, and laid before them a full account of all my proceedings, and the information I had got in my late progress; together with my observations and thoughts relative thereto, which I have already particularized in the course of my narrative. The great and leading point now to be determined was, whether the house should be rebuilt entirely with stone, or entirely with timber; or partly with one, and partly with the other.——One principal matter to be considered, was that of *Time*, upon which subject I was fully examined; and assured the gentlemen, as my mature opinion, that if the building was to be entirely of stone, there appeared to me every degree of probability of my being able, not only to complete it in the like space of time, that the former Lighthouses had taken, which was four seasons; but, if required, to exhibit a light upon the building itself in the course of the third.——That upon the same reasonable grounds, it seemed to be equally practicable to raise a building with a stone base, and a superstructure of wood, in three seasons, and to build one of wood in the style and manner of Mr. RUDYERD (with some improvements) in two seasons.——On being examined respecting *expence*, I observed to the Proprietors, that to make an estimate of a building in each of those ways, was no difficult matter; so far as related to a certain given quantity of materials and the workmanship; but that, as in the progress of the work we should lie so widely open to accidents, I could not undertake to make any calculation of this part, which might not possibly be exceeded *tenfold*; and consequently could not make any estimate of what the whole expence of any structure might amount to, in such a situation as the Edystone. The whole therefore that I was enabled to say with any propriety was, that they being under the necessity of building the house in one of the three ways; whichever they chose, it should be my most earnest endeavour, not only to perform the work in the most substantial manner, but at the least possible expence, consistent with the necessary degree of firmness to give a reasonable expectation of durability.

* It should seem from the printed account of the loss of the *Halsewell Indiaman* in the month of January 1786, which happened in the neighbourhood of these quarries, that the assistance of ropes, &c. given to that very unfortunate crew, would indicate a greater number of quarrymen than would be inferred from the above account of mine; but it must be observed, that I am [illegible] as they appeared to me above 30 years ago.

102. I MUST

122. I MUST here obſerve to the honour of the Gentlemen concerned, that without debate, it was almoſt immediately determined to rebuild the houſe entirely with ſtone, and in the very beſt manner. ——The particular reaſon that induced the Proprietors to prefer that method, which undoubtedly would be the moſt expenſive to them, rather than either of thoſe which would be leſs ſo; as well as attended with leſs loſs of time, it is impoſſible for me to paſs over in ſilence.——It ſeemed very imprudent indeed, as far as their own intereſt only was concerned, that they ſhould think, in the ſituation they then were, of launching out into any expences beyond what was abſolutely neceſſary.——The building which had been lately deſtroyed, had, as already obſerved, ſtood near half a century, and had it not been deſtroyed by *Fire*, might, with proper attention, have exiſted much longer. A building therefore upon a ſimilar conſtruction, would moſt probably laſt for an equal length of time; or at leaſt as long as their preſent intereſt in the duties was to continue, and this would have been ſooner executed, and have coſt much leſs than one entirely of ſtone.——The Proprietors had alſo, with an equal ſpirit of generoſity, excluded themſelves from the reception of all profits, by voluntarily ſtopping the payment of the duties, till a light could be exhibited, as has been already taken notice of.——The Gentlemen were, indeed, ſufficiently ſenſible, that in all probability, the repairs of a ſtone building would be leſs frequent than thoſe of a wooden one; but yet, when neceſſary, might be much more chargeable, and even ſuppoſing they were not ſo, yet as a ſtone building would be much more expenſive, as well as hazardous in erecting, than any other, they would incur a *preſent certain* charge, to prevent a *future uncertain* one; ſo that it could not ſeem prudent, with reſpect to their own intereſt, to lay out 3 or 4,000 *l.* now, with the expectation of ſaving the like ſum in repairs 30 or 40 years afterwards. This therefore was not the ſort of conſideration that determined the Proprietors to erect a ſtone building; but their reſolution was in reality founded on motives wherein ſelf-intereſt did not bear any ſhare. They conſcientiouſly conſidered the intention of the legiſlature, in originally granting the duties, which they conceived were not given to the honourable corporation of TRINITY-HOUSE, and their *Aſſigns*, merely for their own emolument; but granted, through that channel, as the recompence to thoſe perſons, who at a great pecuniary riſque (beſides encountering other hazards) would procure ſuch a degree of ſecurity, as might be the means of ſaving from deſtruction, on this very dangerous rock, not only his Majeſty's fleets, but of preſerving the lives and properties of his trading ſubjects; and at the ſame time afford the like preſervation to the ſhipping of foreigners. This they conſidered as the ſole intention of the legiſlature, and that there might be no deficiency on their parts, in advancing ſo noble, ſo beneficial, and ſo humane a deſign, they determined that this preſervative of trade and navigation, ſhould be rendered as *durable* as *Nature and Art* could furniſh means for doing.——Nor was their public ſpirit confined to this object alone; for they had launched out into another hazardous and chargeable experiment, to ſupply the want of ſo uſeful an edifice, during the time that ſhould be taken up in building a new houſe, and preparing it for the exhibition of a light; and that was, by fitting out a veſſel for a *floating Light*: and though this was only conſidered as a temporary expedient, yet from the nature of the ſervice and ſituation in which it was to be employed, it was requiſite to make the experiment as valid and ſufficient, as if its exiſtence was intended to be of long continuance; and therefore of itſelf was a ſerious concern. This was actually going on at the very time of a new building's being determined upon as above; and had been a conſiderable time before, fitting out under the advice and direction of a committee, or of ſelect members, of the TRINITY-HOUSE: though till the 12th of May then laſt paſt, when the *Merchants* begun a ſubſcription, agreeing to pay the uſual duties, the Proprietors were uncertain, whether there would be a foundation, upon which they might be reimburſed a ſingle ſhilling.——Even by the proſpect which this ſubſcription opened, the Proprietors could not reaſonably expect to receive any great advantage by this undertaking; when the nature and hazard of it, as well as certain charge of the *Out-fit* was duly taken into conſideration; and with regard to the Lighthouſe itſelf, the very utmoſt benefit, that there was any probability might accrue to them, would greatly fall ſhort of reimburſing the difference of expence and time, between erecting a building like the former, and one entirely of ſtone.

Such were the proſpects of thoſe Gentlemen, and ſuch were their determinations at this time; in recording which, I have ſtrictly adhered to matter of fact. Was my pen capable of it, the *Theſis* would admit of great embelliſhment; however it luckily happens for me, that it does not need it: but the pen being

being in my hand, even after this long lapse of time: after all accounts closed; all expectancies ended; and I may say, after all connection and almost all acquaintance dissolved; it would yet be a violence to myself, to refrain from doing the Proprietors justice, so far as I have touched upon this head; by informing the world (that part of it especially which is most nearly interested in navigation and commerce) to whom, and to what principles they owe the present structure of the *Edystone Lighthouse*.

104. THE materials of which the main body of this house was to be rebuilt, being now resolved upon; as well as that its outward form should as nearly resemble that of the former one, as I should find consistent with the different nature of the chief material, and the improvements that offered themselves; to prevent any unnecessary delay in making *Estimates*, &c. the Gentlemen were pleased to content themselves with such general ideas of *expence* and *time* as my observations enabled me verbally to make: I was therefore desired without loss of time, to apply myself to making and providing such models and designs, as should enable me fully to explain my proposition to themselves, and afterwards to such other bodies, as they should think it right to consult: at the same time informing me, that though they were sensible that the season was near approaching in which something *might be expected* to be *done* upon the rock; yet they had such confidence in my judgment, that being now myself apprized of what was to be done, they left both the *Time* and the *Means* of its accomplishment to me.

105. ON this occasion I found myself totally unfettered; and perhaps no resolution of the Proprietors ever more conduced to the ultimate success of the work, than this, which set me so much at liberty. Had they been of the same temper and disposition of by far the greatest part of those who have employed me, both before and since, their language would have been, *Get on, get on*, for *God's sake, get on!* the public is in expectation, get us something speedily to shew, by which we may gain credit with the public! This, however, was not their tone, which I looked upon as a happy earnest from the Proprietors in the outset.

I considered, that though we should have a great increase of tonnage of materials to carry out and fix, beyond what former undertakers had had, yet that the whole bulk and weight, even as the building was now to be executed, would *in reality* be no very great matter; and that, in the present circumstance, the main object was to digest such a scheme as should go *progressively on as opportunity admitted*, without being subject to great derangements, or having the same thing to do twice over, on account of mistake or failure of the parts. It was with this general idea of the matter, that I took so much pains, and spent so much time, in getting accurate dimensions of the peculiarities of the rock, as I have already related; and this part of the work having taken a greater length of time than I expected; which arose from finding the rock more difficult of access; and, from its irregularity, requiring a greater variety of dimensions than I had imagined; yet as I had by perseverance fully accomplished my wish in this respect; the labour so employed would have been of less value, unless made use of to its proper intention; which was, that of having an accurate resemblance of the rock at *all Times* to recur to; in order that, the effect of any operation might, without going upon the rock itself, be judged of, so far as it depended upon the peculiarity of its form.——I further considered, that though I was now upon the verge of the proper season for action; yet as we could not expect to carry out any materials, or do any thing more this year, than *cut the Rock* to such a figure as should suit the building; and as this figure could not be ascertained, without fully considering and determining the form and dimensions of the building itself, so as to shew the manner in which it was to apply to the rock; I could readily see that the time which would be spent in such a mature digestion, would be much more than saved by avoiding unnecessary and improper work, upon a body of so hard a texture as that we had to deal with.——Had it been practicable to have cut the rock down to the level of the lowest part of the intended base of the building, little previous contrivance or consideration, would have been wanted for the purpose: but besides that this would have been more than the work of a full season; the space which had been previously occupied by the rock so cut down must have been made good by *fresh Matter*; and that could never be expected to be so perfectly firm and

 solid,

solid, as the unshaken parts of the rock itself: and besides, we should then have lost the rock as a *Hold-fast*, and *Battery* against the great South-west seas; which, so high as it reached, was of the most effectual kind possible.

It seeming therefore to be a first principle, to cut the rock as *little as we could help*; and for this end, to humour its irregularities as far as we could, so as to get a firm fixing for our work; on this account it appeared necessary, as the first step to be taken (from the dimensions already obtained, and by the methods already specified) to construct a *complete Model* of the rock, in the condition I found it: which being done, a second model might *then* be formed, shewing to what the rock was to be reduced, with the manner of applying the work of the building thereto; and so as to describe the external general form, which would be the whole of what was then wanted, for present determination; and for adjusting the work of the approaching season. These models I determined should be the work of *my own hands*; and this I foresaw, must in its own nature be a work of *Time*.

106. THOSE of my readers, who are not in the practice of handling mechanical tools themselves, but are under the necessity of applying to the manual operations of others, will undoubtedly conclude, that I might have saved much time, by employing the hands of others in this matter: and on the idea of the design being already fixed, and fully and accurately, as well as distinctly made out; that is, supposing the *thing done*, that was *wanted* to be done, it certainly would have been so: and had I wanted a duplicate of any part, or of the whole, when done, I should certainly have had recourse to the hands of others. But such of my readers, as are in the use of handling tools, for the purpose of contrivance and invention, will clearly see, that provided I could work with as much facility and dispatch as those I might happen to meet with and employ, I should save all the time and difficulty, and often the vexation, mistakes and disappointments that arise from a communication of one's own ideas to others; and that when steps of invention are to follow one another in succession, and dependance on what preceded, under such circumstances, it is not eligible to make use of the hands of others.

I had also a further reason for undertaking this part of the work myself; which those who shall peruse this account for the sake of information, may not be displeased to know.—— I have always found in subjects of mechanical invention and investigation, that I can seldom form an original idea so complete, but that by laying it down in its proper dimensions on paper, I could very much mature and improve it; and where the subject is attended with intricacy, it is in a greater degree necessary: but in reducing this to a *solid*, as is the case in making a model, still further corrections and advantages will often present themselves, that did not appear upon *Paper*: and this in a much more eminent degree when the *solid* is produced from the drawing by the artist's *own* hand, than by the hand of another: and still further improvements will occur, by going again over the *detail*, in constructing the work itself at large. Therefore to avail myself of all possible advantages of previous light and information, I determined, from the paper materials that I had brought from Plymouth; as well as those I carried thither; at once to construct the models above-mentioned myself; in which work, though I was closely engaged till the month of July; there was no impatience on the part of the Proprietors; as Mr. WESTON visited me almost daily, and was himself witness of the progress.——It may here be proper to say, that though I thought it necessary to employ my own hands upon the models, yet I availed myself of those of others, wherever I found them applicable: for having considered that I could not avoid having occasion for at least one great *Purchase-Tackle*; I therefore gave out a design to a proper workman, to execute a pair of tackle-blocks, in the style and manner of those I had published the use and figure of in the *Philosophical Transactions*, vol. 47, for the years 1752 and 1753; only that instead of iron or metal plates for forming compartments for the *Sheaves* or pullies, these were constructed with boards, for the sake of lightness, and avoiding corrosion by the salt-water. Plate N° 18. contains the design of these blocks *.

* By afterwards employing the late Mr. DUNSTERVILLE, an ingenious blockmaker at *Plymouth*, upon works of the like nature; a species of new [illegible] of [illegible] blocks has arisen, now, and for a number of years past carried on by the present Mr. DUNSTERVILLE at *Plymouth*, and Mr TAYLOR at *Southampton*.——The term *Purchase Tackle* has of late years been applied to this kind of blocks.

107. IN

107. IN this interval, however, I took a day with the above-mentioned Gentleman to visit the vessel then fitting out in the river, for the purpose of the *floating Light*; and to do this, besides the natural impulse of curiosity, I was desirous of seeing how far its equipment might suit the purposes of a *Store-Vessel* for our building service.——This vessel was called the *Neptune Buss*, having been purchased for this service from a great number of busses, that had been fitted out for the *Herring Fishery*, as a *National Concern*; which project having then failed, the vessels were sold. The *Neptune* was picked out as being remarkably well *found* and roomy, and her burthen, as I recollect, when thus fitted, was about 80 tons.——For this intended service, she had been heightened four *Streakes*; her deck raised, and laid flush *fore* and *aft*; so that if a sea was to break upon her, there would be no lodgment for the water; nor any where for it to enter the vessel, if the hatchways were shut; and those were not spacious: and furthermore in case this vessel was to touch upon the rocks, she would not *sink*, unless broken to pieces; being so far ballasted and loaded with fir timber, that though there should happen to be free admission of the water through the bottom, she still would be *Buoyant*, even with her necessary stores on board. This I thought an admirable contrivance for safety in such a service; and though the timber took up a good deal of room, yet in so large a vessel, there seemed to me a probability of there being room enough, both for the lightkeepers, and such of the Edystone workmen as must in their weekly rotations necessarily remain there. I also found her fitted out with an excellent *Windlass*, and was told, that large mooring chains were preparing: and in every respect, as far as my judgment could carry me, she was exceedingly well calculated for the service intended, and likely to do credit to the Gentlemen who had taken the direction of her works *.

On this occasion I observed to my worthy employer, Mr. WESTON, that it was probable the fitting out of this Buss, would be a saving of at least 4 or 500*l.* in the equipment of a store-vessel, as I had formerly hinted, in case the corporation of TRINITY-HOUSE should think proper to order the Neptune to be moored within a moderate distance from the rocks, any where to the N. or N. Westward of them; and as this might serve both the purposes, it would greatly relieve the heavy expence they were likely to be at, not only in the floating light, but the stone building.——To this he answered, that as the primary intention of a *floating Light*, was the preservation of trade and navigation only; and as the corporation of TRINITY HOUSE, most of whom were bred to the sea, had all along given their advice and assistance in the fitting out of this vessel; so it was presumed they were the proper judges, *where* it ought to be moored to answer the end best; and that for his part in particular, though he had presumed to suggest a hint to their more mature consideration, yet he by no means wished to bias their judgments, from an attention to the public welfare, by any reasons which might appear to be blended with a principle of self-interest. ——However, though thus fully answered, as I was sure it would be no very material impediment to the works, I was determined not to be precipitate in purchasing, or agreeing for a proper store-vessel, till I should know for a certainty, where the floating light was intended to be moored; and by that means give the Proprietors a chance of saving 500*l.* which I judged might be about the sum which a store-vessel fitted separately for our use would cost.——Upon the 8th of July I was informed that the buss with all her men, tackle, and furniture, sailed down the river for Plymouth, but the account of her arrival there (which was on the 17th of the same month) was not returned, while I staid in town.

108. MY models and preparatory matters were now so far brought forward, that Tuesday the 13th of July was appointed by the Proprietors for receiving my explanation of what I had to lay before them. I accordingly attended, and submitted to their inspection a complete model of the *house-rock*, in the state in which I had found it; and representing all the iron branches broken and whole, of which model, Plate N° 7. contains a reduced plan and elevation: and this was accompanied with another model of the same rock, cut to the intended shape for receiving the building; and therewith connected, a model of the building itself; shewing distinctly how the work was to be adapted to each separate step in the ascent of

* Those descriptions and anecdotes concerning the *Neptune Buss*, I should have entirely omitted, as being themselves of little consequence *now*; had it not happened to me afterwards, to have even more connexion with her than I then expected; and as this will save so much explanation and description hereafter, I therefore give this part of it in the order of time.

the

the rock, as high as I proposed to continue it; and particularly exhibiting the construction of the first entire course, after rising to the level of the upper surface of the rock; to which a solid being fitted, this model shewed the external form of the whole building, including the lantern; and by a complete section of this on paper, to the same scale, the rooms and conveniencies on the inside were fully expressed: and I must beg leave on this occasion to observe, that it was by now working in the solid, in forming the model for the building, I perceived that for the security of the ground joint, which would be subject to a superior action of the sea, to any other (as lying in the internal angle) it would be necessary, not only that the bed of every stone should have a level bearing; but that every outside piece should be grafted into the rock, so as to be guarded by a border thereof, at least three inches in height before it; which would in reality be equivalent to the founding of the building in a *socket* of three inches deep in the shallowest part.

109. THE whole having been now fully considered by the Proprietors, the greatest part of whom attended this meeting; they were pleased after a full explanation and discussion to declare unanimously, their entire approbation of, and satisfaction in the whole of my proposition; and therefore desired me to shew my models and draughts, and explain my scheme to the lords commissioners of the ADMIRALTY, and to the corporation of the TRINITY HOUSE: and one of the Proprietors undertook to give intelligence of this to the *Admiralty* and *Trinity House* respectively, which he did the next morning; also intimating, that I was then ready to depart for *Plymouth*, and proposed to do so in a few days; and would wait upon them with my *models*, &c. when they chose to appoint: and the Proprietors having adjourned their meeting to Saturday the 17th, they concluded that in this time those exhibitions would be over, and the sentiments of those respective bodies known.

The gentleman immediately received an answer in writing from the ADMIRALTY, that their Lordships would be glad to see the models at two o'clock the next day; at which time I accordingly waited on them, accompanied by one of the Proprietors; and must own I was not a little flattered by the thorough approbation their Lordships were pleased to express of my scheme*.

Saturday came without any other thing intervening, except my own preparations for my journey. I met the Proprietors at the time appointed; but as nothing had then been received from the TRINITY HOUSE, and the season was so far advanced, that all delays were dangerous, in a case where winds and tides were concerned, and the present season in hazard of being in some measure lost; therefore as the Proprietors could not answer it to the public, nor to the corporation of TRINITY HOUSE, if they kept me in waiting; it was determined that I should set forward early on the Monday morning following.

110. DURING the whole of my stay in London, I had kept a constant and regular correspondence with Mr. JESSOP, concerning the forwarding of such preparatory matters as I should stand in need of on my return to Plymouth; so that, in that respect, no time was lost.——During this interval, the Proprietors had also appointed a clerk to assist me in all matters of account and correspondence, and in whatever other business I should think proper to employ him. They then proceeded to give me their ultimate instructions, which in one sense might be said to be as *particular*, as in another they were *general*; and were nearly to the following effect.——To commence and carry on the works with all possible dispatch.——To employ what persons, and what number of men I should think fit.——To retain, dismiss, or reward them at such times, and on such occasions as I should judge right or convenient.——To agree or contract on their behalf, with any person or persons on any account whatever, relative to the rebuilding of the *Edystone Lighthouse*.——To direct the whole business and all persons I employed, and to exercise my discretion in the largest extent.——And, in short, that I was to command without controul except from themselves.

How much soever I was flattered by the thorough trust and confidence that those gentlemen now appeared to have reposed in me; yet I was not less pleased at their delegating one of the Proprietors to

* Lord ANSON was then at the head of that Board, who together with Sir WILLIAM ROWLEY were members of the corporation of TRINITY HOUSE.

act

act for them in the business of holding a correspondence with me, and managing and directing all such matters as I should have occasion at any time to resort to them for, of what nature soever: and this judicious measure certainly tended to the speedy advancement of the works; for in many instances while this work was carrying on, had I unfortunately been under the necessity of waiting for a resolution till the individual opinions of all, or a majority of the Proprietors had been taken, much time would have been lost, and possibly seasons; for whatever wisdom there may be in numbers, yet it is a trite and just remark, that they are generally tardy in their resolutions; and delays ought always to be avoided, when it is possible, in matters the execution of which depends on *Tides, Seas,* and *Winds:* different judgments and different ideas there must naturally be expected to be among many; but, in such a case, to enter into a debate, as to the propriety of taking any step, perhaps *absolutely necessary*, and possibly at the very time when that step should be *taken*, could have no other tendency except to delay and to increase the expence; from the fatal consequences of such circumstances, I was however happily relieved by the resolution of the Proprietors above-mentioned.

111. I AFTERWARDS understood that a verbal message was delivered by the secretary of the Trinity House, appointing the Wednesday following for my waiting upon them with the models, &c. but as this would necessarily have created a further delay of some days, the remainder of the season now growing precarious, the Proprietors did not think it proper to countermand my departure; I therefore set out according to appointment, very early on Monday morning the 19th of July for Plymouth; but not without greatly regretting the not having had the opportunity, as well as the advantage, of exhibiting my designs to the *Elder Brethren* of Trinity House: whose approbation as professional men, I was sensible would have greatly contributed to dispel the surmises, and that kind of distrust which must ever hang upon the minds of those who feel their own judgment incompetent; and who yet think themselves called upon to decide on so material a subject as I now had before me, though without having had the opportunity of its being properly laid before them: those, by way of security to their own, generally fall in with the popular opinion; which was, *that nothing but WOOD could possibly stand upon the Edystone.* However I consoled myself with the expectation of having a future opportunity; and that as the whole purport of the present remaining season, was nothing more than cutting the rock to a shape that must in every event, render it more apt for the reception of any structure whatever; I could not fear that any labour would be lost, by any difference in judgment that could possibly happen afterwards.

112. THE models that were prepared and exhibited as above related still remain in my hands, and Plate N° 7. is, as already mentioned, taken therefrom; for being professedly an exact representation *of* the rock, in the condition I first found it; this admits of no change: but the other model and section, containing the design *for* the Lighthouse (which as I have before hinted, was subject to some change in entering on the detail of the work at large) no longer remains an exact model of what was executed: nor at the completion thereof, had I any perfect design of it in that finished state; but having taken memorandums of the alterations, I have been enabled to make out a due representation of the work as it *now* stands: and as the original models, &c. served very well for many years to explain the nature of the work that *had been* done; the difference not being very considerable, in like manner the present representations of the work as really executed, will equally explain, what was formerly exhibited; first to the Proprietors themselves, then to the lords of the Admiralty, and afterwards to the honourable board of Trinity House; who to my great satisfaction entirely approved thereof.

Plate N° 8. contains the elevation or present appearance of the Lighthouse, as seen from the south. ——Plate N° 9. contains a section of the whole as seen from the same quarter.——Plate N° 10. contains the plans of the rock as cut into dovetails, with all the courses up to the top of the rock.——Plate N° 11. contains the plans of the first whole or ground course, and of all the courses above it.——And Plate N° 12. is an enlarged plan and section of the lantern.

B O O K III.

Containing an Account of Proceedings, from the COMMENCEMENT *of the* WORK *upon the* ROCK *in* 1756, *to the Beginning of the Second Seaſon in June* 1757.

C H A P. I.

Narrative of the PROGRESS *of the Work done upon the* EDYSTONE *from my Arrival at* PLYMOUTH *in July* 1756, *to the Time of mooring the* NEPTUNE BUSS.

113. I ARRIVED at Plymouth on Friday the 23d of July 1756, having been met by Mr. ROPER at *Dorcheſter*, with whom all neceſſary matters were ſettled; among which, the price of the ſtone, the mode of admeaſurement, the number of feet (16) per ton, and the method in which we were to receive a regular ſupply, were not the leaſt material. On my arrival, I found that Mr. JESSOP had completely fitted up, for preſent ſervice, *Hancock's Sloop*, which I had before made uſe of as an attendant; alſo, the Edyſtone boat; and a large yawl with ſails and oars; and had likewiſe got other things in forwardneſs that had been committed to his charge; and I immediately entered another able ſeaman, which, with our former crew that I had left on half pay, made the number ſix.

The *Neptune Buſs* I found was arrived, and lay in *Stonehouſe* creek; but without any order for the exhibition of a temporary light: on the contrary, I now underſtood, that ſome difficulties had ariſen between the Trinity Board, and their leſſees of the Lighthouſe*; and that in conſequence of this, two of the members of that corporation were then in the country, preparing another veſſel for that purpoſe. It ſeemed therefore to me moſt likely, that the Neptune Buſs, if not applied as a floating light, would be deſtined to be a ſtore-veſſel for the ſervice of rebuilding the Lighthouſe; and this occaſioned me ſtill to ſuſpend all orders for the preparation of chain moorings, till I ſaw the event of this buſineſs: but that our immediate ſervice might not be hindered, I ordered the ſloop's cable to be very well *wormed* and *ſerved* †, and a new one to be prepared in addition, in the ſame manner.——The weather proved not ſuitable to go out to ſea when I came, and I was informed, that the ſeaſon had never been very favourable for our ſervice ſince my departure from Plymouth in May: however, Sunday the 26th appearing promiſing, though there was but little wind, and being deſirous to reconnoitre the place, as our ground cables for the ſloop could not yet be got ready, I determined to try what we could do in rowing out in our new yawl, with the aid of ſuch breezes as might happen: the ſloop being ordered to follow us as ſhe could; that in caſe a freſh

* [illegible] of the *Merchants* of *London* to that Corporation, that they would take the propoſed temporary [illegible]

† [illegible] to fill up the ſpiral furrows between the *Strands* of the cable, and to bring the ſurface [illegible] the cable, but enables it better to endure friction againſt the ground: and the *ſerving* of a cable [illegible] other, like the baſs ſtring of a *Violin*; and to render this ſtill more [illegible] with canvas, and then the [illegible]-rope wound tight upon it, which was done in the preſent caſe.

of

of wind ſhould ariſe from the north, which would be very unfavourable to our return, ſhe might then get out to ſea, and bring us back, or make her courſe good to land us at *Fowey*, or ſome other convenient port.——We went out about eight in the morning; and with four oars, without aſſiſtance from the wind, got to the Edyſtone. I landed there, ſtaid an hour, found every thing exactly as I had left it; and after making ſome remarks relative to fixing the center of our propoſed building, got back to Plymouth at four in the afternoon. In our return we met the ſloop in the entrance of the Sound, ſhe not having been able to get any farther.

114. AFTER this day the weather came on bad and rainy, and continued ſo till Tueſday the 3d of Auguſt; which a good deal retarded our work in preparing the cables, &c. However, the interval was of ſo much length as to allow us to prepare every thing fully for the ſea.——I made uſe of this time alſo in preparing and eſtabliſhing our working companies upon the plan I have already mentioned, § 85. ——I made choice of and agreed with Mr. Thomas Richardson, a maſter maſon of Plymouth, of good reputation, to act as foreman to one of the companies; and alſo with William Hill, who had been ſome time foreman to another maſter maſon of the ſame place, to act as my other foreman. I likewiſe entered three maſons and nine tinners*, as a company to go out with Mr. Richardson to take the firſt turn or week, commencing from Saturday the 31ſt of July.——Mr. Jessop I appointed my general *Aſſiſtant*. The wages of the foremen, while out at ſea, were to be 5s. per day certain; and for every hour ſpent upon the rock, the further premium of 1s. But when employed in the work-yard, or otherwiſe on ſhore, their wages were to be 3s. 6d. per day. The wages of the maſons were to be 2s. 6d. per day certain at ſea, with a premium of 9d. per hour; and the tinners 2s. per day certain at ſea, and 8d. per hour. In the work-yard or on ſhore, the maſons were to have 20d. and the tinners 18d. per day; and to be paid for over time, when required to work, at the rate of double the price per hour, that their day wages came to, as propoſed in my original plan: and that the ſeamen might not want inducement to do their utmoſt in landing the workmen at the Edyſtone as early as poſſible at every opportunity, and ſupply them with what was neceſſary for keeping them at work; over and above their weekly wages, which were ſettled at 8s. per week, they were all to receive a premium for every landing upon the rock; the maſter ſeamen of 2s. 6d. and the ordinary of 2s. to make their advantage equivalent to that of the other workmen, in whatever ſervice the ſeamen (who were *conſtantly* on duty) might be employed.——Mr. Jessop as general aſſiſtant was to have 10s. 6d. per day at ſea, and 5s. per day at land, as he had been uſed to be paid; and every one was to ſupply himſelf with victuals.

In this interval I alſo agreed with Mr. Delacombe for half an acre of ground for a work-yard; being part of a field lying on the weſt ſide of Mill Bay (as before deſcribed, ſee Plate N° 17, Fig. 1.) which he rented of Lord Edgcumbe, and which by permiſſion of his Lordſhip, was to be applied to this uſe; and I marked out the yard and agreed for the fencing it with boards†.——Within this time Mr. John Harrison, the perſon made choice of as clerk to the Edyſtone works, arrived from London, with whom I digeſted a plan for the keeping our accounts and correſpondence, and for the diſtinct noting of ſo great a variety of articles as muſt neceſſarily occur, we found it expedient to open no leſs than 14 different books.

115. MATTERS being thus put in a train on ſhore, and the weather having become more promiſing, on Tueſday morning the 3d of Auguſt, Mr. Richardson and company embarked in the ſloop with her ground tackle‡ on board; attended by myſelf and Mr. Jessop, and alſo the yawl properly manned: the wind was favourable at N. W. on ſetting forward, but preſently changing to W. and afterwards to S. W. our progreſs towards the rock was not ſo ſpeedy as we all earneſtly wiſhed. Having got within

* The Corniſh miners, as the general produce from the mines in *Cornwall* for ages paſt has been *tin*, are commonly called *tinners*; and at this time many of them came to Plymouth to work as labourers.

† Upon this ſcite the *Baths* and *Long Room* have ſince been erected, as alſo the *Marine Barracks*.

‡ The general term for cables, anchors, and all other ropes and furniture for *mooring* or anchoring of veſſels.

two miles of the Edystone, and the weather being moderate, I went into the yawl attended by Messrs. Jessop and Richardson, and by the help of oars landed on the rock at half past four, where having brought some tools with us for that purpose, I proceeded to fix the center, and to lay down the lines of the intended work upon the surface of the rock; and being followed by Mr. Richardson, he with sharp picks left indelible traces of those lines, so as to be proceeded upon by the workmen whenever they should be able to land. This work however could not be further prosecuted for the present; for at six the sea began to be so unquiet, as to make it advisable to quit the rock, and return to the sloop: and before the sloop could gain a proper place for mooring, the sea became so rough, that it was judged impracticable to moor her that evening, or even to lie safely at anchor; we therefore went to *Cawsand Bay* in hopes of better weather the next morning.

Wednesday the 4th, the wind having continued to blow fresh all the preceding night, and still more so at four in the morning, I returned with Messrs. Jessop and Richardson to Plymouth in the yawl to expedite matters on shore, leaving the company on board the sloop.——Still the uncertainty of weather seemed to pursue this undertaking; but comfort arose from the reflection that as there *had* been opportunities to former undertakers enabling them to fix and complete their respective works, it was by no means to be doubted but that circumstances would again occur either sooner or later, so as to allow us effectually to pursue the present intention; and that, whenever we could get a vessel well moored near the rocks, many opportunities would be found of landing and pursuing the work, which otherwise must be lost by our being obliged to proceed from the shore, as was in reality the case in the instance just given.

116. THURSDAY the 5th, the wind being moderate at W. I went on board the yawl at seven in the morning attended by Messrs Jessop and Richardson, and on reaching the sloop in Cawsand Bay we immediately weighed and sailed; and arrived off the Edystone at two, when we again proceeded towards mooring the sloop; but before we got our moorings down, the wind again came on so fresh, that we had only the choice of dropping them in a situation not quite eligible, or experiencing a further delay: the former was chosen, as the less of two apparent evils; and upon doing this we found ourselves too near the S. E. reef, in which situation, in case of a hard gale at N. W. and any failure in the moorings, the vessel would be upon the rocks before her sails could be got up and set: however, being free from present danger, and every one anxious to make a beginning, as the tide now served, the whole company landed upon the rock, and immediately began the work, which was pursued for about four hours, when the sea advancing upon us, we quitted the first tide's work at half past eight, with which we had reason to be satisfied. The yawl was then dispatched home with the blunt picks, with orders to return immediately; as the sloop being left with only her small boat, the yawl's service would be wanted the next tide, if favourable to land the company: and to avoid delay, directions were given, that the Edystone boat was to bring out the tools when sharpened.

Friday the 6th, the yawl being returned in due time, all hands landed before sun-rise and worked that tide six hours: in the afternoon's tide, the company landed again, and continued the work, by the light of links, till ten at night. At seven in the evening the Edystone boat arrived with the sharp tools, and was immediately sent back with the blunt ones: and this day I got nearly the whole of the work laid out, as is particularly expressed in Plate N° 10. Fig. 1. which shews the dovetail recesses, and two new steps which were formed below all the former, according as it was ultimately finished for the reception of the stone-work: only that (to save a figure) the first course of stone is here expressed as laid; the doing of which was in reality the beginning of the work of the next season: the whole object of the work of this season being to get the surface of the rock converted from the shape and condition in which we found it, according to Plate N° 8. *Fig.* 1. to that of the figure just referred to: we also made good dispatch with the cutting of the rock, considering the exceeding toughness as well as hardness of it.

117. IT might seem at first sight, that a greater dispatch would have been made by the use of *Gunpowder* in blasting the rock, in the same manner as is usual in the mines, and in procuring limestone from the marble rocks in the neighbourhood of Plymouth: but though this is a very ready method of working hard

hard and close rocks, in proportion to the dispatch that could be made by picks and wedges; yet as a rock always yields to gunpowder in the weakest part, and it is not always easy to know which part is weakest; it might often have happened, if that method had been pursued, that instead of forming a dovetail recess such as was required, the very points of confinement would have been lost.——Besides, the great and sudden concussion of gunpowder might possibly loosen some parts that it was more suitable to the general scheme should remain fast. For these reasons I had previously determined to make no use of gunpowder for this purpose.

118. SATURDAY the 7th, the company again worked six hours in the morning's tide, but this being the day established for the change of the company, they had been but half an hour at work, when WILLIAM HILL and his company arrived in the Edystone boat, with sharp tools, and landed, taking up the tools that RICHARDSON's company had in hand.

Having now completed the lines upon the rock*, I returned with RICHARDSON and company, leaving Mr. JESSOP to attend HILL and his company for the following week. Our establishment respecting seamen was as follows: three of the seamen being left with the *Rock* or *Out-company*; one of them constantly remained in the store sloop; and the other two attended the workmen with the yawl, lying along side the rock at the landing-place in the Gut, to carry any thing that might be wanted to or from the sloop. The other three attended the Edystone boat, being now a passage-boat from the sloop or rock to the shore; and though such a kind of boat was easily managed by two men in ordinary, yet, as expedition was most necessary in the calmest weather, we now allowed three, that two might row, and the other steer.

119. I SHALL in this place take the opportunity of observing, that fine settled weather in these parts is almost constantly attended with *Land* and *Sea Breezes*: for about sun-set, or often before, the wind begins to blow a fresh breeze from the northerly points, which is from the land towards the sea; and in one, two, or three hours after sun-rise, it changes to the opposite direction, and blows a fresh breeze from the southerly points, that is, from the sea towards the land: and this circumstance proved in reality one of the greatest advantages towards helping forward our work; as by this means, the Edystone boat was enabled to make one regular *trip* every twenty-four hours; it being so contrived that she should depart in the evening, and return some time in the forenoon of the next day, sooner or later as the wind and tides served.

120. HAVING given this specimen of the mode of our operations in good weather, it is unnecessary to proceed with the account by way of journal, though I am sufficiently enabled to do it, having kept a regular one from the 23d of July, the day of my arrival at Plymouth to begin the works, to the completion of the same: a copy whereof was made out and sent weekly to Mr. WESTON, for the information of himself and the rest of the Proprietors. I shall therefore now only remark that from the first tide upon the rock, which was the 3d of August, the work was incessantly pursued at the average rate of about five hours per tide, with very little interruption, till Sunday the 15th, when the wind began to blow fresh at S.E. and shall content myself with remarking such occurrences as were more particularly deserving of our notice during this interval.

121. THE very evening I sailed with RICHARDSON, &c. for Plymouth, the seamen on board the sloop discovered a difference in the riding of the vessel, and that in all probability one of the anchors had dragged; and getting sufficient help from the other seamen and company, to heave up the ground cable, they found, that not only the *service* and *worming* were cut, but the cable itself was so greatly injured by the sharpness of the rocks, though it had been down not much more than twenty-four hours, that had the weather been rough, it would scarcely have borne to have been heaved up.——Had this not been disco-

* Here may be observed the great utility of the time employed in getting dimensions, and forming accurate models of the rock, and of the work immediately connected with it, before the operation was actually begun; for had the *contrivance* been to make out, while the workmen were upon the place, it is easy to judge of the loss of time, and number of mistakes and incongruities, that must have attended it.

 vered,

vered, as the wind in the night came on to blow fresh from the N.W. the cable would in all probability have parted, and the vessel gone upon the S.E. reef of rocks; the consequence of which might have been fatal to all on board. Mr. JESSOP, however, after getting the cable refitted in the best manner possible, determined with the assistance of HILL's company, to weigh the anchors and shift the moorings, so that the sloop might have the chance of riding in a more safe situation; that is, at about 100 fathoms to the north of the Gut, where it was judged the rocks might be less sharp, as the soundings were tolerably regular; and where also, in case of breaking loose, a north-west wind would *shoot* the sloop clear of the house reef. This in reality was every thing that could be expected under such a circumstance: for as a north wind proceeding from the nearest land is productive of the least swell, there would in the distance of 100 fathoms be a probability of hoisting a sail, and steering the vessel clear of rocks, through some of the passages (see the Plan, N° 3): yet after all, without *some risque* to every individual, there was no prospect of re-erecting the Edystone Lighthouse. This operation having been performed the same evening, there was little or no time lost to the work upon the rock.

122. ON Friday the 13th, which was in the course of HILL's company's week, the vessel fitted out as a *floating Light* by the TRINITY-HOUSE, sailed from Plymouth; and being got out to the vicinity of her place of destination, exhibited a light the same evening. Saturday morning the 14th, being the day of RICHARDSON's company going out to change, I went with them at seven, and arrived at the rock at twelve: when I found the seamen on board the sloop busily employed in piecing the ground cable, which this forenoon had again parted, having been cut by a rock in the same manner it had been on that day se'nnight. As soon as the cable was refitted, the moorings were replaced, and at four P.M. I landed upon the rock with Messrs. JESSOP, RICHARDSON, and C°, and staid an hour to examine the work that had been done; HILL's company having worked every tide in the preceding week, amounting to 64 ½ hours: and having found the work properly executed, I returned on board the Edystone boat with Messrs. JESSOP, HILL, and C°, and landed at Plymouth the same evening.——From this view of the work upon the rock, I judged that nearly one third of the whole was already dispatched.——The great wages that had been made this last week by HILL's company (amounting to above three guineas *extra* by the foreman, as also by the workmen in proportion) had the good effect of producing so much spirit in them, and that of emulation in RICHARDSON's company to do the same, that we now looked on the performance of the work of this season as quite within our power: provided, that we got a vessel in due time with *chain* moorings, which could better contend with the rocks, and keep her in her due situation: and as this day the *Corporation*'s vessel compleated her moorings, I judged it would not be long before the *Neptune Buss* would be delivered to my use. This was the more desirable, because the floating Light lying as we judged at the distance of two miles, in a direction W. by N. by the compass, the vessel could not in that situation be of any use to us in carrying on the building, notwithstanding the Light might be in a very proper situation to give timely notice to homeward bound vessels from foreign voyages, they being most likely to be out in their reckonings, in coming into the Channel in foggy weather.——This however occurred, respecting the position of the floating Light; that in case we should happen in our yawl to be caught with a fresh of wind from the Easterly points, so as not to be able to reach our store vessel from the rock, we might find a place of refuge in the floating Light.

123. ON Sunday the 15th, the wind was so fresh at S.E. as to put a stop to the work upon the rock; and in the course of the day the sea became so rough, that at five P.M. Mr. RICHARDSON, and the seamen on board, fearing some greater damage might happen to their moorings, slipped their *Bridle Cable* *, having put a sufficient buoy upon it, and brought the sloop into Cawsand Bay, where she lay till Monday at midnight; but the weather then mending, they got back to their moorings on Tuesday morning at four, and soon after made a landing; but could stay only half an hour.——This day I dispatched draughts to Mr. [illegible], according to which the Portland stone for the two first courses above the rock

* When a vessel is moored by laying down a cable upon the ground, with an anchor at each end, then another cable attached to the middle of [illegible] is called the *Bridle Cable*.

were

were to be rough *scappelled* [*]; it being agreed on my former interview with him at *Dorchester*, that in order to save time, draughts for the present would be sufficient.

In the afternoon of the day (Tuesday) that Mr. RICHARDSON and C° regained the moorings, they were able only to work a couple of hours upon the rock, before they were glad to get on board their vessel, and soon after they were obliged to quit their situation, and come again into Cawsand Bay; where adverse weather caused them to remain till Thursday evening; when it becoming more promising, that matters might be expedited as much as possible, I went on board the sloop, and sailed with the company to the Edystone; but found the weather there too violent to attempt any thing upon the rock, or even to lay hold of the moorings; we therefore judged it prudent again to return to Cawsand Bay with the sloop on Friday morning.

Saturday morning the 21st, HILL's company, who had been employed at Mill Bay during the past week in clearing away the mud, and deepening the channel, went in the Edystone boat to Cawsand Bay, and the companies at this time shifted there. In the afternoon HILL's company attempted to go out to sea; but the wind proving too fresh at South, they were obliged to put back. Sunday morning they again attempted it, got out to, and laid hold of the moorings, and landed; but after staying half an hour, were obliged to quit the rock; and in the afternoon, though the weather was fine, and apparently favourable at Plymouth, yet there was so much sea at the Edystone as to prevent their attempting to land. That no time might however be lost, on Monday noon Mr. JESSOP went out in the Edystone boat; but the wind being contrary, after attempting to beat out, he came to an anchor in Cawsand Bay in the evening; and in the night the sloop returned to the same place, having found the ground cable cut a *third* time.

124. THE next day I received an order from the Proprietors to make use of the *Neptune Buss* as a store vessel, for expediting the work of the house: I therefore determined to lose no time in getting her out to proper moorings; and having inspected her along with Mr. JESSOP, and found room sufficient in her for the men, without unloading any part of the timber that was in her for buoying her up in case of accident (as has been already mentioned § 107.) we determined to moor her without alteration, except *unshipping* the tackle belonging to the lantern; which, however, was preserved entire, so that it could have readily been replaced, in case any accident had made it necessary to apply this vessel to the purpose for which she was originally intended.

On Friday the 27th the wind came fair, and the weather moderate; so that HILL and C° went out in the sloop from Cawsand Bay, and got to the Edystone; but the buoys being driven away, they were not able to regain the moorings; they therefore came to an anchor, which enabled them to work every tide while they staid; though on account of the ground swell from the S.W. they made but short tides. During this time the moorings were recovered by *sweeping* for one of the anchors, and the sloop was once more established thereat.——It was not till Sunday the 29th that the Buss was cleared of unnecessary stores, and fitted for the service of the building; but the weather not suiting to carry her out, RICHARDSON and C°, who were to have gone in her, went out in the Edystone boat. The wind being then moderate, and there being apparently good weather for working upon the rock; finding they made but little way towards it, as the wind was right ahead, the whole company, eager to get upon the rock, took to the yawl which attended them, and making a great exertion, rowed out, and landed about noon, and received the tools from the hands of HILL and C°.

125. TUESDAY 31st. This morning the wind being favourable, the Buss was brought out of *Stonehouse Creek*; but all, that from circumstances we were able to do this tide, was to *warp* her out to one of the *Transport Buoys* belonging to His Majesty in *Hamoaze*. In the mean time, that no opportunity might be lost to the Out-company on the rock, sharp tools and other necessaries were dispatched in the yawl, along with Mr. JESSOP; who returned the same evening, reporting all well; RICHARDSON and C° being close at work.——Wednesday morning, 1st of September, I went on board the Buss with Messrs. JESSOP, HILL and C°, and four of the seamen. There was a fresh breeze, which not being quite

[*] A term for such work as could be done with the *Kevel* before described. See § 93.

in

in our favour, we proposed, by making a *tack*, to get the buss fairly out into the Sound; but in attempting to tack, we found our vessel would not *stay*, and after endeavouring at it twice more, we were glad to let go an anchor to prevent falling upon the rocks; and thus we lost this day, to our no small mortification: and this was the first of a train of incidents that gave me a less favourable idea of our new vessel than I had pre-conceived; and in the end satisfied me, that however completely the *Neptune Buss* was fitted for the service for which she was intended, yet she was not at all adapted to our *particular* service, insomuch that I had every reason from the sequel to say, that she proved not only the greatest clog and impediment we met with in the whole course of the work, but the real source of almost every disastrous event that happened to us: so that had the Proprietors disposed of her in any way, rather than destined her to our use, the charge of a new vessel constructed upon the plan proposed § 77, would have borne no proportion to the difficulties, disappointments and losses the service in reality suffered from her.

Thursday Sept. 2d. This morning the wind being at N.E. and of course favourable for carrying the Buss out of the Sound, at the proper time of tide we weighed, and sailed about nine in the morning; but before we got out to sea the wind became Easterly, and as we got without the Heads, it came to S.E. so that the wind was then nearly upon our beam, and consequently still fair; but as it was not very fresh, we made but little way; and our way was still less, on account of our vessel being so heavy a sailer: we continued however moving through the water; and as we had reason to suppose the work was going briskly forward upon the rock by RICHARDSON and C°, delays of every other kind seemed within the bounds of patience. About five o'clock in the afternoon, judging the Out-company would be in need of sharp tools, I went in the yawl with one of the seamen and two of HILL's men, got to the rock, landed, and had the pleasure to find RICHARDSON and C° at work, and proceeding properly. In the mean time the Buss came forward, and at eight in the evening, when she was about 2 ½ miles from the rock, the wind dying away, and the tide being against her, she came to an anchor; and soon after I returned to the Buss with the blunt tools, and dispatched them with HILL, and four of his men in the yawl to Plymouth, with orders to return as soon as they were sharpened.

Friday the 3d, there being a fresh breeze at N.E. we got under way this morning at five; but it soon becoming Easterly and gentle, it was nine o'clock before we got near the rock: we then dropped anchor, the rock being E.S.E. distant about half a mile. RICHARDSON's company leaving the rock soon after, I sent for some of them to assist in warping the Buss to a proper position for dropping one of the mooring anchors: and being at that time joined by the hands in the yawl, who were now returned from Plymouth, we proceeded to the business of mooring; which to *us* was a considerable operation: but to make it intelligible to the reader, it will be necessary to describe the nature of the *ground-tackle* our vessel was furnished with for this purpose.

126. WE had two mooring chains of 40 fathoms in length each; and the *bolt*-iron of their links being about 1 ¾ inches diameter; every fathom of this chain weighed 120 lb. so that each chain amounted to the weight of 2 tons 2 ¾ cwt. and consequently the two chains to 4 ton 5 ¾ cwt.; this, with the two mooring anchors of 12 cwt. each, made the weight of anchors and chains together 5 tons 9 ¾ cwt. and with the farther addition of a large swivel, with shackles and bolts, the weight of iron in this set of moorings might fairly be accounted six tons. The laying these down properly seemed so formidable a business, that I was told by my friends at Plymouth, the force of hands and purchases we had, would never be sufficient for the purpose; but that I should be under the necessity of getting it done by the *Master Attendant*, and proper people from the *King's Yard*, with their *Mooring Barges*, &c. and to this I was seriously advised. I had no reason to doubt of the good will and best assistance of the Commissioner, whenever it was in reality wanted; but always wishing to be master of my own operations, and foreseeing how much delay might arise from the carrying out the *King's* Mooring Barges so far to sea, where they could not *live* but in *fine* weather, I was desirous that the moorings might be put down from the *buss* herself; and being clear in the operation, and having the assistance of six able seamen, together with that of the two companies of stout hands, and the advice and experience of Mr. JESSOP, I proceeded to the business without apprehension of difficulty.

According

According to the manifest intention of these moorings, the two 40 fathom chains were to be joined together by one of the loops of the large swivel, the other end of each chain being attached to its respective mooring-anchor; one of the anchors therefore being laid to the westward (or down channel) from the swivel, and the other anchor as much to the eastward, or up channel from the same; the *bridle* cable proceeding from the bows of the vessel, being *bent*, or annexed to the upper loop of this swivel, the vessel would ride thereby fairly in the middle between her two anchors. It occurred to me, however, that according to this construction, either a considerable part of the two chains must be hoisted, and kept suspended above the ground by the bridle cable, and hang continually upon the bows of the vessel, or else, if the swivel, in the up and down motion of the vessel by the waves, was suffered to strike the ground, that there would be danger, not only of cutting the cable, but of breaking the swivel, by its violently pitching upon the rocks in storms and hard gales of wind. To prevent this, I considered, that the sea being liable to come much more heavy and violent from the western than from the eastern points of the compass, if 40 fathoms of chain were competent to the strain from the West, 40 fathoms would be more than sufficient to resist the strain from the East; and consequently five or six fathoms of it might be spared to act as a bridle; so that, instead of having the two chains joined by the swivel, the western chain should be joined to the eastern at five or six fathoms from its extremity, by a bolt and shackle, and the swivel be applied to the end itself. Thus the western chain of 40 fathoms lying upon the ground, and 34 or 35 fathoms of the eastern also, and the bridle cable being attached to the upper loop of the swivel, when the vessel was riding at her moorings, there would be five or six fathoms of chain, besides the swivel, between any part of the cable and the ground; whereby not only the swivel itself would be preserved, but the cable would be prevented from ever touching the rocks. Having prepared our ground tackle according to this plan, we proceeded to lay them down as follows.

127. OUR vessel was anchored too much to the westward. Soon after RICHARDSON's company came on board, it became tide of flood; and the water having risen half its height, agreeably to what was mentioned, § 3. it would then begin to run from West to East; and therefore, lest when we weighed anchor we should drive eastward with the tide, and overshoot our mark, we immediately let go another small anchor or *Catch*, and *paied* out the *Hawser* * by which we were riding; at the same time paying out the hawser of the catch-anchor; by which means the vessel drove eastward till the whole of the first hawser was run out: we then weighed our first anchor (by means of its buoy-rope with the yawl) and heaving in its hawser short, we again dropped the first anchor, and paied out the hawser of the other; and thus alternately, weighing and paying out, the Buss drove to her proper place, to the north of the rock; where, at the distance of about 300 fathoms, we found 20 fathoms water.——At this depth I thought it imprudent to drop our mooring-anchors, in such manner as with their chains to run *amain*; as this might break the anchor by its fall upon the rocks; or by cracking it we might afterwards be deceived: so I took the resolution (in order to prevent damage) to lower the anchors and chains leisurely and gradually.

The windlass of our Buss, though a very good one for general use, was totally unequal to such a purchase; and here indeed we should have been at a stand, or obliged to run some risk in case we had not been better provided than my friends at Plymouth were aware of. This furnished the first occasion of using the large *purchase tackle* of 20 sheaves, that I got prepared while in London, and which is mentioned § 106. Those blocks being *reeved* and brought together, we fixed the standing block to the stern timbers of our vessel, and discharged from one of the bows one of the mooring anchors, attached to its chain, which went over a strong iron roller very well fixed, and secured upon a *Davit* †, in place of the *Hawse* hole, intended for the bridle cable to bear upon, and facilitate the getting in of the cable, or weighing the moorings. The anchor thus discharged remained suspended by about two fathoms of the chain,

* A rope of a smaller size than the cable, and *laid* or twisted in a less degree, so as to become more soft and pliant.

† A piece of strong timber overlaying the bows of a vessel, containing sheaves, or a roller for purchasing the anchor; its tail being securely fixed upon the Deck.

which, after having passed the roller, was stopped from running further out by strong *Salvagees* *; then bringing the chain along the deck to the moveable purchase block, and hooking it to one of the Links, we lowered the anchor perfectly at our ease, again stopping the chain with the salvagees, when the moveable block was come near the *Davit*; and then extending the chain upon the deck as before, the block was again hooked; and in this way we proceeded *flitting* the tackle and lowering till our anchor was grounded. As we foresaw that the tide running eastward would be far spent before the first anchor was got to the ground, we previously determined to put down the eastern anchor first: and it was grounded somewhat before the turn of the tide to the West.

In this position we staid till *Still* water, and then having got the hawser of the small anchor through the stern opening, and forward to the windlass, we were thereby enabled to heave the vessel astern westward; in which we were soon assisted by the tide: and thus, the chain being paied out, under the command of the great blocks, and the vessel being heaved westward by the hawser, the whole of the chain was laid upon the ground in a straight line East and West: and it is obvious, that after the whole of the eastern chain was let go, as far as its junction with the western chain, and that junction was completed, then the five or six fathoms of the eastern chain reserved for a bridle, as well as the bridle cable affixed thereto, must be *paied* out, or let go with the other.

We proceeded as above till the whole of the western chain was gone out, except as much as was necessary to reach to the ring of its intended anchor; which being upon the bow of the vessel, and necessarily at some distance from the davit-roll, here occurred a difficulty in getting the whole grounded in the same leisure manner, without the risk of letting the anchor and 20 fathoms of the chain go over board all together.——For this purpose, we got the anchor as near the bowsprit of the vessel as possible; and passed a small rope several times round the arms of the anchor, and round the bowsprit of the vessel, as close as possible to the stem upon which it rested, and made it very secure: we then let go the anchor from the bow, which of course became suspended by the bowsprit, with the *Peck* upwards, and just above the water's surface. We now lowered the western chain till it became suspended by the anchor; which, with the chain down to the ground, now hung at the bowsprit. In this situation a strong hawser, of a sufficient length to reach to the bottom double, being *passed* under one of the arms of the anchor, and the two parts being brought together over the davit-roll, and to the main blocks, the whole suspension was in that manner *purchased*; and the small rope being loosened, the anchor and chain were then let down by the double hawser: and still heaving the vessel westward, this western anchor was quietly laid upon the ground; and both ends of the double cable being on board, we were enabled, by letting one part go, to free it of the anchor.—We were so fortunate as to have an exceeding fine and calm day for this operation; by which means the whole was performed without the least accident.

128. ON Saturday the 4th of September I landed at six A. M. and found the work to be in the following state. The two new steps at the bottom, and all the dovetails were roughed out, and some of the beds brought to a level and finished; and I judged that full one half of the work I intended to be done on the rock this season was completed.

While I was upon the rock, Mr. JESSOP, the seamen, and HILL's company were employed on board the buss, heaving in the stray cable, weighing the anchors, and getting the buss to rights at her moorings. The tide's work being done at ten, I returned to the buss with RICHARDSON and Company, and in the yawl to Plymouth; which passage, being in a calm, was rowed in four hours.——On Monday evening the 6th the sloop was brought home, and the seamen reported, that on weighing her anchors, they found the ground cable almost cut in rags from end to end.

* Salvagees or Selvagees are ropes made with the yarns laid parallel and untwisted; being slightly bound together by passing a single yarn [illegible], which renders them not only the most pliable of all others, but the strongest possible to be made with that number of yarns. [illegible], they are in the form of loops, or endless ropes; being made by passing a yarn round two fixed pins, as many turns [illegible] necessary for the strength intended; the distance of the pins regulating the length of the loops according to their use.

CHAP.

CHAP. II.

Sequel of the OPERATIONS *upon the* ROCK *of the First Season of* 1756.

129. OUR Buss being now satisfactorily moored, and a regular intercourse established between her and the shore, there was nothing to hinder the companies from changing regularly every Saturday, except bad weather; nor from working upon the rock, whenever the least interval of good weather concurred with a proper time of the tide to render it practicable: it will therefore now be only necessary to recount such circumstances as happened out of the usual course of proceedings; or such as may deserve particular notice.

On Tuesday the 7th I dispatched to *Portland* the draughts for the six *foundation* courses, that were to be employed in bringing the rock to a level; which, with the draughts for eight that I had before dispatched, compleated the order for the whole quantity of *Portland Stone* to be used in the *solid* up to the entry door; being all that we could expect to set in place, the next season. The rock was not indeed yet ready for compleating the exact moulds for those stones that were to fit into the dovetails made in it: but by ordering the stones *large enough*, and being scappelled something near their proper form, it would prevent loss of time in waiting to get the true figure from the rock, as well as unnecessary waste.

130. NOTHING happened to prevent the companies from working every tide from the 27th of August till the 14th of September, in which time they had worked 177 hours upon the rock.——In this interval, having procured a carpenter to be applied to that purpose, I began to make the moulds for the exact cutting of the stones to their intended shapes. This was done by laying down in chalk lines upon the floor of a chamber the proposed size and figure of each stone, being a portion of the plan at large of the intended course; and the carpenter having prepared a quantity of *Battens*, or slips of deal board, about three inches broad, and one inch thick, *shot* straight upon the edges by a plane; those battens being cut to lengths, and their edges adapted to the lines upon the floor, and properly fitted together, became the exact representatives of the pieces of stone whose figure was to be marked from them, when their beds were wrought to the intended parallel distance.

It is obvious that there was no necessity for making moulds for a *whole* course after the work became regular; as was the 7th course, after the six foundation courses brought the rock to a level; it was sufficient to make one mould to each circle of stones, beginning with the center stone; but as the six foundation courses were adapted to the particular irregularities of the rock, and consequently could not be strictly regular, it was necessary that a separate mould should be made for every separate stone, composing that part of the work.

131. DURING this interval I visited the rock, and on arriving there the 8th of September, was informed by Mr. Jessop that the preceding evening, there being a very strong tide, and no wind, a *West Indiaman* homeward bound, and a man of war's *tender* were in great danger of driving upon the N.E. rock; but that he timely perceiving their danger, though they themselves were not aware of it, ordered out the seamen and hands, who towed them off.

On

On this visit I staid two days; for as the working company had begun to take down the upper part of the rock, it was necessary to concert, and put in practice the proper means of doing that, without damage to what was destined to remain. I have already mentioned my resolution of not using *gunpowder*; yet it was necessary, for the sake of dispatch, to employ some means more expeditious, than the slow way of crumbling off the matter, by the blunt points of picks.——It has been already noticed, that the *Laminæ* composing the rock were parallel to the inclined surface: and it was very probable that the chasm, into which Mr. WINSTANLEY's chain had been so fast jambed that it never could be disengaged, extended further into the rock than the visible disunion of the parts: this made me resolve to try a method sometimes used in this country, for the division of hard stones, called the *Key and Feather*; in order to *cross cut* this upper *stratum* of the rock. The construction and operation of the key and feather is as follows. A right line is marked upon the surface of the rock or stone to be cut, in the direction in which it is intended to be divided. Holes are then drilled by a *Jumper* at the distance of six or eight inches, and about 1½ inch in diameter, to the depth of about eight or nine inches; the distances however of the holes and their diameters, as well as their depth, are to be greater or less, according to the strength of the stone, in the estimation of the artist directing the work. The above dimensions were what we used on this occasion. The *Key* is a long tapering wedge of somewhat less breadth than the diameter of the holes, and so as to go easily into them; the length being three or four inches more than the depth of the holes. The Feathers are pieces of iron, also of a wedge-like shape; the side to be applied to the key being flat, but the other side a segment of a circle, answerable to that of the holes; so that the two flat sides of two feathers being applied to the two flat sides of the key; and the thick end of the feathers to the thin end of the key, they all together compose a cylindric, or rather oval kind of body; which in this position of parts is too big to go into the holes by at least one eighth of an inch; that is, in the direction of a diameter passing through the three parts; but in the other direction is no broader than to go with ease into the holes. A key and a pair of feathers is made use of in each hole; and the feathers being first dropped in, with the thick ends downwards, the keys are then entered between them; the flat sides of all the keys and the feathers being set parallel to that line in which the holes are disposed: the keys are then driven by a sledge hammer, proceeding from one to another, and being forced gradually, as in splitting of moor-stone, the strongest stones are unable to resist their joint effort; and the stone is split according to the direction of the original line, as effectually, and much more regularly and certainly, than could be done with gunpowder, and without any concussion of the parts. Had our rock been entirely solid, this way of working might not have been applicable, on account of the crack's going too deep; but here, when it arrived at the joint where the chain was lodged, the split part became entirely disengaged from the rest; and in this way we were enabled to bring off the quantity of several cubic feet at a time: and thus the chain was released after a confinement of above *fifty* years. The impossibility of disengaging it before now appeared very evident; for the pressure had been so great by the rock's closing upon it, as before suggested, that the links in their intersections were pressed into each other, as compleatly as if they had been made of lead; though the *Bolt* iron composing the chain had been at least five eighths of an inch in diameter.

132. ON Tuesday evening the 14th of September there came on a hard gale of wind at the S. W. and on Wednesday the 15th, though the weather was moderate, yet the ground-swell, raised by the S. W. wind the night before, prevented any landing upon the rock. This being the first fresh of wind since the *Buss* was moored, those on board were not a little attentive to her.——On Thursday the 16th I again went off to the rock, and landed, finding RICHARDSON and Company at work, though it was the first tide they had landed, since the 14th: they acquainted me that the Buss had rode perfectly easy in the gale of wind they had had, and that there was no occasion to veer out any more cable than she usually rode with; which at first had been hawled in so tight as to keep the swivel from the striking ground, when right up and down. I found the work now in the following situation.——The lowest new step (the most difficult to work upon, because the lowest, with its dovetail, quite compleated.——The second step rough bedded, and all its dovetails *scappelled* out.——The 3d step (being the lowest in Mr. RUDYERD's work) smooth bedded, and all the dovetails roughed out. The 4th in the like state.——The 5th rough bedded, and dovetails scappelled out.

out:—And the fixth fmooth bedded, and all the dovetails roughed out.—Laftly, the top of the rock, the greateft part of the bulk whereof had been previoufly taken down by the *Key* and *Feather* method as low as it could be done with propriety, was now to be reduced to a level with the upper furface of the fixth ftep; the top of that ftep being neceffarily to form a part of the bed for the feventh or firft regular courfe; fo that what now remained was to bring the top of the rock to a regular floor by picks: and from what now appeared (as all the upper parts, that had been damaged by the fire, were cut off) the new building was likely to reft upon a bafis even more folid than the former ones had done.

133. FROM the time of the hard gale upon the 14th, we found ourfelves got into a feries of unfettled weather; yet the feafon did not feem fo far fpent, but that we might reafonably expect a return of the land and fea breezes, which conftantly attended our works whenever they went on uninterruptedly upon the rock; we therefore kept ourfelves in conftant readinefs to feize the lucky minutes, that the works of this year, now brought very far forward, might be *perfectly* compleated.——I attempted to go off feveral times, but was as often forced to return, until Thurfday the 30th, when I landed on the rock with RICHARDSON and his company; but as only about 20 hours work had been done upon the rock fince I was there before upon the 16th, I could not expect to find much change in the appearance. However I traced the outlines upon the upper part of the rock for the border of the feventh courfe, all within which was to be funk to the level of the top of the fixth, and all without to be left ftanding as a border for defence of the ground joint of the work with the rock; and meafuring the height of the top ftep above the bed of the firft, I found it to be eight feet four inches; which would now be the difference of level, between the weft or loweft fide of the new building and the eaft or higheft.——On the company's returning on board the Bufs after this tide's work, the yawl's grapling got fo faft among the rocks, that it could not be weighed; but in the attempt, it *parted* the grappling rope: we therefore now laid down the Bufs's catch or *Kedge* anchor a little to the North of the Gut, that is, about 40 fathoms without the mouth of it*; and having *bent* to it a part of a fufficient *Hawfer* with a large buoy at the top, that when any veffel went in, fhe might make faft to this buoy, inftead of dropping her own anchor, or grappling; this for the prefent completely anfwered the purpofe of the *Tranfport Buoy*, mentioned § 86. as intended to be placed there.

134. ON Saturday, 2d October, there being a hard gale at S. W. RICHARDSON and company having no fharp tools, or weather to work in, came home in the great yawl, leaving the Bufs to the care of the three feamen. In their way home they met Mr. JESSOP with HILL and Company in Cawfand Bay; who had fet out that morning to relieve them; and where, after this attempt, they remained wind-bound for two days, and then were forced to return to Plymouth; fo that now both companies were at home together, and employed upon the works in Mill Bay.

THE unfavourablenefs of the weather retarded our operations upon the rock for fome time, infomuch that, upon the 8th of October, the three feamen who had been left in the Bufs (having firft fecured every thing on board in the beft manner they could) returned to Plymouth in the *little* yawl; having put up an oar for a maft, and a blanket for a fail. This they were under a neceffity of doing; for as no boat had been able to get out to relieve them, fince the departure of RICHARDSON's company, they had nearly exhaufted all their provifions. In their paffage home they met the Edyftone boat going out with HILL and Company, who got on board the Bufs that evening.

135. THE equinoctial winds that now were reigning afforded me but little profpect of doing much more work upon the rock this feafon; for though a more moderate interval of weather might be expected, after thofe winds were fpent, before the winter came on; yet as this might probably be exhaufted in finifhing the rock compleat for receiving the ftone the beginning of next feafon, we might find it a difficult matter to get the Bufs's moorings weighed, after that was done; as it would require the fame good weather to take them up, as to lay them down; I therefore began to confider whether this

* Near where the founding 15 (fathom) is marked on the general plan of the rocks; Plate, N° 3.

 operation

operation might not be dispensed with; conceiving that if a chain was affixed to the swivel, of a sufficient size to support so much of the main chains, as must be raised from the ground, by bringing the swivel to the surface of the water; then a large buoy (which would next year serve for the intended *Transport Buoy*) being fastened to the top of this subsidiary chain; the main chains, on taking away the bridle cable, might be lowered to the bottom by this buoy chain; and the buoy thus riding all winter by its own proper chain, would afford us an easy means, not only of unmooring the Buss this autumn, but of mooring her again the next spring.

After advising with Mr. Jessop on the practicability of this method, and probability of its success, I immediately bespoke the buoy chain; which, as it must be made at Plymouth, would take some time; to save which, by reducing its length, Mr. Jessop proposed that we should be content with eleven fathoms of buoy chain to be attached to the swivel, and the rest of the necessary length for riding the buoy, to be of cable; which never coming to touch the ground, he conceived, that the buoy might ride out the winter just as well as if it was attached to a chain only. He farther proposed to fix an under-buoy at the top of the buoy chain, which would in part support it, and being eight or nine fathoms under the surface of the sea, would be in a region of much greater quietude than the surface, in time of storms; on account of which the upper or *floating* buoy might be the less, and therefore be less subject to any misfortune: and also if by any mischance the floating buoy should break loose, or be carried away, still the under buoy would support its chain, so as to ride some fathoms from the ground, and in that case it might easily be recovered by *Sweeping**.

136. ON the 13th of October, the wind blowing very hard, the great yawl in riding at the stern of the Buss broke loose, having parted a double hawser, and driving away at the rate of four miles an hour, it was impracticable to follow her in the little yawl, which was then on board; and notwithstanding the speediest, and most diligent enquiries after her, we never could hear of her again. This was a real loss, as it had proved a boat particularly adapted to our use.

The weather continued so variable and uncertain during the whole month of October, that the out-companies had worked only 23½ hours.——It was Wednesday the 27th before I saw any chance of going off to examine the state of the work; and this day, the weather being moderate, I went off, and got out to the Buss, but could not land. Richardson acquainted me that his company had worked only 2½ hours this turn; for though they had tolerably fine weather over head, yet the sea had become so long in settling at this advanced season, that they were obliged to return to the Buss, after two strenuous but unsuccessful attempts to land. He further reported, that there was now very little wanting to finish the work of the season, but the levelling of the top of the rock. He also acquainted me, that the seamen, by the help of the company on board, had heaved up the bridle chain, till they could see the *Clinch* of the cable to the swivel; and found it somewhat damaged, as they judged by having touched the rocks; but the weather coming on rough before they could do any thing at it, they were obliged to lower it as it was; two days after however they again heaved it up, and repaired the clinch. The Buss in all the past bad weather had indeed rode it out to admiration, having never shipped any water, or needed the bridle to be veered out.

137. I NOW considered, that nothing remained to be done of this season's work, that could possibly hinder the beginning to set the foundation courses, at the commencement of the next season; as the top of the rock could be brought to a regular floor, and the dovetails in the upper steps corrected, in the intervals that would necessarily happen, while the lower courses were setting. It therefore seemed unprofitable to continue the companies longer in a state of hardship, merely for the sake of having it to say, that the *Year's Work* as *intended* was *entirely completed*; in consequence I was much inclined not to send out any more hands this season; and ordered Mr. Richardson to return with his company at the conclusion of their week, though the other company should not go out to relieve them; which he did on Saturday the 30th, and brought word that they had worked four hours the day after I had left

* The operation of [illegible] will be fully explained hereafter.

them;

them; and I could not but notice, that on this day it was remarked at *Plymouth*, how very unpromising the weather was for our business; such difference is there, in our climate, in a small space between the land and the sea; and such especially between *Plymouth* and the *Edystone*; and this shewed still more strongly the great advantage of doing our work by a *Store Vessel*, in preference of separate voyages.——Mr. RICHARDSON also reported that both the buoys had broke loose from the mooring anchors, but that every thing else was well.

138. HAVING received advice from Mr. TUCKER that three vessels were ready to load with stone as soon as the weather would permit them to go to the pier, we now pushed forward the completion of the work-yard, with its machinery, and conveniences, (See Plate N° 17.) as also the channel up to the Jetty Head, so as to be ready to receive the *Portland* vessels: and that we might have an assurance of the strength, and sufficiency of our shears, and tackle for heaving the stones they should send us, I made the following trials.——First, I tried them by a strain from the *Capstand* equal to what would be required in heaving the largest stones intended for the Lighthouse: then by a strain double the former; after that by one treble; during all which every thing stood firm; but on applying a quadruple force, a great hook upon which the large purchase blocks were hung, gave way, by becoming straight, as if it had been a piece of lead; but no other damage was done: so that I was now well assured of the firmness of all the material parts, as relative to the force to be employed, when in proper use: for from the above trials every thing stood fast with eight ton weight upon the tackle-blocks: and now the work-yard was ready for receiving the stone.

139. THE month of November setting in with a better appearance of weather, HILL's company desired to take another turn, which was granted.——On Sunday the 7th, I went off in the Edystone boat with Mr. JESSOP, and carried out battens, and the carpenter, to mould off the dovetails from the rock: but there being but little wind, it was evening before we arrived at the Buss. HILL informed me that they had worked Thursday night and Saturday afternoon tides, that they had had violent weather on Friday, but rode it out without fear or danger; not having veered out any more cable, or shipped any water; agreeing with what had been reported by RICHARDSON. At twelve o'clock at night I landed with Mr. JESSOP, HILL and Company, and the mould-maker, with the battens; the Company staid 2½ hours, but the night not proving favourable to make much progress with the moulds, I fully explained my meaning to Mr. JESSOP; and left full directions with him about that business, which I doubted not, but his known care and exactness would complete to my satisfaction, if the weather gave leave after my return. On landing upon the rock this tide, I found the work as follows: viz. four or five of the dovetails in the upper steps wanting some small amendment, that would employ as many men at each for about four or five hours. The greatest part of the top of the rock was now brought to a regular floor, but some part of the N. E. side wanted bringing down to a level.

140. ON the 12th of November the buoy-chain for our Buss's moorings was completed; and upon a trial thereof by means of our purchase tackle at Mill Bay, in manner as before, I found it to bear a strain of six tons without any appearance of giving way, which I deemed fully sufficient.——Supposing that HILL's Company, who were now going on in a second week, might want provisions, as also Mr. JESSOP who was with them; the next morning (Saturday the 13th) I ordered out the Edystone boat, but meeting with bad weather, after *beating* all day and night, it was obliged to return upon the 14th.——On the 15th I ordered the Edystone boat to make another attempt early in the morning, and to get out, if possible; she failed, but the wind coming South, and continuing to blow hard, she could not get out to sea; and at three o'clock this afternoon we were surprized by the arrival of the *Buss*, which came to an anchor at the mouth of Mill Bay. Mr. JESSOP informed me, that having scarcely one day's provision on board, and the weather then being, and seeming likely to continue so bad, that no boat could come off to them, and the wind standing fair for bringing them in (not having any boat, in which they could venture home) they all agreed to slip their cable and carry the Buss into harbour, lest the wind should come foul upon them,

them, after their provisions were all spent.——Accordingly, after having fixed buoys upon the cable, and secured them as well as they could, they set sail for Plymouth this forenoon: but though the wind blew a hard gale, and they came in right before it, they could not sail at a greater rate than *three* miles an hour. When they came abreast of the Ramhead, they met the Edystone boat endeavouring to beat to windward, which was able to make but little way; and the purpose of the voyage being now over, they returned in company with the Buss.——Mr. JESSOP further reported that the weather had never permitted them to go upon the rock since the night of Sunday the seventh, when I was there; which, notwithstanding all the bad weather, was the only entire week since the commencement of the work, that one company or the other did not land; and it appeared by the account, that since the 2d of October, being 40 days, the whole of the landings amounted but to 38½ hours. Considering therefore the rock-work to be now as good as finished, I was thankful that we had in reality got through what might be justly esteemed the most laborious and difficult part of our work.——Every thing was said of the case and buoyancy of the Buss's riding at her moorings in all weathers, though nothing could be said in favour of her as a *Sailer*.

141. THE Buss being thus prematurely arrived, there was a necessity of carrying her out again for the purpose of fixing the buoy-chain of the moorings: we therefore determined to warp her up to our Jetty Head in Mill Bay, that her bottom might be cleaned, previous to another voyage; and indeed on laying her upon the ground, she appeared very much to need it; for though she had been out of harbour but eleven weeks, the foulness her bottom had contracted was amazing; for it was found to be grown over with a kind of sea-weed, resembling *Hog's Bristles*; which in some places were near six inches long. From hence I could not help concluding, that though vessels while under sail in performing their voyages, do in time get much foulness, yet in fact, their motion through the water rubs off many of the tender filaments of the weeds, which prevents their growing so rapidly as when a vessel lies in the water, with a much less degree of relative motion; as is the case with those at moorings, though in a *Tide's-way*.

142. ON Sunday morning the 21st of November, the Buss being cleaned, and prepared for the sea, and the wind fair for going out, I sailed in her at four in the morning with Mr. JESSOP, HILL and Company, and four of the seamen; the other two with a part of RICHARDSON's Company being in the Edystone boat. As the wind was moderate at E. though our Buss was now cleaned, and the Edystone boat had us in tow, yet it was twelve o'clock before we arrived at the moorings: we had however a hindrance in our passage of about half an hour, by an accident to one of the seamen, who in endeavouring to climb up the mast of the light yawl to rectify something, as he had been used to do in the large one, the boat oversetting he fell into the sea: as the weather however was moderate, nothing further than a wetting was the consequence.

In getting in the bridle cable by means of its buoys; it being a ten-inch cable, having been very hard *laid* at first, and having become harder by lying in the water, it was found to be so excessively stiff and troublesome to manage, that it was the work of all the hands for the whole afternoon. In one place we found it damaged by fretting against the rocks, but being much longer than experience shewed to be necessary for us, we cut it at the damaged place.——After refreshing ourselves, we began in the evening to heave up the ground chains by the bridle, which employed all the hands for several hours; for though the operation of our large purchase-blocks was very sure, yet having so many times to stop, overhawl, and *flit*, (as described in laying down the moorings) to get in above 20 fathoms of bridle, the work could not go on very speedily; and indeed without the purchase-tackle, we could not have done it all: however, at three o'clock in the morning of the 22d, the swivel was got above water.——At this time the wind blew a smart breeze at E. which gave us so much motion, that we found it exceedingly difficult, especially as it was very dark, to get the forelock of the bolt and shackle clinched, by which the buoy chain was attached to the great swivel: this was however effected; and as much depended upon it, I did it myself: but as from its stiffness, we found it equally difficult to get the bridle cable unbent from the swivel, and the men being much fatigued by the previous operations, it was thought best to let all stand as it was till day-light.

At

At daylight the 22d, the wind blew very fresh at S. E. so that it was with great hazard, that the Edystone boat lay alongside the Buss to deliver the great buoy on board: this was however done without mischief; but it then came on so very fresh, that it became expedient for the Edystone boat to return home for her preservation; first receiving orders to come out again as soon as the weather would permit, in case we did not follow her. The wind being now equally favourable for carrying in the Buss, and still increasing, to save time it was agreed to cut the clinch of the bridle cable, and lower down the ground chains by the buoy chain, in the same gradual manner in which they were heaved up; and by twelve o'clock we had lowered it twelve fathoms: while this was doing, one of our yawls broke loose, and before we were aware that it was gone, had driven away too far for us to attempt to recover it.——On driving a bolt through one of the links of the buoy-chain (intended as a stop to the *under-water* buoy as before mentioned) we discovered a flaw in that link, which, though it did not appear of great consequence, yet deserved consideration, and, if possible, amendment: but as no *extempore* remedy, that could there be applied, offered itself, and we found the wind had not increased since morning, and that the Buss rode very well, as she was then circumstanced; our solicitude that nothing should be left in an exceptionable state, prevailed upon us to abide where we were, till the Edystone boat should return, when we might send her back for something proper to secure that link.——This over-precaution, as the wind was fair, and quite enough for us, cost us dear; for at three o'clock the wind and sea had so much increased, that it became unsafe to ride any longer by the buoy-chain; we therefore had no other alternative, but to launch the large floating buoy, and cast ourselves loose.

143. WE found the Buss go much better since her cleaning; yet the wind having by this time veered to the North of the East, which was but one point before our beam, and therefore in the common estimation of sailing *fair* for us; we found in stretching some length on our course, that we could not fetch *Plymouth Sound*; and an attempt to make a tack with *our* vessel, as we before had *proved*, would have been to no purpose. We therefore unanimously agreed to steer away before the wind for *Fowey*; and as it then blew a hard gale and was quite in our favour, we expected to reach our port before it was *dark*; which however we esteemed of the less consequence, as almost every one on board had been there before; and though we must expect the night to be dark, this being the day of the new moon, yet the headlands being bold, we concluded ourselves under no difficulty; insomuch, that for my own part having been up most of the former night, and a good deal fatigued in lending a hand to the forenoon's operations of this day, I went down to my cabin, and as it had been rainy, as well as stormy, I disencumbered myself of my wet clothes, intending to repose till I heard we were come to an anchor in *Fowey Harbour*.

The persons on board were, four seamen, HILL's company, Mr. JESSOP and myself; in all 18 hands. ——For a space of about three hours, I had the satisfaction to hear every thing going on well over head; and it was no small addition thereto, when I heard those on deck were altering their course, in order to run into the harbour: but suddenly an universal *alarm* and *clamour* arose, insomuch that I ran upon deck in my shirt, it then raining hard, and blowing quite a storm. It being very dark, the first thing I saw was the horrible appearance of *Breakers*, almost surrounding us; JOHN BOWDEN, one of the seamen, crying out, For God's sake heave hard at that rope, if you mean to *save your lives*. I immediately laid hold of the rope, at which he himself was hawling, as well as the other seamen, though he was also managing the helm; I not only hawled with all my strength, but calling to, and encouraging the workmen to do the same thing, in as little time as I have been describing our situation, the vessel's head was brought round, so that we no longer faced the breakers, which, from the darkness of the night, were almost the only objects we could see; the vessel was then heaved down by the stress of the wind, her gunnel to the water; but as we soon found she answered her helm, we concluded she was making way. It would require a pen of a different sort from mine, to describe the jeopardy of our present situation, while we were uncertain whether or not we should escape the rocks, on which the seas were breaking with a tremendous noise; we had been but a little time in this situation before our *Jib* was split to pieces, and to prevent our mainsail* from suffering the same fate, we were obliged to lower its yard so much down the

* It has already been noticed that the Buss was *Ketch* rigged, that is, with a large square mainsail.

maſt, that the ſail did not preſent above half its ſurface to the wind; yet in this poſition the gunnel of the veſſel was frequently dipped under water. Finding however our veſſel to obey her helm, her head being South by the compaſs, the wind about E. N. E. we began to collect ourſelves ſo far as to conſider what was beſt to be done; ſome ſaying we had overſhot our port; whilſt others alledged that we were ſhort of it: in this uncertainty it appeared to me, that our beſt chance was to ſtand out to ſea, upon the point we then were; which though two points behind the beam (or *large*) we found was as near to the wind as, under the circumſtances we were in, we could make way to advantage. We knew our veſſel would float like a cork upon the water, till ſhe was daſhed to pieces upon the rocks. We could now ſee nothing of land on our lee ſide, yet the extreme darkneſs of the night, rendered ſtill greater by the rain, and the confuſion of the elements produced by the violence of the wind, made it uncertain whether we ſhould be able to ſee the boldeſt ſhore, if of a dark colour, at the diſtance of 50 fathoms. Our danger therefore ſeemed to be that of falling upon the rocks that ſtretch away from *Trewardreth* Bay towards the *Deadman**. In this perilous uncertainty we continued nearly two hours, when having kept upon our point (S.) and meeting nothing, we concluded that we muſt have weathered *Deadman's Point* †; however we had ſtill a violent ſtormy night to contend with, and having ſplit our foreſail alſo, we were now under our mainſail only, and though it was lowered as above deſcribed, yet even ſtill we frequently dipped our gunnel in the water; ſeveral times the ſea broke over us; yet our deck being fluſh *fore* and *aft*, and our veſſel very buoyant, as before deſcribed, we ſhipped no water.

144. AT daylight on Thurſday the 23d we were out of ſight of land, and having had the laſt of our yawls in tow all the night, in which time ſhe had gradually filled by the ſpray of the ſea (the ſtorm being not at all abated) we found ſhe greatly retarded our way, without any poſſibility of clearing her of water; we agreed therefore to cut her adrift; which indeed nothing but the apparent neceſſity of the thing could have induced us to do, as the yawl might be the means of ſaving our lives, though the Buſs had been loſt: but the neceſſity of this meaſure will appear, when it is conſidered, that in our preſent condition we might poſſibly do better than yield to the violence of the wind, which we found was driving us at a great rate towards the Bay of *Biſcay*. On being freed from the incumbrance of the yawl, we determined to *wear* the veſſel, and make the beſt point we could by ſtanding in for the land; and the veſſel's head was now pointed to N. W.——About noon we got ſight of the coaſt on our weather ſide, which on a nearer approach we judged to be the *Lizard*; and could alſo diſcern land almoſt right ahead. By this time the ſtorm began to abate; we therefore purſued our courſe, and before night perceived that the land we had before ſeen right ahead was the *Land's End*, and that we had been driving ſo much to the leeward of our courſe, that the weſternmoſt point of land we could ſee was now upon our weather bow; we could therefore form no expectation, as the wind then ſtood, of fetching any port of *Great Britain*.——Towards evening it became more moderate, and as we had on board a ſpare fore ſail, a mizen, and a ſtorm jib, we determined to ſet thoſe ſails, put the veſſel about, and make one great effort to beat to windward, and flattered ourſelves that with ſome aſſiſtance from the tide *of Flood*, we might be able to get into *Mount's Bay*.

We ſtood off the land at night, lying as cloſe to the wind as we could make any way, our ſhip's head being about S. E. by E. wind at N. E. At two o'clock on Wedneſday morning we again wore the veſſel, and ſtood on for the land at N. W. by N. which we ſaw ſoon after it was daylight; we ſtood on this courſe till noon, when we found that our veſſel had not altered her ſailing properties; for that, ſo far from having gained any thing to Eaſtward, ſince the preceding day at the ſame hour, we had now got as much to the Weſtward of the *Land's End*, as we were yeſterday of the *Lizard*: the Land's End bearing from us N. E. by N. diſtance by eſtimation eight leagues.——We were now fully convinced, that in this veſſel, as the wind ſtood, we could not make any thing Eaſtward by ſailing: we therefore *lay to* and

* [illegible] Eaſt of the *Lizard*. See the general chart, N° 1.

† [illegible] we had not overſhot our intended port, but had fallen ſhort of it, having got into *Lantippet Bay*, to the [illegible] we really overſhot our port, and got into *Trewardreth* Bay, as then apprehended, we could ſcarcely have eſcaped being wreck'd on the rocky ſhore between that and the *Deadman*.

founded,

ſounded; and finding 40 fathoms water, bottom fine ſand mixed with fragments of ſea-ſhells, we let go an anchor, in order that we might conſider what to do.——The wind though now moderate but freſh, ſeemed invariably fixed to the N. E. we had therefore to conſider, whether we ſhould attempt to croſs the Bay of *Biſcay*, and get into ſome port of *France*, or *Spain*; lie where we were, as long as we could, in expectation of a ſhift of wind in our favour; or endeavour to get into ſome port in the iſlands of *Scilly*.——On muſtering our hands, and our ſtores, we found we had not amongſt us all above a week's proviſions, at ſhort allowance; and this ſeemed inadequate to the attempting to croſs the Bay: for, if the wind ſhould change, when we were almoſt over, we ſhould be obliged, in obedience thereto, to return back again. In ſtaying where we were, we might expend the whole of our proviſions, and at laſt be left to make ſuch ſhift as we could: we therefore were unanimouſly of opinion, that the laſt propoſition, though attended with the moſt immediate *apparent* danger, from the rocks ſaid every where to ſurround thoſe iſlands, yet, as it would put the matter to the ſhorteſt iſſue, was the beſt to be adopted. We therefore reſolved to ſhape our courſe for *Scilly*; but, having neither maps, charts, books, nor inſtruments on board, we could none of us tell (having never been there) what point to ſteer upon from where we were, ſo as with certainty to get within ſight of the iſlands, eſpecially ſhould it come on *foggy* or *hazy* weather.

145. WHILE under this dilemma, we ſaw a ſail to the Eaſt, ſteering directly to us; we therefore made a ſignal of diſtreſs, concluding, that if an enemy, the ſervice we were upon would protect us; yet the ſtate of anxiety we were then in was ſuch, that we would have compounded for being carried to *France* rather than lie there with our preſent proſpects.——The veſſel bore down upon us, and proved to be the *White Hart* of *Pool*, bound for *Guinea*: we told them our ſituation, and ſervice; but we having loſt all our boats, and her's being ſtowed under deck, we could neither of us go on board the other; we learnt from her, however, what ſeemed very material to us to know, that our courſe for Scilly was W.N.W*. We therefore determined to lie there till four o'clock the next morning; that by getting early under way, we might have it daylight by the time we could reach within ſight of the iſlands; and that by having the day before us, we might have the better chance of making ſignals, and obtaining a pilot. ——This evening the wind became more gentle, and at midnight it was a calm.

146. ON Thurſday morning the 25th of November at two o'clock, the hands began to heave in our cable; for, anchoring in 40 fathoms, this was likely to take up ſome time: while it was doing, between three and four o'clock, a gentle breeze ſprung up at N. N. W. The joy and ſatisfaction wherewith this inſpired the whole company, tended greatly to expedite the getting up of our anchor; and by the time it was got to the *Bows*, the breeze was ſo much freſhened at the ſame point, that we did not heſitate in abandoning our propoſed viſit to *Scilly*; and in lieu thereof directed the head of our veſſel towards the *Lizard*.——The place where we anchored is referred to in the general map by the mark ⚓ 40, South-Weſt of the Land's End. As the day came on, the wind ſtill freſhened at the ſame point; and we not only ſet our uſual ſails, but a topſail; and brought out every yard of canvas we could muſter, as well as ſome of our blankets, which we contrived to ſet to ſome advantage as *ſtudding* ſails. Early in the day we paſſed the *Lizard*, and made our courſe good, ſo that at nine in the evening we were abreaſt of the *Deadman*. Soon after midnight we began to get ſight of the *Floating Light*; at four on Friday morning the 26th, we once more eſpied our old acquaintance the *Ram Head*; and at ſix came to an anchor in *Plymouth Sound*; not without thankful hearts for this deliverance, and to the inexpreſſible joy and ſatisfaction of all our friends, who had concluded we had either been caſt away or carried to *France*. And indeed ſuch concluſions were not unreaſonable; for the Edyſtone boat having been ſent out on Wedneſday (which was the firſt day ſhe could look out to ſea) and not finding us, returned with the melancholy tidings; and going out again on Thurſday to make enquiry at the floating light, where they met with a very unſatisfactory account of us, our friends were not without great reaſon alarmed concerning us.

* This was indeed nearly the courſe by the *true meridian*, or rather N. W. by W. Had we therefore ſailed upon a W. N. W. courſe, as directed us, by the *compaſs*, as we then *underſtood it*, we ſhould probably have paſſed by the iſlands without ever ſeeing them.

A few

A few days after, the Buss was brought into Mill Bay, and laid upon the Beach, near the Jetty Head, that she might be in daily view of those employed in the work-yard.

147. HAVING now completed the relation as to the work of this season, I cannot in justice avoid paying that tribute to a deserving poor man that I think due to him.

I found my mind very forcibly struck with the distinguished activity and presence of mind of our seaman JOHN BOWDEN, upon the occasion of our missing the harbour of *Fowey*. I was fully convinced that had he not been on board, the Buss would certainly have gone ashore, most probably been dashed to pieces upon the rocks, and in the confusion and darkness of the night, several of us would in all probability *have* lost our lives: and therefore that the safety of the vessel, as well as ourselves, was owing to his expertness as a seaman. He had on all occasions shewn himself to be an active, sober, modest, obedient man; and in the light of a *foremast* seaman, he appeared to be quite a *Genius*; for, if any thing went wrong with the tackle on board, his readiness of thought, and invention, accompanied with an expeditiousness in the application of something for supplying defects, and remedying, if not preventing, disasters, was beyond any thing I had ever had the opportunity of observing amongst others of his class; and he was the only seaman in that station I have ever met with, who never swore an oath, drank a dram, or was seen disordered with liquor of any kind. Had I been an admiral, I could not have done less than signally have rewarded his services: but though my employers had generously left it to me to reward merit wherever I found it, I was obliged to be contented to do on this occasion what was *properly* in my own power: I therefore put him upon the same footing with WILLIAM SMART, who was master of the *Edystone Boat*, and had long been employed in the service of the Proprietors; paid him the difference of the wages, and emoluments, from the time of his entry; and further promised him the command of the first vessel that should be built in addition for our service: which boon I know not whether he had more satisfaction in receiving, or I in bestowing; but I was sure he could not be better satisfied with it, than I was convinced that he deserved it.

C H A P. III.

Containing the Transactions of the WINTER *of* 1756, *and of the following* SPRING 1757, *to the Commencement of the* Outwork *of the ensuing Season.*

148. DURING this period, my operations were so numerous, diversified, and blended together, with respect to the time in which the several transactions were performed, that though I suppose a minute detail thereof was very interesting and satisfactory to the Proprietors at the time they were carried on, yet now such a particular relation would be unworthy of their attention, and much less that of the public: for which reason I shall only recount the leading or most interesting facts, without always regarding the precise days on which they were performed; unless it should appear proper in some instances so to do.

I have already mentioned, that our work-yard at Mill Bay was ready for the reception of stone, and the employment of stone-cutters: but though I found that Messrs. RICHARDSON and HILL were very well qualified for the *Outwork*, yet as they had been but little used to the working of *Portland* stone, upon the exact performance of which the *Frame* (if I may so call it) of our building depended; I was on that account induced to accept of the services of WILLIAM TYRRELL, who had been one of the masons concerned in the preparation of the stone at *Portland* for *Westminster Bridge*, and who, on the recommendation of Mr. RICHARDSON (on whom I found I could always rely,) offered himself as foreman over the stone-cutters, and to overlook the works of the yard.

149. THE

149. THE general defign and contrivance of our *Work-Yard* will appear by Plate N° 17, and the detail will be fully underftood by the technical explanation of the plate; but to render it fufficiently intelligible for the prefent, I take this opportunity of explaining the principal properties thereof: and though the plan of a mafon's work-yard may not appear to be a matter of much concern, or fufceptible of much invention, yet in our particular cafe, the fuccefsful carrying on, and expediting of our works, depended more upon a convenient difpofition of this, than can readily be imagined.

From the beginning I always laid it down as a *fundamental* maxim, that on account of the precarioufnefs of weather to fuit our purpofes, (and without its being favourable, I think it has already fufficiently appeared, that nothing is to be done upon the Edyftone) if we could fave one *Hour's* work upon the *Rock* by that of a *Week* in our *Work-yard*, this would always prove a valuable purchafe; and that therefore every thing ought to be done by way of preparation, which could tend to the putting our work together with expedition and certainty, in the ultimate fixing of it in its proper place; and for this purpofe, it was neceffary to make ufe of as large and heavy pieces of ftone as, in fuch a fituation as the Edyftone, were likely to be capable of being managed without running *too great* a rifk.

150. THE common run of modern buildings, even of the largeft fize, are compofed of pieces in general not exceeding five or fix hundred weight, except where columns, architraves, cornices, and other parts are to be formed that indifpenfably require large fingle pieces; becaufe ftones of this fize and bulk are capable of being handled without the ufe of *Tackles*, or *Purchafes*, unlefs where they are to be raifed perpendicularly: yet it appeared to me, that this choice of general magnitude refulted only from the workmen's not having commonly attained all that expertnefs in the management of the *mechanic Powers* that they might have; in confequence of which, they avoid, wherever they can, the neceffity of employing them. This arifes not from the real nature of the thing, when properly underftood; for a ftone of a ton weight is, when hoifted by a proper tackle, and power of labourers, as foon and as eafily *fet* in its place, as one of a quarter of that weight; and in reality, needs much lefs hewing than is neceffary for the preparation of four ftones to fill up the fame fpace; nor needs this reafoning ftop at ftones of a ton weight, but it might proceed even to as large fizes as are faid to be found in the ruins of *Balbec**; if there were not inconveniences of other kinds to fet on the oppofite fide of the queftion, as well as the want of quarries in this kingdom to produce ftones of that magnitude.

151. THE fize of the ftones that could be ufed in the Edyftone Lighthoufe feemed limited by the practicability of landing them upon the rock: for as nothing but fmall veffels, that were eafily manageable, could poffibly deliver their cargoes alongfide of the rock, with any reafonable profpect of fafety; fo no fmall veffels could deliver *very* large ftones, becaufe the fudden rifing and falling of the veffels in the Gut amounted frequently to the difference of three or four feet, even in moderate weather, when it was very practicable for a veffel to lie there; fo that in cafe, after a ftone was raifed from the floor of the veffel, her gunnel fhould take a fwing, fo as to *hitch* under the ftone, one of fuch a magnitude as we are now fuppofing, on the veffel's rifing, muft infallibly fink her; and hence it appeared, that much of the fafety in delivering the cargoes would depend upon having the fingle pieces not to exceed fuch weight, as could be *expeditioufly* hoifted, and got out of the way of the veffel, by a moderate number of hands, and by fuch fort of tackles as could be removed from the rock to the ftore-veffel each tide: and on a full view of the whole matter, it appeared to me very practicable to land fuch pieces of ftone upon the rock, as in general did not much exceed a ton weight; though occafionally particular pieces might amount to two tons†.

The general fize of our building ftones being thus determined upon at a ton weight, thofe would have been far too heavy to be expeditioufly transferred and managed, even in the work-yard, unlefs our

* There are three ftones lying contiguous in the plain part of a wall, that from the meafures amount together to upwards of 1,500 tons. See Wood's account of the ruins of *Balbec*. Defcript. Plate 3d. Page 19.

† In the courfe of the building we have had inftances of the boat's gunnel hitching under a ftone in the tackle, and fo as to unhook it: yet we fortunately never fuffered any damage by lofing the ftones, as they always happened to fall from the gunnel into the boat.

machinery rendered that easy, which would otherwise be difficult, without too great an expence of labour: and as the moving and transferring the pieces of stone in the work-yard would be greatly increased in quantity, by the very mode of attaining a *certainty* in putting the work together upon the rock; this consideration made it still the more necessary, to be able to load upon a carriage, and move the different pieces from one part of the yard to the other, with as much facility (comparatively speaking) as if they had been so many bricks: for, that we might arrive at perfect certainty in putting the work ultimately together in its place upon the rock, it did not appear to be enough, that the stones should all be hewn as exactly as possible to moulds that fitted each other; but it was further necessary, that the stones in every course should be tried together in their real situation in respect to each other, and so exactly marked, that every stone, after the course was taken asunder, could be replaced in the identical position in which it lay upon the *Platform*, within the fortieth part of an inch.——Nor was this alone sufficient; for every course must not only be tried singly together upon the platform, and marked, but it must have the course next above it put upon it, and marked in the same manner, that every two contiguous courses might fit each other on the *outside*, and prevent an irregularity in the outline: and this indeed, in effect, amounted to the *platforming* of every course twice: so that, in this way of working, every stone must be no less than six times upon the carriage; 1st, When brought into the yard from the ship, to carry it to the place of deposition till wanted to be worked.——2ndly, When taken up and carried to the *Shed* to be worked.——3dly, After being wrought, to be returned to its place of deposition.——4thly, When taken up to be carried to the platform.——5thly, When finished on the platform to be returned to its place of deposition.——6thly, When taken up to be carried to the Jetty, to be loaded on board a vessel to go to sea.

It might at first sight appear superfluous, to try the courses together *upon* each other, as the under and upper sides of all the courses were planes: and, in case the work could have been put together upon the rock in the same way that common masonry generally is done, it would have been so: that is, if we could have begun our courses by setting the outside pieces first, then it would have been very practicable to have regulated the inside pieces thereto; but as our hope of expedition depended upon certainty in every part of our progress, this required us to be in a condition to *resist a Storm* at every *Step*: the outside stones therefore, unconnected with the inner ones, would have scarce any fastening besides their own weight, and would be subject to the most immediate and greatest shock of the sea; and after compleating the outward circle, the inner space would be liable to become a receptacle for water: the necessity therefore of fixing the center stone first, as least exposed to the stroke of the sea, and of having sure means of attaching all the rest to it, and to one another, rendered it indispensable that the whole of the *two* courses should be tried together; that if any defect appeared at the outside, by an accumulation of errors from the center, it might be rectified upon the platform *.

152. THE second week in December three vessels arrived from *Portland*, and their cargoes (amounting to about 120 tons) were landed, and stowed away in the yard with all possible facility; and on Monday the 13th, the masons first began to work the stone, under the inspection of Mr. TYRRELL, who that day entered as foreman of the yard.——I now found there was a likelihood of meeting with difficulties and delays in getting the moorstone; for having some time since given course XI. to be roughed out by WALTER TRELEVEN, he came to Plymouth to inform me, that he had prepared the same, according to the moulds and my directions; but having engaged a master of a vessel to bring it to Ply-

* From a view of Plate N° 17, the reader will perceive that a vessel to be unloaded of stone being laid *athwart* the Jetty Head, a pair of *Parib[illegible] Blocks* being suspended from the top of the *Shears*, and the tackle *fall* (or running rope) carried to the small *Capstand* in the yard, the stones, being hoisted sufficiently high, can be delivered upon the four-wheel carriage that runs along the timber road, commonly called at the *Collieries*, where they are used, a *Rail Road*: and being landed upon the carriage, any stone can be delivered upon any of the *Bankers* in the line of the work-sheds on either side: or the carriage being turned a quarter round upon the *Turnpike*, or *Turn-table* T, it can be carried along the road that goes up the middle of the yard, and be delivered upon any part of its area destined for [illegible], all the stones marked for the same course being deposited together; from which place they can be again taken up upon the carriage, run along the road, and be delivered upon any *Banker* in the line of sheds, or upon the *Platform*, and afterwards returned back to their place of deposition, ready to be carried to sea in their proper order: the particular modes for the performance of which are explained in the description of this Plate, N° 17.——N. B. A *Banker* in a mason's yard is a square stone of a suitable size, made use of as a work-bench.

mouth

mouth that ſpring tide, he had been diſappointed by him, as he had been twice before by two others; all the three excuſing themſelves from their engagement, on account of the largeneſs of the ſtones, which they alledged were *unmanageable*, the larger ſort of them weighing (to them the aſtoniſhing weight of) *one* Ton! And therefore, unleſs I could myſelf induce ſome perſon to fetch them, they muſt ſtay where they were. Finding nothing but difficulties and diſappointments likely to ariſe from that quarter, I again hired *Hancock's Sloop*, and the next morning diſpatched J. Bowden and three other ſeamen, with one of our ſmaller purchaſe tackles, in the ſloop to *Parr*, with which the ſtones were got on board with all imaginable eaſe, and in three days depoſited in our yard; and our moorſtone hands began immediately to work upon them.

153. THE moorſtone, though very hard with reſpect to its component parts, yet being of a friable nature, is extremely difficult to work to an *Ariſs* (or ſharp corner) or even to be preſerved, when ſo wrought by great labour and patience, that is, with ſharp tools, and ſmall blows; it therefore ſoon appeared to me, that we ſhould make very rough and coarſe work of it, if the finiſhing of the pieces were left to the workmen of the country where produced; for, though carefully wrought there in their place, yet in loading and unloading from their carriages, and again putting on board, and unloading from the veſſels, the *Ariſſes* would be very ſubject to damage. Therefore to have as much done in the country as poſſible, and to ſave weight in carriage, (leaving the finiſhing part to be done at home) rough moulds were ſent for each ſize and ſpecies of ſtone, which were to be worked by them to a given parallel thickneſs, and with length and breadth enough, when ſo *bedded*, (as it is called) to be cut round all the ſides to the true figure of the finiſhing mould: but they were to reduce them as near the ſize as they could ſafely do it by the hammer; and that they might not leave on unneceſſary waſte, they were to be paid no more for either ſtone or carriage, than what the *mould* meaſured upon the thickneſs given *; and if they were *wanting* of ſubſtance ſufficient to make the figure compleat, it ſhould be at our option to reject them when they came home.

According to this plan I ſoon after agreed with Mr. Box for 200 tons of moorſtone; 100 tons of which were to be delivered by *May-day* next enſuing, and the remainder in the courſe of the following ſummer, to be laid down in our yard at the price of 20*s.* per ton †, clear of all charges, and 7*d.* per foot ſuperficial for working the beds as before-mentioned. I alſo agreed with Walter Treleven for 40 tons of ſtone, conditioned as above, at the price of 25*s.* per ton, cubic meaſure of the moulds, and 4*d.* per foot ſuperficial for working the beds, to be delivered by *May-day* at *Parr*; we undertaking the water-carriage.

There was ſome difference in the price, upon the whole, between the two contractors; but this was the leaſt material part of the conſideration: however as the terms with Mr. Box were not only the loweſt, but his ſtone was leſs friable and better coloured, and would give us no trouble in getting home, it may reaſonably be aſked, why I did not get the whole quantity wanted from Mr. Box? The reaſon was, 100 tons were not ſufficient for the ſervice of the approaching ſeaſon, and he could not undertake for more in due time. I might indeed have made 100 tons ſuffice, could I have been ſure of its delivery; but as accidents and diſappointments might happen, as well to Mr. Box as to Mr. Treleven, it appeared to me, that the way to be ſafe was, to order a quantity from both; beſides, I found, that had I not before given an order to Walter Treleven, I had not had the offer upon ſo low terms from Mr. Box; who now plainly ſaw, that if he did not agree with me, the order for the whole would go to his rival.

154. AS ſoon as the works of the yard commenced, I conſtantly viſited them twice a day; and as I laid down all the lines myſelf upon the mould-room floor, I was not without a regular ſeries of daily buſineſs.——It was judged neceſſary, for the ſervice of the next ſeaſon in carrying out our ſtone and materials, immediately to ſet about the building of additional veſſels: the making of proper deſigns therefore for thoſe veſſels, and the ſurveying the conſtruction thereof, with occaſional duty in the yard,

* There was to be no deduction from the contractor, on account of the contracted *ends* of the moulds.

† The ton was to meaſure 14 cubic feet.

furniſhed

furnished a fixed employment also to Mr. Jessop.——It has been already observed, that it was wholly impracticable to carry vessels of any considerable burthen into the *Gut* to deliver their cargoes; it therefore appeared, that our service would be best performed by multiplying small vessels, of such a size as to be tractable when lying to unload therein, and which could readily be hauled in and out by a small number of hands. It appeared also impracticable to make use of vessels decked over the hold, where the stone was to lie; for any thing being in the way of their rising would be subject to hitch upon the stone, so as to occasion the breakage of the tackle, and the fall of the stone; so that in this view, they would require particular dimensions and constructions.

It appeared, however, that we might make use of vessels somewhat larger than the Edystone boat, which was about 12 tons; but we judged 16, or at the utmost 18 tons, was as large a vessel as could well be managed in the Gut. Mr. Jessop judiciously advised their being built unusually *bold* in their *Bows*, and to have a sufficiency of height, or depth, to render them very *floaty* and lively in a rough hollow sea; though by this mode of construction they might not be so speedy sailers. It also appeared, that as there could be no taking in of ballast, when they had delivered their cargo at the Edystone, they must necessarily always be in sailing *trim*; and consequently, that the necessary tonnage of the ballast must be so much to be subtracted from the whole burthen of the vessels, the remainder only being the tonnage of materials that could be put on board them. But this was not to be the only deduction from their whole burthen; for we judged it would much contribute to the general safety, not to load them more than within one-fourth or one-fifth of their full capacity, which would not only render them buoyant upon the water, but be a sufficient allowance for an occasional addition by carrying other building materials, as also the companies.

To form some estimate therefore of what we should want; suppose from the whole burthen of 18 tons, we deduct four tons for ballast, and allow each vessel to be four tons underloaded, then an 18 ton vessel would carry a cargo of ten tons. How many of these vessels we might probably want, was determined as follows:——We could not expect in the approaching year to get the building higher than the completion of the *entire* solid; and as the plan of every part thereof was already fixed, we could easily determine, that the tonnage of this part of the work would be about 450 tons. Now supposing our working season to be, the months of *June*, *July*, *August*, and *September*, and that during this season, we could at an average operate with full effect for two days in the week; then in this space we might expect 35 working days, and this would amount to about 13 tons that should be carried out per day.——The Edystone boat's burthen being about 12 tons; admit her to carry three tons of ballast, and to be three tons light, then her cargo would be six tons, which, with a new boat's cargo of ten tons, would make 16 tons, that is, three tons more than the quantity required: but as things of this hazardous nature seldom come up to calculation; as here is too little to make up deficiencies, or possibly *the loss of a boat*, we judged it requisite, in order to guard against accidents, that two new boats of 18 tons each, should be built.

155. IN regard to our *Yawls*, having lost them all, the experience of the last season taught us what we should want, and what best answered our service; and having now not only the opportunity, but time also, we provided ourselves accordingly. We much regretted the loss of our original large yawl, which was of Mr. Jessop's providing, while I was last in London; as it completely answered the service for which it was built: but being too large, and too heavy, to get upon the deck of the Buss after every tide's work, we were obliged to let it lie at her stern, and in the hard gale of the 13th of October, it gradually filled by the broken seas driving into it; and there being at that time far too much sea to haul it up and clear it of water, it became by degrees heavier and heavier, and at last broke the *Painter* *, and went adrift as before-mentioned.——The yawl that we lost in the last storm, when we were driven out of the Channel, was one procured from *Deal*, which place is famous for the building of this kind of boats, both for lightness and ability to bear the sea: this boat, when not in use, was commonly hawled upon the deck of the Buss, but as in our passage from the Edystone to Fowey, we were almost right before the

* The *Painter* is the rope which is fastened to the *Stem* of a boat, and by which it is either detained or hauled in.

wind,

wind, the getting her on deck, while we were thus failing, was thought unneceffary, as we fhould immediately have wanted her in the harbour: and afterwards it became impracticable.

As there was now upon fale a veffel and her equipments, in different lots, we purchafed her long boat, being a ftout broad boat, much of the fize and model of the great yawl we had loft, and which would anfwer for her *occafional* fervice; we called her the *Sea Horfe* yawl from the name of the fhip to which fhe had belonged. However, as we faw very plainly that we fhould be frequently lofing our boats on the out-fervice, unlefs we could take them all on board the Bufs, we determined to build two light yawls, of fuch fize and conftruction, as that both might be ftowed upon the deck of the Bufs at once, and alfo to build them at home; becaufe, though for want of time, Mr. JESSOP had ordered the former light yawl from *Deal*, and fent the builders there the dimenfions and fort of veffel; yet they confiding that their experience in this branch needed no directions from any one, fent us a boat much about our fize, and fufficiently light, but confiderably narrower in proportion to her length, as well as fharper both before and *aft*: which though perhaps better adapted for rowing in *moderately* rough water, (and which doubtlefs would anfwer very well at *Deal*) yet was not fo well adapted to the hollow diftracted feas that are frequently encountered among the Edyftone Rocks, as we evidently found the bold full-breafted boats to be. As all the veffels built by Mr. JESSOP's directions fully and completely anfwered their intentions in our fervice, I am forry that I have it not in my power, for the fake of thofe, who may happen to have a work to perform in *rough Seas*, to give the delineations of them; for though the defigns were regularly made out by Mr. JESSOP, yet by being worn out in the builders hands whilft they were in ufe, they were not preferved; I happen however to have by me the original draught for one of the fmaller yawls that Mr. JESSOP produced to me for my approbation, and Plate N° 15, contains a tracing thereof from his own drawing, which will indeed ferve for every fize of *Yawl*, by altering the fcale; but our large boats for carrying out the ftone, though much of the fame kind of mould, were confiderably deeper in proportion. The figure of the boat reprefented as lying in the Gut delivering her cargo, Plate N° 14, though only fketched from memory, yet may ferve to give fome idea of what they were, efpecially if attention be given to the real defign of the yawl, Plate N° 15. The principle of all our veffels, as far as they differed from common ones, was, that they were confiderably broader in proportion to their length, and remarkably full in their bows; which, though not adapted to make way fwiftly through fmooth water, yet enabled them to float much more *lively* upon the furface, when a fharper veffel would almoft bury itfelf in the water; they were therefore not only fafer, but even made better *Way* in a rough fea.——Accordingly, one of the large boats of 18 tons, and a light yawl were immediately put in hand.

156. IN this refpite from fea operations, I ferioufly began to confider the great importance that it was likely to be of to our work, to have a *Cement* the moft perfect that was poffible, to refift the extreme violence of the fea. And on a confideration of this matter, it appeared, that nothing of the refinous, or oily kind, could have any place in our work, as it would require the furface to be *dry*, to enable it to make a compleat adhefion; whereas the getting any thing *compleatly dry*, was one of our greateft difficulties. It feemed therefore that nothing in the way of Cement would anfwer our end, but what would adhere to a moift furface, and become *hard*, without ever becoming compleatly *dry*.

157. I began now to forefee that before I could have a compleat fample produced of every part of the work, that might be wanted for the operations of next feafon, it would be pretty far advanced in the fpring; and as I propofed beginning the outwork as early in the feafon as poffible, I determined to winter at Plymouth (without returning to my refidence in London, as I had before intended) though to the detriment of my own private concerns; laying every confideration afide in favour of the Edyftone. I therefore refolved to take every opportunity in the evenings and intervals of my attendance on the work-yard, mould room, &c. to go through a compleat fet of experiments on *Cements*, fo far as it concerned the fubject I had in hand: for I plainly faw from the manner of working the moorftone, already defcribed, that not only much of the beauty and neatnefs of the work, but its real folidity too, would depend upon getting a Cement that would, in defpite of water almoft continually driven againft it with every

degree of violence, become of so firm a consistence in itself, and adhesion to the stone, that it should lie fair and *flush* in the joints, and so as to compose one even regular surface with the stone; and without needing *Hoops* of *Iron* or *Copper* to surround the horizontal joints, as seems to have been the expedient of Mr. WINSTANLEY. I was so fortunate as to succeed in this part of the business entirely to my satisfaction; and perhaps in a degree unknown before: and having made much use since of the experience which I then acquired; having had frequent occasions and opportunities of communicating it to others; and having been asked many questions concerning it; I trust that my reader will forgive me, if I am diffuse enough to enter into a full explanation of the subject, so far as I know it. I mean not however to tire him with recording all the particular experiments, as this would be almost endless, they having been pursued through the whole of this winter; but only to state the principal scope and design of them, with the results: nor do I propose to enter into a chemical disquisition upon them, which I leave to the learned in that science. But as what I have to say on this subject will carry me to some length, I shall reserve it to a distinct chapter, in order to keep the matter together.

158. EARLY this spring I thought it expedient to make a journey to the West, not only to survey the moorstone works that were then going on, but to acquaint myself with *Mount's Bay*, in case we should have a future occasion to take refuge there.——I must however premise, that on the 25th of January, in returning from *Mill Bay* at five o'clock in the evening, I observed four flashes of lightning towards the West, within the space of six or seven minutes, but heard no noise of thunder. A few days after, I was informed, that the same evening the lightning had shattered the church of *Lostwithiel*, in a very surprizing manner: and though from the many relations I had read, I could not doubt, but that the effects of lightning were very great; yet as this was the first opportunity that had occurred to me of seeing them with my own eyes, I was very solicitous not to lose the opportunity. I therefore on this journey called to visit this church, not only as an object of curiosity, but as a matter very interesting to my own work; and I communicated a particular account of these effects to the ROYAL SOCIETY, which, as it stands recorded in the 50th volume of the *Philosophical Transactions*, for the year 1757, page 198, I shall take no further notice of here, than as it immediately applies to the subject I am upon.

The steeple of the church of *Lostwithiel* before this accident was 113 feet high, whereof the lower part was a square tower of 49 feet, finished above with an elegant Gothic octagon lantern, 12 feet high, and above it a stone spire of 52 feet, of which a portion of 20 feet of the upper part was entirely burst, and dispersed in all directions; and some of the stones that composed it were found at the distance of 200 yards.——The masonry, as is usual in ancient and well-built spires, was very light, the stones composing the shell of it being no more than seven inches thick; so that the single stones of it could not in general exceed one hundred weight: yet as they were all curiously joined together at the ends, *mortoise* and *tenon* fashion, and appeared to have been exceedingly well cemented together, nothing, as it should seem, but a great power of some elastic vapour, similar to the sudden explosion of a considerable quantity of gunpowder, could have burst and dispersed the materials of the spire in the manner it had done: for besides the part entirely destroyed, to six feet further down, one half of the shell was thrown down, and the other half left standing, in so perilous a state, that it was judged necessary to take it down; and on doing this, the work was found so disjointed and shattered, that it was thought necessary to take down six feet more. It was in this situation when I viewed it, the beginning of March; and I found that the whole of the spire left standing, as well as the lantern, was greatly cracked, and damaged. Many other circumstances occurred which shewed the effects of an elastic vapour, that wanted to get at liberty by expansion, somewhat similar in its most obvious effects to that of gunpowder; and under this idea, I might have been tempted to suppose, that had the shell of the spire been rendered stronger by cramping the stones together, as well as *tenoning* the ends, it might have sustained the elastic pressure outwards, without being torn to pieces: but there were some attending circumstances which convinced me, that the action had not been altogether in the way of an included elastic vapour, endeavouring to expand itself; upon which principle, the *weakest part* would have given way, and have afforded an opening to the vapour: for, at the bottom of the steeple, at the level of the ground, an hole had been pierced entirely through the wall, and through an opposite

opposite buttress, whose compound thickness amounted to eight feet; whereas at the distance of a foot side-way it might have got through by piercing the wall alone, which was not more than five feet thick.—— This circumstance, beyond all the devastation that had been made, both in the steeple and the body of the church, convinced me, that there could be no certainty of making any wall so strong as to withstand the action of *Lightning*; and consequently that no security against the effects of it, that human sagacity had either discovered, or could suggest, ought to be omitted in any building of consequence. Therefore, however strongly I was disposed, before I saw this example, to adopt the proposition of *Dr.* (then Mr.) FRANKLIN, for the preservation of buildings from the effects of lightning by means of a *Conductor* (which had had not at that time become popular) this instance applied itself so closely to my feelings, that I determined to put his method in practice in my proposed building, in the best manner I was able: and the particular mode in which this was done, will be fully explained when we come to that period of the building.

159. DURING the time the experiments on Cement were making, and the works of the yard proceeding vigorously, I was very desirous to find an opportunity of going upon the rock to compleat our moulds for the foundation courses; but it was very seldom at that time of the year that the weather, even in appearance, was promising. However, Wednesday January the 12th, there having been some days of frost, with moderate breezes, this morning the water in Plymouth Sound was very smooth, and I went on board the Edystone boat with Mr. JESSOP and the mould-maker, the Sea-Horse yawl attending. All continued promising till we got out of the Sound, but without the Ram Head we met with a swell from the South, which increased as we came nearer the Edystone, so that when we came there, we found the sea beating over it with great violence at low water: we ran within twice our boat's length of it, on the West side, to have a view of the work, in which we could not perceive any injury from the late storms, nor change, except that the new surface was of the same colour as the old; being all grown over with dark coloured green sea-weed. We also ran alongside our buoy upon the moorings, and had the great satisfaction to find it floating, and in good order.

We made several expeditions of the same nature in the course of the spring, and with no better success; so that it was not till the 23d of April that we got a landing. We then went out in our first new boat, which was launched on the 22d of March, and was called the *Weston*, JOHN BOWDEN, master. There being little wind, we were obliged to row almost all the way. Between twelve and one, when we were now about a league from the rock, it became calm; and as we were not soon likely to get out with the great boat, we betook ourselves to the Sea-Horse yawl which attended us, and in an hour landed, and got a tide's work of four hours; in which time having marked a durable middle line upon the rock, we got the moulds compleated for courses I. II. and VI. except that a right line was wanted to be drawn upon them, to enable us to join them together again on shore, in the same position exactly in which they lay upon the rock; and for this particular use a ruler had been provided, which being too long to carry in the yawl, was left on board the *Weston*, to be brought forward by her: but as she did not arrive at the moorings till we were obliged to quit the rock, this was a sensible disappointment; however it did not prevent us from compleating for use the courses we had framed: for, by stretching a piece of packthread over the moulds, we were enabled to bore two small holes in every piece; so that when the parts of the moulds were laid together in contact upon a level floor, and those holes brought into a right line, they would then be in the same position as they were upon the rock.——As it remained calm, we determined to stay in the Weston all night, but, on examination, finding the carpenter had neglected to bring off an additional paper of nails that he was expresly ordered to bring, and *reminded* of, this trifling incident, however small in itself, was yet likely to put a stop to our farther proceedings; for not being able to form any expedient to do without the nails, the carpenter and three seamen were dispatched in the yawl for Plymouth to bring out this necessary article. The weather continued calm all the night, but in the morning it began to blow fresh at S. which brought on a swell; and not only prevented us from landing, but obliged us to return to Plymouth.——Upon the 30th, we got a very good landing

landing in the yawl, and had the good fortune to compleat the whole of the moulds that were wanting, just in time to quit the rock when the wind and sea would very soon afterwards have obliged us to do so.

160. THE accomplishment of these moulds, (an object much desired ever since the conclusion of the last year's work) having been thus happily effected, after much delay, disappointment, and danger; the next thing was to procure a room, upon the floor of which we could lay them together, and, by laying down chalk lines, form the rest of the pieces that were wanted to make up each course, to which they formed, as it were, the *Roots*. This requiring a larger room than any we had at our command, I applied to the Mayor of Plymouth for the use of the floor of the *Guildhall*: and I am very sure the present magistrates will blush for their predecessor, when they are told that his Worship had so little feeling, or attention to the public service, that I was absolutely refused, on pretence that the chalk lines would spoil the floor. I afterwards applied for the *Assembly Room*, but there I succeeded no better. These unexpected rubs were not however insuperable; for by removing a partition between two rooms, which were the garrets of our cooper, I got a floor large enough to hold each course at *twice*; and to this, though attended with a considerable addition of trouble, yet as it would only occur in the third, fourth, fifth, and sixth courses, I determined to submit, rather than subject myself to any more Denials.

161. IN considering at leisure the various impediments to which our work was liable, it behoved us to endeavour to remove every thing of that sort possible. Though our predecessors, to prevent annoyance from an enemy, had a vessel of war upon the station to protect the workmen, yet the generous behaviour of the *French King* on a former occasion, (mentioned § 51,) gave us assurance that we should have nothing to fear from the enemies of the state. But yet we had experienced, during the course of the last season, a good deal of hindrance and interruption from our *Friends*; for our boats were frequently stopped and boarded by the men of war's cutters, to impress the seamen; and notwithstanding they were furnished with *Admiralty* protections, yet there occurred some instances of the officers being so indiscreet as to pay no regard either to the protections, or the service they were upon. And though our men were always released with politeness, when the matter was represented to the *Commander in Chief*, yet all this produced delays and hindrances incompatible with the urgency of our business. And as it plainly appeared, that nobody would molest us, provided it could be made clearly to appear, without collusion, that our men were really and *bonâ fide* employed in the Edystone service, it occurred to me, that if a large figure of the Lighthouse was painted upon the mainsail of our boats, it would be an evident mark of distinction at a distance, and prevent their being stopped. But yet, that after all, the seamen, when on shore, would still be liable to be detained, when absent from their boats. To prevent this, I considered, that if I had a stamp, which could not readily be counterfeited, with which one might at pleasure stamp a piece of silver, each man employed by us might thus be furnished with an evident token in his pocket of the service to which he belonged. This idea having been communicated to Mr. WESTON, he soon got a sufficient number of silver medals made for the purpose, of which Fig. 7, Plate N° 18, is the representation: and after the distribution of these, and the painting of the sails, we never had any further interruption.

162. A HINDRANCE of another kind however arose; for about the middle of February, we had advice from Mr. TUCKER, that the frequent appearance of French privateers had intimidated the masters of the Portland vessels so much, that they were afraid to stir out: and this gave me the more solicitude, as all the stone we had received from Portland was then nearly worked up. On communicating this, Mr. WESTON immediately applied to the *Lords* of the ADMIRALTY, who dispatched an order to the commander in chief at *Portsmouth*, to send a convoy upon notice from Mr. TUCKER, of any vessel being ready to sail that was freighted with stone for the *Edystone*. However, before any convoy was sent, two vessels thought good to *run it*; and arrived with a fresh supply of stone from Portland the 8th of March, and carried back to Portland the moulds for all the stone that could possibly be wanted in the course of the ensuing Summer.

163. AS

163. AS we had been for feveral days without any unwrought ftone in the yard; the mafons were employed in detaching fufficient pieces from the neighbouring marble rocks, and forming out of them cubes of one foot each fide, for inlaying between the different courfes; as will be more particularly defcribed hereafter in its proper place: and the labouring tinners were employed in drilling a couple of holes through the outward end of every fingle ftone; by which they were intended to be *trenailed* down to the courfe below. For, though I could not eafily conceive, when each block was fixed in its place, by oak wedges in the dovetail fpace cut out of the rock, or furnifhed by the work already fixed, that any thing could move it; yet, confidering the unmeafured violence of the fea, I determined to omit nothing that could tend to keep the whole firm together, while the cement was frefh and unhardened; as that feemed the beft way to prevent derangements and difappointments, while things were going on: and foon after, we purchafed 300 *trenails*, of the beft quality, and the fame fize that I underftood was ufed in building the firft rate men of war; being 2½ feet long, and two inches fquare, in the rough.

164. IN carrying on a work of this fort, I have always found it more difficult to manage the workmen employed, than to controul the elements. High wages and encouragements may have the effect of *inducing* men, in cafes where they cannot be *compelled*, to enter into fuch fervices, which no other kind of perfuafion would be able to accomplifh.——This mode, however, by no means teaches them *Submiffion* and *Obedience*; on the contrary, it leads them to fuppofe that every fuccefs, in the operations they have been concerned in, is owing to their own perfonal merit and addrefs; and that, had they not been employed, the thing could not have been done by any other perfons: of this I had feveral examples in the courfe of the outworks of the laft feafon; having difcovered a ftrong tendency to *Mutiny* and *Combination*.——WILLIAM HILL, though as a foreman he received one fhilling per hour *extra* pay, and had in one week of the preceding feafon intitled himfelf to the receipt of near *five Guineas*, (including his conftant wages,) yet this by no means increafed his *gratitude* for being taken into the employ, or his attachment to the fervice. In fhort, having found him irregular and diforderly, and privately a fower of difcord among the workmen; and having always in fuch cafes experienced it to be the moft effectual method to lay the axe to the root of the tree; I difcharged him the fervice for *difobedience of Orders*, as an example to lefs offenders.——This tranfaction being upon a Saturday, on Monday following, HILL came into the yard to fetch away his tools, and claimed the fulfilling of their promife of all thofe who had worked with him upon the rock; which was, "that if *he fhould be difcharged they would all follow him*." Upon this I inftantly called them together, and defired that whoever had any dependance upon, or attachment to, WILLIAM HILL, would take away his tools and depart the yard immediately; which one of the moorftone mafons did, all the reft prudently chufing to ftay where they were.

165. THIS tranfaction gave an opening to rectify what I had plainly perceived to be an evil to the fervice of the *Outwork*; that is, that the *Premiums* with refpect to the inferior workmen were not only too near that of the foremen, but in reality higher than neceffary to countervail the rifk, in their own *Opinions*: and indeed every encouragement *more* than that tended only, as we have feen, to make the men diforderly and untractable: wherefore after confideration, the following Saturday I called together in the yard all the workmen that ferved upon the rock during the laft feafon, and reprefented to them, that in proportion as the houfe was raifed, the number of hours they would have opportunity of working thereon would increafe, and the work become eafier and lefs hazardous; and that therefore they *ought* not to expect the fame *premium* by the hour, the enfuing year, that they had had the laft year; and that in confequence I intended to fettle fuch a price at the beginning of the work of this feafon, as I propofed to hold to till we could make a *lodgement* thereon; for then, they would be able to make regular days works; and that the price I fhould now fix would be fix-pence per hour for the mafons and carpenter, and four pence per hour for the tinners; their weekly wages to be the fame as laft year: and under thefe conditions every individual might take his choice, either of working conftantly in the yard, or of going off to the rock by rotation every other week. Whereupon every one without hefitation declared his readinefs to ferve upon the rock, upon the terms offered: an event which gave me particular fatisfaction, as it would

 not

not only be a conſiderable ſaving to the proprietors, but the work itſelf would be quite as well and expeditiouſly done. And, though it is not an eaſy matter to *reduce* emoluments, with the *Conſent* of parties; yet I have always found amongſt mechanical artificers, as I ſuppoſe it is with other denominations of men; that firmneſs, juſtice, equality, and a *fair alternative*, will always carry the point.

166. IN the month of May I received a letter from Mr. TUCKER, importing that in conſequence of the ADMIRALTY's order, he had ſometime ago applied to the *Commanding Officer* of the *Fleet* at *Portſmouth*, to have a convoy for the *Edyſtone* materials to *Plymouth*; that he had regularly got an anſwer from the commanding officer, that a convoy ſhould be ſent; but that no convoy *had come*. This was repeated, and anſwers regularly received; but the fact was, that no convoy did ever attend this duty: ſo that the favourable ſentiments which the *Lords* of the ADMIRALTY, and their principal commander had of the importance of our work were yet defeated; as it happened not to appear in that light to thoſe who were appointed to the ſervice: ſo that we remained equally unſerved, as if we had never had any order of aſſiſtance. Doubtleſs on proper repreſentation, this neglect would have been duly adverted to; but as the delays, before they amounted to a matter of complaint, had been ſuch, as to oblige us to run *all riſks*; and nothing in reality had happened adverſe; we thought it unneceſſary to trouble the Admiralty for a kind of redreſs that could *then* no ways conduce to the *re-erection* of the Edyſtone Lighthouſe.

167. IN the courſe of the month of May we received from London five fathoms of additional main chain propoſed to be added to the ſix fathoms that already acted as a bridle, which, as it would make us eleven fathoms of bridle chain, and this was more than half the depth of the water at the place of our mooring, would prevent the neceſſity of lifting ſo conſiderable a part of the ground chains from the bottom in mooring or unmooring, and thereby prevent a loſs of time, that might in effect prove conſiderable: for in many caſes we had ſeen, that the want of an hour, to the accompliſhment of ſuch points of our buſineſs, as depended upon winds and ſeas, might prove a delay of weeks, which might ultimately occaſion the loſs of a ſeaſon in the finiſhing of the building.——Theſe neceſſary preparations having been made, and a quantity of *Plaſter* received, ready prepared for uſe in London, and cloſe rammed into five caſks, to prevent the bad effects of the air upon it; we were now ready for commencing the operations upon the rock as ſoon as the ſeaſon would give us room to ſuppoſe we were likely to have ſucceſs in carrying them on: but previouſly to my relation of the works of the approaching ſeaſon, I ſhall now perform my promiſe of giving an account of my experiments and obſervations reſpecting the *Cement* we uſed, which was referred to a ſeparate chapter.

C H A P. IV.

Containing EXPERIMENTS, *to aſcertain a compleat Compoſition for* WATER CEMENTS; *with their Reſults.*

168. ON this ſubject, I was already apprized that two meaſures of quenched or ſlaked lime, in the dry powder, mixed with one meaſure of *Dutch Tarras*, and both very well beat together to the conſiſtence of a paſte, uſing as little water as poſſible, was the common compoſition, generally uſed in the conſtruction of the beſt water-works both in ſtone and brick; and which, after being *once ſet**, would afterwards become hard, without ever being compleatly dry; nay, that it would in time grow hard, even *under* water. This therefore ſeemed to be the kind of cement adapted to our uſe; and what

* This is the term uſed in the application of calcareous mortar, which denotes its firſt ſtep, or degree of hardening; but in this ſtate, though it has loſt its ductility, it is a very friable ſubſtance.

I had

I had yet to learn, was, the beft materials, and mode of treating and ufing them. I was ignorant at this time, whether there would be any difference in the firmnefs of the mortar, on account of the lime being made from different kinds of lime-ftone, provided the proportion of the ingredients was fuitable. I found it indeed commonly afferted by *Mafons*, that the harder or ftronger the *Lime*-ftone was, the ftronger would be the *Lime*; but whether this maxim chiefly regarded the ufual compofition of lime and fand in common buildings (with which they were chiefly acquainted) or whether it held good alfo in *Tarras Mortar*, did not appear.——It was alfo generally agreed by mafons, that mortar, if mixed up with falt water, would never harden in fo great a degree, as the fame kind of compofition would do if made with frefh water.——I could readily conceive, that if mortar was mixed with falt-water, and ufed for the plaftering, or even the walling, of a dwelling-houfe, the wall fo built would never become fo perfectly dry, but that when the atmofphere was in a humid ftate, the fea falts, by this means conveyed into the compofition of the mortar, would attract the moifture of the air, and render the wall vifibly and palpably moift: Nay I have been told, that if a houfe be covered with plafter which has fea fand in its compofition, though it is mixed up with frefh water, or even if fea fand is made ufe of in the joints of the walls, it will fhew its affection to moifture in very damp weather, and the plafter over thofe joints will become evidently difcoloured. But as it appeared to me, that in the cafe of *Tarras* mortar, *drying* and *hardening* were diftinct properties, not evidently dependant on each other; it might be, that though *Tarras* mortar made up with falt-water, might equally difcover its fenfibility of moifture, if ufed for the *fame purpofe*, as common mortar made up with fand only; yet this circumftance might not impair its hardnefs, or *firmnefs* of *Adhefion*, where perfect drynefs was not wanted; confequently it would be no injury, in the fubject of *Water Building*: and as the neceffity of carrying out, or not, from the land all the water we fhould have occafion for in this building, was a matter of moment, the full inveftigation of this queftion became very material.

169. THE firft object of enquiry, as I had heard much complaint from the workmen, of limes not being *well* burnt, was, whether good or bad burning affected the *Quality*, or the *Quantity* of the lime produced from a given quantity of ftone, or both? Therefore, in my firft effays, I did this part of the bufinefs myfelf; the refult, as it then appeared to me, was, that if the ftone was not expofed to a certain degree and duration of fire, according to its original hardnefs and compactnefs, it remained ftone, without becoming lime; or was converted into lime to a certain depth from the outfide only, the parts near the center remaining ftone: the diftinction between *Lime* and *Lime-ftone* being (fo far as I have had occafion to enquire into it) that lime-ftone, after it has been expofed to a fufficient degree of fire, will, on throwing water upon it when in large heaps, or plunging a fingle lump into water, and quickly drawing it out again, become hot, fmoke, and fwell fo as to be refolved into a dry impalpable powder, in which ftate it is called *flaked Lime*; I fuppofe, to diftinguifh it from that foft, moift, earthy fubftance, which it becomes on fuch a further addition of water, as muft be ufed to prepare it for making mortar. Now if the lime-ftone is imperfectly burnt, it only in part falls into flaked lime; the refidue not being capable of being reduced to that kind of mealy powder, which, with a further addition of water, and a little beating, becomes a tough kind of pafte; and which is capable of firmly uniting into one mafs, with any kind of hard, fandy, or gritty matter, that may be introduced as a mixture with it, in the compofition of mortar for mafonry: whereas, the part that will not fo fall down, inftead of a foft pafty fubftance, becomes in general rather more rigid and hard by the addition of water.

I therefore tried a quantity of powder-lime that had fallen from a ftone imperfectly burnt, and an equal quantity of lime from one that was thoroughly burnt; and having in other refpects treated them in the fame manner, both with falt water and frefh, I found the former to work fomewhat more harfh, but that ultimately there was no material difference in the quality of the mortar: and from hence I formed this conclufion, that the complaints of workmen on this head were rather founded upon the *great wafte*, and *fmall produce*, from imperfectly burnt lime, than from a real difference in the quality of what is produced. It is however to be noted, that I took none of the flaked lime, that was produced from the imperfectly burnt ftone, but what would pafs the *fineft* fieve; becaufe I conceived, that a degree a degree of burning may be so much in the confines of what is enough, and what is not enough, as that the stone may fail to such a degree of fineness as to pass a coarser sieve, and yet not fall to that impalpable powder necessary to form a compleat paste. For though, when passed through a coarser sieve, there may be enough of the finer parts to form a paste, yet in this way a comparative experiment would be rendered inconclusive, because the small parts of unburnt stone must be considered as so much admixture of *Sand*, or gritty matter, and this at least alters the intended proportion between the quick-lime and the gross matter. The result of this experiment however, though it shews that the use of imperfectly burnt lime is not only wasteful, but in every sense of it ineligible, when applied to a work in large; yet it sufficiently secured me in the course of my experiments, from any doubts that might be formed, of the results of such as were made with slaked lime, which was neither of my own burning, nor of my own quenching; because it was always easy to get enough passed through the *finest sieve*, for the purpose of an experiment, though it might prove impracticable to get enough so passed to answer the demands of a real building*.

170. BEFORE I proceed any further, it will be necessary to explain the mode in which I compounded, and made up my mortar for trials. I took as much of the ingredients, as all together would ultimately form a ball of about two inches diameter.——This ball, lying upon a plate till it was set and would not yield to the pressure of the fingers, was then put into a flat pot filled with water, so as to be covered by the water; and what happened to the ball in this state, was the *criterion* by which I judged of the validity of the composition for our purposes.——The measure I used was a common small chip box, taking as many measures from each ingredient, as I meant to try.——I constantly put down the lime upon the flat bottom of a common pewter plate, and with as much water as would sufficiently wet it, worked it upon the plate, with a broad pointed knife, till it was become a tough but a pretty soft paste. I afterwards added the quantity I intended of tarras, or other gross matter, gradually; working it after each addition till it was become tough; and in this way, adding the gross matter at three or four different times, I was generally enabled to get in the whole quantity, without any addition of water, more than had been necessary to bring the lime only at first to a proper consistence. The whole was thus worked till it acquired a tough and stiff ductility; but if it happened, by the addition of too much water, to become too soft, I let it stand till it began to set, which might be quickened by putting it a few minutes upon a dry stone, or brick, and when it was a little hardened by partially setting, I worked it till it was brought to a stiff paste; the whole of which operation took up generally above a quarter, and sometimes near half an hour, to make a single ball.

171. IN making up balls of mortar in this way, however well they were worked, if made up of no other ingredients but common lime and sand; though this might be denominated excellent mortar for the common purposes of building, yet upon being immersed in water, I found none of them which would not dissolve; and therefore I judged such sort of mortar, however hard it might become by being gradually dried, was totally unfit for our work.——Balls even of the common composition of *Tarras* mortar (two parts slaked lime to one of tarras) I found would not always stand this test: but balls made up with *equal* measures of lime and tarras would in general stand it. This degree of information, though in itself very material, was soon attained; but as many points seemed to want investigation, I regularly proceeded to determine the following questions.

Question 1st. What difference in the effect results from lime burnt from stones of different qualities, in point of hardness?

* T[illegible] conclusions then; about which time the learned Dr. BLACK discovered that lime-stone by burning would lose [illegible] of [illegible], by the expulsion of *fixed Air*, which is driven off by the force of fire. And since him, Dr. HIGGINS has discovered [illegible] of the *Gas* is driven off by a less force of fire, *however long it is continued*; and that when compleatly driven off [illegible] *above, or nearly so*, the lime then falls the most freely in quenching, or *slaking*, and to the most impalpable [illegible] of experiments, that lime so burnt makes the best and hardest composition of *mortar*: but how far [illegible] *mortar for water* building, which has not the advantage of induration by drying, (as those specimens had [illegible] of the Doctor's experiment) it is still out of my power to determine.——*Higgins on Calcareous Cements*, §. 2 and 4.

Chalk

Chalk lime is generally confidered by workmen as the weakeft of all; and it is accounted for in general, by its being burnt from one of the fofteft of all limeftones.——The marble rocks near Plymouth are of fo hard a nature, that the ftone obtained from them to be burnt to lime (and which is the common lime of that country) is, by far the greater part of it, blafted off with gunpowder. From obfervations of the buildings about Plymouth that had been conftructed with this lime, at different periods of time, it appeared to me to be very nearly of the fame nature with chalk lime; not only being of the brighteft white, but of the fame weak crumbly nature. I therefore made a couple of balls of tarras mortar of each fort of lime in the above ftated proportions of two to one; and alfo equal parts; and the refult of feveral trials of the fame kind was, that there was no apparent difference in the ftrength thereof for the purpofe of water building *.——Hence it appeared, as the effect of two limes was the fame, from one of the ftrongeft and one of the weakeft fpecies of limeftone; that the ftrength of the lime muft depend upon fome other quality, than that of the *hardnefs* of the ftone. So far, my experiments had proceeded with frefh *Water*.

Q. 2d. What difference refults in the ftrength of the mortar when made up with *frefh*, or with *Sea Water*; the compofitions being immerfed in the fame water?

Balls were made up in the former different proportions; one pair with falt and the other pair with frefh water, and this was feveral times repeated; the refult was, that as to what happened immediately, or within the compafs of a few days, there was no apparent difference; but of the balls which remained entire, when kept under water for two, or three months, thofe made up with falt water appeared, if there was any difference, to have the preference. Hence I concluded, there was no need to burthen ourfelves, with carrying out *frefh* water to the Edyftone for making the mortar: and in confequence all future trials, except it is otherwife mentioned, were made with falt water †.

Q. 3d. What difference refults from different *Qualities* of limeftone, fo far as I could procure the fpecimens?

Having heard of a lime produced from a ftone found at *Aberthaw*, upon the coaft of *Glamorganfhire*, that had the fame qualities of fetting in water as *Tarras*, I was very anxious to procure fome of the ftone; which I did, and burnt it into lime. I found it to require a good deal of fire to make it, by quenching, fall into a fine powder. This ftone, before burning, was of a very even, but dead fky blue, with very few fhining particles; but when burnt and fifted, it was of a bright *buff colour*. Having made up a couple of balls, according to each of the former proportions; and alfo a couple of balls with common lime (by which I mean Plymouth lime) the difference of hardnefs after twenty-four hours was very remarkable: the compofition of two meafures of *Aberthaw* to one of *Tarras*, confiderably exceeded in hardnefs that of common lime and *Tarras*, in equal parts: the compofition of Aberthaw and Tarras in equal parts was ftill confiderably harder, and this difference was the more apparent, the longer the compofitions were kept.

172. THUS encouraged, I was willing to try farther; and particularly to examine the validity of the notion entertained by workmen, refpecting *Tarras Mortar*, that the longer it was kept and the oftener it was beaten over, the ftronger it would fet: for, as it would be likely to prove a very great incumbrance, in our fituation, to keep our mortar in a ftate of beating for a length of time, and from one time of ufing to another, it was very material to be thoroughly known, how far this was really the cafe; and if fo, whether, for faving of time (to us *moft* valuable) a greater proportion of tarras might not anfwer the fame end as a longer beating: for it was evident, we fhould have every *moveable* thing to carry to and from the rock each tide, along with ourfelves.

Q. 4th. Whether *Tarras Mortar*, after having been once well beaten, becomes better by being repeatedly beaten over again?

* This, though very contrary to the common opinion of workmen, is fupported by the experiments of Dr. HIGGINS, which fhew, that *Chalk Lime* well burnt was fully equal to the beft fort of *Stone Lime* he ufed; which he efteemed that made from *Plymouth* marble, for the purpofe to which his enquiries were directed; viz. Buildings in the *Air*. *Higgins* on *Calcareous Cements*. Sect. 24.

† In a compofition of mortar for *Water-building* that BELIDOR gives from M. MILET DE MONVILLE, he ufes *Sea Water* for making the mortar of fuch works as are expofed to the *Sea*. Belidor, Arch. Hydraul. part 2. tom 2. p. 186.

To

To prove this, I made up a couple of balls of *Aberthaw* lime, one in each proportion above mentioned, and laid them in a damp place upon a water soaken brick, sprinkled them with water, and covered them with a wet cloth; so that they might be as slow as possible in setting: these I broke down, and beat over again, every morning and night for three days: and then prepared a couple of balls of the same materials afresh, and beat them very well. These balls were, when set, put all together in salt water. Between these, where the composition was equal parts, there was *no discernible* difference: but of those in which the lime predominated, the preference seemed due to such as had had the repeated beatings; though the difference was not very remarkable.——The same experiments being tried with common lime, the preference was evidently more in favour of repeated beatings, in that composition in which the lime predominated (that is, the common one) than in that of equal quantities. Hence though the practice of workmen is very right, where common lime, and the smaller quantity of tarras, as in the common case, are used; yet where the tarras is not spared, and the lime is of superior quality; the repetition of beatings appears not to be material: and therefore for *our use*, where nothing was to be spared, that could save time and labour upon the rock, the composition of equal quantities of Aberthaw lime and tarras seemed adapted in the best manner possible to the purpose.

173. I HAD heard that *Shell Lime*, that is, *Cockle* or other shells burnt, set very hard and made an excellent mortar for under-drawing, and inside work. It is mentioned in WREN's *Parentalia* as having been made use of in *St. Paul's* Cathedral for this purpose, and found excellent. On trying some of this mortar I found it to set hard, and readily, without any admixture of sand, tarras, or other matter. In short, for water work, tarras scarcely appeared to improve its natural quality. On being put into water, after it was set, it did not dissolve, but did not acquire an additional hardness; on the contrary by degrees it macerated and dissolved, not internally, but gradually from the surface inwards; and hence I concluded it totally unfit for our use. I was afterwards informed, that a part of the work at *Ramsgate Pier* had been done with this kind of lime, but was afterwards obliged to be taken up, on its dissolving quality in sea water being discovered.

174. HAVING observed how very speedily *Plaster* of *Paris*, from a semi-fluid state would set into a hard substance, I conceived it might probably be of some use in our work. On making up a ball as I did with the mortars, but without beating, it very readily set; and did not dissolve on putting it into water; but I soon found that, while in a moist state, it had little firmness, and did not acquire any additional hardness under water; and by continuance, it became less firm: though I do not remember in the time I had it in trial (perhaps two or three months) that it re-dissolved, either throughout its substance, or by maceration of its surface, like the shell lime*. I tried many experiments to improve its qualities by admixture, but did not find that either sand or tarras was of any use: I also tried to beat it while in a pulp, which would for a little time prevent its setting, but this did not appear to produce any good effect, either alone, or with admixtures. Indeed I did not find that any thing was likely to give it solidity beyond what it naturally has; unless that after it was dry, it would then drink up linseed oil plentifully; and which, if dried in its pores, would doubtless give it a considerable degree of solidity: but this treatment not being applicable to my purposes, I did not pursue the experiment any further.——However, the great readiness wherewith I observed plaster to set to a *moderate* degree of firmness, suggested to me this thought, which afterwards proved to be useful; that when there was not time for our cement to set, before it was subjected to the violence of the sea, if it was coated over with plaster, it might thereby be defended till it had time to set; and then, if the plaster should be washed off, it would be of no consequence.

175. THE last species of lime I had an opportunity of trying in these my original experiments, was a kind that was much commended for water-works, and which is produced in the county of *Devon*,

* I am lately told, that Plaster of Paris is liable to be perfectly dissolved in a large quantity of water, if suffered to remain in it for a length of time, and especially if the water is frequently changed or much agitated.

at

at a place called *Bridiſtow*, about thirty-five miles north from Plymouth.——I procured a piece of this ſtone and burnt it: its appearance, both before and after burning, was much like that of Aberthaw, and on a ſimilar trial it anſwered pretty much in the ſame manner; but the compoſition formed with it appeared to be ſomewhat inferior in hardneſs: however, it ſeemed capable of becoming a ſubſtitute, in caſe I met with any difficulty in procuring that of *Aberthaw*.

176. HAVING now found a ſpecies of materials, and a method of compounding them, very competent to our purpoſe; and having plainly ſeen, that there was a great difference in the effect, ariſing from the different *nature* of lime burnt from different kinds of limeſtone; and that its acquiſition of hardneſs under water did not depend upon the hardneſs of the ſtone; inaſmuch as *Chalk* lime appeared to be as good, as that burnt from *Plymouth* marble; and that Aberthaw lime was greatly ſuperior to either, for the purpoſe of aquatic buildings, though ſcarcely ſo hard as Plymouth marble; I was very deſirous to get ſome light into ſome of the *ſenſible* qualities, that might probably occaſion the difference, or at leaſt become a *mark* of diſtinction. I therefore applied to my friend Mr. Cookworthy, whom I had found at all times ready to afford me his aſſiſtance, wherever his knowledge could be of uſe to me. He taught me how to *analyze* limeſtones: and though my *chemical* friends will be at no loſs upon this ſubject; yet as it is very poſſible, that ſome of my readers may be no more acquainted with chemiſtry than myſelf; for the ſake of theſe I will deſcribe the proceſs, as being uſeful for all thoſe who are concerned in building to know.

177. I TOOK about the quantity of five penny weights (or a *guinea*'s weight) of the limeſtone to be tried, bruiſed to a coarſe powder; upon which I poured common *aqua fortis*, but not ſo much at a time as to occaſion the effervеſcence to overtop the glaſs veſſel in which the limeſtone was put; and added freſh aqua fortis after the effervеſcence of the former quantity had ceaſed, till no further ebullition appeared, by any addition of the *acid*. This done, and the whole being left to ſettle, the liquor will generally acquire a tinge of ſome tranſparent colour; and if from the ſolution little or no ſediment drops, it may be accounted a *pure* limeſtone (which is generally the caſe with white *Chalk* and ſeveral others) as containing no uncalcareous matter: but if from the ſolution a quantity of matter is depoſited in the form of mud, this indicates a quantity of uncalcareous matter in its compoſition. When this is well ſettled, pour off the water, and repeatedly add water in the ſame way, ſtirring it and letting it ſettle till it becomes taſteleſs. After this let the mud be well ſtirred into the water, and without giving it time to ſettle, pour off the muddy water into another veſſel: and if there is any ſand or gritty matter left behind (as will frequently be the caſe) this collected by itſelf will aſcertain the quantity and ſpecies of ſabulous matter that entered into the texture of the limeſtone. Letting now the muddy liquor ſettle, and pouring off the water, till no more can be got without an admixture of mud, leave the reſt to dry; which, when it comes to the conſiſtence of clay, or paſte, make it into a ball and dry it for farther examination.

178. ON treating common white chalk in this manner, the whole diſſolved into a tranſparent ſolution; and Plymouth marble, when free from apparent extraneous mixtures, did the ſame: but, as I found *Plaſter* would not effervеſce with the acid, I therefore concluded that it was a peculiar ſubſtance diſtinct from limeſtone, having nothing calcareous in its compoſition*; and therefore that its cementing property depended upon ſome different principle.——On trying *Aberthaw* lime in this way, it was diſſolved in the aqua fortis; but the ſolution appeared very dark and muddy, and on examination I found a ſmall quantity of undiſſolved ſandy particles at the bottom, *ſome* of them tranſparent like cryſtals, but moſtly very minute, and of a dirty appearance. The muddy *reſiduum* being brought into an argillaceous ſtate, was very tough and tenacious while ſoft; and when ſufficiently hardened, being worked into a little ball, and dried, in that ſtate it appeared to be a very fine compact dark blue clay, and weighed nearly one-eighth part of the original maſs. One of theſe balls having been burnt became a good compact *brick*,

* Plaſter or *Gypſum*, as I have ſince been informed, is an earthy ſalt compoſed of calcareous matter diſſolved in the acid of *Vitriol*.

which

which being of a reddish colour, it from thence appeared, as I was told was the case, that it had an admixture of iron in its composition. On weighing it, I found that it had lost near upon one-fourth part of its former weight in burning. *Bridistow* limestone, by the same mode of examination, exhibited nearly the same appearances.

179. FROM the experiments now related, I was convinced that the most *pure* limestone was not the best for making mortar, *especially* for building in water: and this brought to my mind a maxim I had learnt from workmen; that the best lime for the *Land* was seldom the best for *Building* purposes; of which the reason now appeared; which was, that the most pure lime affording the greatest quantity of *Lime Salts*, or impregnation, would best answer the purposes of *Agriculture*: whereas, for some reason or other, when a limestone is intimately mixed with a proportion of *Clay*, which by burning is converted into *Brick*, it is made to act more strongly as a Cement*.——This suggested to me the idea, that an admixture of *Clay* in the composition of limestone, when treated as above specified, might be the most certain index of the validity of a limestone for *Aquatic Buildings*: nor has any experience since contradicted it; as all the limestones in repute for water-works, that I have met with, have afforded this mark; even the *Darking* lime much esteemed for these uses at *London*, and in the country round about, is plainly nothing but a species of chalk, impregnated with clay, of which it makes one full seventeenth part of the original weight.

180. HAVING thus satisfied myself in respect to limestone, that, if I had not arrived at the best in the world, I had found one so competently good, as to answer every idea of what I could possibly want for the purpose of mortar for the Edystone Lighthouse: I considered that though *Tarras* was really endowed with those qualities, which had justly obtained it a reputation for water building; yet it was generally admitted to have some properties, that for our use were not quite so eligible.——In the first place, though it will cause most kinds of lime to set and become hard *under* water, as we have seen by several examples; yet if the Cement grows dry by a gradual exposure to the air, it never sets into a substance so hard as if the same lime had been mixed with good clean common sand; but is very friable, and crumbly: and if, after it has acquired a considerable degree of hardness by immersion in water, it is then exposed to the air, it *loses* a considerable part of its firmness, and also becomes crumbly: though according to my observation, it never becomes so much so, as if it never had acquired a greater hardness by a submersion in water.——For this reason, though there is no necessity for using it where the work will *always* be dry, or subjected only to the rain; and though it may be considered as being always wet, where it is in the joints of a massive work immersed every tide; yet in our case, those parts which were above the ordinary swell of the tide and sea, and liable to be wet only in storms, and hard gales of wind; and which, properly speaking, could never wholly be immersed, so that the pores might be thoroughly soaken with water; in such a state, between wet and dry, or of being wet and dry by intervals, tarras is known not to answer well. The knowledge, that in parts so circumstanced, the mortar is the most liable to fail, and to be affected by the frosts, whatever its composition may be, has put artificers upon trying other mixtures; one of the principal of which was communicated to me by *Lord* MACCLESFIELD in his letter as under†.

181. ANOTHER

* It is not to be wondered at, that workmen generally prefer the more *pure* limes for building in the *Air*, because being unmixed with any uncalcareous matter, they fall into the finest powder, and make the finest paste, which will of course receive the greatest quantity of *Sand* (generally the cheaper material) into its composition, without losing its toughness beyond a certain degree, and requires the least *labour* to bring it to the desired consistence: hence mortar made of such lime, is the least expensive; and in *dry work* the difference of hardness, compared with others, is less apparent.

" London, 14th April, 1757.

† " SIR,

" I was favoured with yours in due time, and should have sooner returned my thanks for it, had I not waited for a more " particular account of the manner of making the *Ash Mortar*, than I could give you merely from my memory: and for which I " therefore sent into the country, and received it only yesterday. It may not, however, be improper to inform you, that the lime " that

181. ANOTHER property of tarras mortar is, that when kept always wet, and consequently in a state most favourable to its cementing principle, it throws out a substance something like the stony concrescences in caverns of limestone *Strata*, called *Stalactites*; which substance from the tarras comes to a considerable degree of hardness, and in time becomes so extuberant as to deform the face of the walls; and when smoothness and regularity of surface is wanted, as in navigable *Sluices*, mill *Conduits*, &c. it becomes necessary to remove its roughness by tools; for otherwise the tarras mortar will *grow* so much in the joints of these conduits, as to knock off the *Floats* or *Ladle-boards* from the wheels. I was therefore desirous to try the properties of other substances, said to be useful in making calcareous mortar to set in water; one of which I had found mentioned by BELIDOR*; and that is the *Terra Puzzolana* found in *Italy*.——In making enquiries how some of this might be procured from thence, I very fortunately learnt, that there was a quantity of it then in the hands of a merchant in *Plymouth*; which had been imported as an adventure from *Civita Vecchia* during the time *Westminster Bridge* was building; and which he expected to have disposed of for that work to a good advantage; but failed in his speculation: for having found that tarras answered their purpose, neither *Commissioners*, *Engineers*, nor *Contractors*, would trouble themselves to make a trial of it, and therefore refused it. This proved a lucky circumstance to me; for it might otherwise have been many months before I could have got any for trial; and afterwards as many more, after finding it to answer, before I could have got a quantity from *Italy* for actual service.

182. ON trial of this, I soon found it in every respect equal to *Tarras*, as far as concerned the hardening of water-mortar, if not preferable to it. And the merchant having had it long by him, and the keeping it being an inconvenience, he declared himself desirous to get rid of it, considerably under the price of tarras; I therefore made no hesitation in purchasing the whole quantity; and had the satisfaction to find, so far as time would give leave, antecedent to my actual use of it, not only that it appeared fully to answer every good end of tarras; but in letting it dry immediately, or keeping the balls sometimes under water, and sometimes in the open air, in which latter state they were suffered to become perfectly dry; I perceived that in every state of it, if made into a mortar with *Aberthaw* lime, it exceeded in hardness any of the compositions commonly used in dry work; and in *wet* and *dry*, or wholly wet, was far superior to any I had ever seen or experienced; for, when the balls were immersed in water, they appeared to acquire hardness *progressively*; which progress, while they were out of the water and became dry, was indeed suspended, but yet they retained the hardness they had there acquired.——With respect to those balls that were kept constantly under water, they did not seem inclined to undergo any change in form, only to acquire hardness gradually, insomuch that I did not doubt but to make a cement that would equal the best *merchantable Portland Stone* in solidity and durability.

183. ALTHOUGH, in my main object, I had by degrees succeeded to my wishes; yet there was still one circumstance more that required investigation.——My reader will perceive from the nature of the bond that I proposed in my work (see Plate N° 13.) that one half of each piece of stone, being lodged in a dovetail recess, wherein it was locked fast on three sides, there was no way to get them into their places, but by letting them down perpendicularly: in consequence of this, mortar beat up and prepared in a manner

"that is generally made use of in my neighbourhood is made from chalk, of which we have great plenty: though I am sensible that *Stone Lime* is much stronger, and better; and that the strength and goodness of the Ash Mortar depends, in a great measure, upon its being well beat, in which there is no danger of excess. The manner of making it (as sent to me from the country) is as follows.

"Take of lime that is *very fresh*, two bushels, and take of wood-ashes three bushels. Lay the ashes in a round trench, and the lime in the middle of the trench; then slake the lime, and mix it well with the ashes. Let it lie thus till it is cold, and then beat it well together; and so beat it for three or four times before it is used.

"This mortar thus made is reckoned, by our bricklayers, to be much more strong than that prepared with tarras, in places that are at some times wet, and at others dry; though they acknowledge, that the tarras mortar is better in work that is constantly under water.

"It will give me much pleasure if this communication should be of any service to you at any time, and especially in carrying on the work you have now in hand, which is of so great importance, and of such public utility."

* Architecture Hydraulique, Part II. Tom II. p. 186. This indeed, is pointed out by VITRUVIUS in his Architecture, B. II. Ch. VI.

fimilar to what has been fpecified, could only be applied to the *ground* joint, or *under-bed* of each ftone: the upright, or fide joints (fuppofing the work to be clofe put together) could not be lined with any quantity capable of filling the whole joint; for if that was attempted, the ftone, in being *lowered* into its place, would carrry down the mortar, upon the fides, along with it; leaving fo little, as not to make thofe joints folid and full. It therefore muft become neceffary, to confolidate the upright joints, by pouring in *liquid* mortar, commonly called *Grout*, in fo fluid a ftate, as to run into every cavity and crevice.——The common way *then* in ufe of doing this was, by putting as much flaked lime into water, as when ftirred would be fufficiently fluid to anfwer the end; which is called *puttying*. And the *beft* way then in practice was, to put the ingredients together according to the due proportion, to make the fpecies of mortar intended, and with as much water as would render them fluid; and after *ftirring* them well together, to pour the mixture into the joints.——Seeing therefore of how much importance it was to the folidity of our work, to attain the beft method of *grouting*; and perceiving how great a degree of folidity was attained by the well *beating* of mortar, in comparifon of that which was only fparingly *beaten*; it occurred to me to try the following experiment.

184. I TOOK about three times the quantities of materials, that were neceffary to make a ball of the common fize I ufed in my other experiments, and beat them well together, as I ufed to do for the beft mortar; I then took the like quantities, and put them well mixed, but unbeaten, into a quart mug, with as much water, as that, when well ftirred, the compound might be capable of being poured, like metal, into a mould. I then gradually added water to the beaten mortar, fo as to reduce it by beating to fo foft a pulp, as to require a veffel to contain it, and put it into another quart pot, adding water by degrees, and ftirring it well, till this, like the other, was alfo capable of being poured into a mould.—— Both the pots, with their contents, were then depofited where they might be at reft; and within an hour the grofs matter of both had feparated from the water by fubfiding to the bottom, leaving the water clear at top.——The next day I perceived fo entire a feparation of the materials from the water that it had become perfectly clear in both. On putting down my finger to the fediment of the unbeat materials, I found it quite loofe and muddy, but making more refiftance underneath than at the top. The diffolved mortar made a refiftance equal to that of foft clay at the top, and of ftiff clay underneath: and afterwards examining them both from day to day, with a blunt-pointed ftick, I found them to acquire a progreffive firmnefs: for, in a week the unbeat ftuff was become clayey, being foft at top, but of a ftronger confiftence below; while at this time the diffolved mortar was fcarcely penetrable with the ftick at top, and feemed to have acquired a ftony hardnefs below. In the compafs of a month both mixtures were grown fo hard as not to be eafily feparable from the veffels: I therefore broke the pots, and found the contents of both had acquired a ftony confiftence, each hardeft at the bottom: that of the diffolved mortar being confiderably harder than the other, that is, of a moderate *ftony-hardnefs*; not indeed equal to that of balls of the fame age and compofition, yet of a degree of hardnefs very fatisfactory, and competent to my purpofes. And as it appeared that thofe compofitions, notwithftanding their being originally in a liquid ftate, and always having had water upon them, yet acquired a ftony hardnefs gradually; and that though they did it in a flower degree than undiffolved mortar; yet in *length* of *time*, the grout made of the diffolved mortar might become as compact as the undiffolved mortar; I had therefore no doubt of being able to unite the whole of the materials of my building into one *folid mafs of ftone*.

To avoid prolixity, I have mentioned thefe experiments as fingle trials; but they were all repeated, and fome of the principal ones feveral times. I alfo made trials of other compofitions, which for the fame reafon I think it unneceffary to mention; particularly feveral mixtures of lime with *Plafter*; and though I am aware that the plafterers ufe fome compofitions of this kind with advantage in their works, yet when fubjected to the teft for water-works, that I had eftablifhed for the conduct of my own experiments, I found nothing ufeful in all the mixtures of lime with plafter, nor even of tarras and puzzolana with plafter; as the refult was, that they rendered the plafter lefs fpeedy in fetting, and the plafter rendered the compound, that would have refulted from the other ingredients, lefs firm, and more crumbly.

185. THE

185. THE inquifitive reader will undoubtedly be defirous to know the nature of the two fubftances of fo much confequence in water building; viz. *Tarras* and *Puzzolana:* and I wifh I was able to fatisfy him in this refpect, as well as I truft I have been in the *application* of them to ufe. But if I tell him what has come to my knowledge and information, as this may incite the learned *Naturalift* and *Chemift* to enquire further, fo as to give us more accurate accounts of their origin, natural compofition, and properties, what I have to fay on this head may have its ufe.

When I was in *Holland* in the year 1755, I made it my bufinefs to enquire, as particularly as I could, concerning the *Tarras.* I there faw the tarras ftones, and was informed that they were brought down the rivers from *Germany,* (if I remember right, from the province of *Liege)* where this material is dug in mines under ground, and lies in regular *Strata.* I found it in lumps of various fizes, from the bignefs of a pea to that of a middle-fized turnip. This ftony fubftance is called in *Holland* the *Duif Steen,* fignifying the *Dove Stone,* as I was told: it is of a light greyifh colour, or afh colour, is rather tender than hard, and is very *porous,* fomewhat refembling a pumice-ftone. It is brought to Holland in the fame ftate as it is taken out of the earth, and the only art that is there employed in preparing it for ufe is, to reduce it to a coarfe powder, by means of mills for that purpofe, which I faw. It is beat by iron-headed *Stampers* upon an iron bed, till it paffes through a fieve of a certain finenefs, equivalent to one of ours, having about eight wires in an inch; it is then ready for ufe, and is generally fent from Holland in cafks.——There feems to be nothing calcareous in its compofition, for aqua fortis dropped upon it only wets it like water: to me it much refembles fome *petrifactions* that I have feen; but my more learned friends feem to be of opinion that it is a *Lava* *.

186. THE Puzzolana is alfo a *porous* fubftance, and, like the tarras, produces no effervefcence with aqua fortis: it has much the appearance of being a *volcanic* production, is of a brown colour, and, as my friend Mr. COOKWORTHY told me, contains iron; it has the look of an iron ore rendered porous, or burnt to a cinder by fire. It is faid to be found in large quantities in the neighbourhood of Mount *Vefuvius* and in feveral other parts of *Italy.* That which was the fubject of my experiments, as well as the beft of what I have fince caufed to be imported, or have feen, was from *Civita Vecchia:* I have feen a kind of puzzolana faid to be brought from *Naples,* of a lefs ruddy and more grey colour, but on trial I did not find it to be near fo ftrong as the former; for, one half of the quantity from *Civita Vecchia* would caufe a compofition of calcareous mortar to fet harder in water, than that from *Naples* would do. ——It is faid, that the ancient baths and water-works of the *Romans* were built with this kind of mortar; and their duration has, it feems, proved the validity of the compofition: but I apprehend, unlefs they have the *Lyas* limeftone in Italy †, it was referved to the *Edyftone,* to have thofe two materials firft combined; and of confequence, fo far as has yet appeared, the perfect compofition of water mortar was now firft afcertained to be a proper mixture of blue *lyas* lime and puzzolana.

187. SEEING that both tarras and puzzolana agreed in two of their obvious properties, porofity, and refiftance to the action of aqua fortis, as well as the hardening of calcareous mortar under water; and alfo, as *volcanic* fubftances, in having paffed the fire ‡, I was induced to try experiments on feveral porous fubftances, that appeared to have fome fimilarity to them; fuch as *Pumice Stone, Coal Cinders, Brick* and *Tile Duft,* and fuch like. I found them all poffeffed of an abforbent property, which caufed the mortar made with them to fet fomewhat more quickly, than when made up with fand only: fo that where hardnefs is expected from *drying,* and time is wanted to produce the effect fully, they may be ufe-

* I now underftand that this fubftance, when prepared for ufe, is by the *Dutch* called *Tras,* from which our appellation of *Tarras* undoubtedly originates. It is by fome faid to be brought from *Andernach.* It is fuppofed to be the fame as the *Peparino* of the *Italians*; which, as I underftand, according to BERGMAN, is a concretion of *Volcanic* Cinders.

† *Lyas* is the general term for *ftrata* of ftone of the fpecies of *Alertbaw,* in feveral counties.

‡ If *Tarras* and *Puzzolana* are much of the fame nature, it would be curious to know why one fubftance caufes the mortar to alter its form, or, as the workmen call it, *grow* in the joints under water; and the other to lie quiet.

ful

ful to this end, in procuring it to be done more *speedily*; but being, when set, immersed in water, they did not appear to possess any powers of resistance to their dissolution, more than the same lime would do with common sand, if, by a little *more* time, the composition was become equally set.

188. HAVING made up my mind, that the proper composition for our mortar was, lime of *blue Lyas*, and *Puzzolana*, in equal quantities; and having procured a sufficient quantity of puzzolana; it was now time to think of securing to ourselves, a sufficient supply either of *lyas* lime, or lime*stone*.—— In making enquiries on this head, I learnt that, for doing such water building as they wanted at the city of *Exeter*, they procured the *blue lyas* lime ready burnt, from *Watchet*, a small sea-port of *Somersetshire*, lying upon the *Bristol Channel*, almost right across the *Peninsula*; but which, though near forty miles north from *Exeter*, they were obliged to carry on horses backs: for if they waited to have it brought by sea, round the *Land's End*, it would, in the length of time thus necessarily expended, attract so much moisture from the air, that it would be reduced again to the state of *Limestone*; after which, it would not fall into powder by *quenching*: and even if it got wet in the land carriage by the fall of rain, this would happen in such a degree, that they were obliged to quench it with boiling water; and if that would not do, it was concluded to be spoilt.——Upon this information, it appeared to me, that the best way of procuring it in a sufficient quantity for our use would be in the stone, and to burn it in our works at *Mill Bay*: but as the right management, and a thorough knowledge, of this article appeared of the utmost consequence; that I might get all possible information concerning it, I determined to take a journey for that purpose to the country where it was produced, and in common use.

189. I SET out therefore on the sixth of April, and first went to *Minehead*, another small port upon the Bristol Channel, a few miles farther west than *Watchet*; having been informed, that the *Pier* of Minehead had been built partly with lime from *Watchet*, and partly with that of *Aberthaw*; which lies also upon the Bristol Channel, nearly opposite to it, upon the *Welch* coast.——On examining the works of this pier, it appeared to me, that those done with *Watchet* lime were quite as good, or even preferable to those done with that from *Aberthaw*; the parts so done being pointed out to me by a workman upon the spot, that had been employed in the erection: but as all agreed that they were the very same *Strata* of lyas-stone, that were found on each side the *Channel*, though at the distance of twenty miles; what difference there was, might very easily arise from a difference of treatment in making the mortar, or a more favourable season of the year when the work was executed.

In passing through *Dunster*, from Minehead to Watchet, as all the buildings in that part of the country were erected with lyas lime, I took care to remark the appearance of every kind, both wet and dry. And though the workmanship in general appeared but coarsely performed, yet the mortar bore to me the evident marks of being excellent; for, wherever I saw it, however coarsely it was done, yet it appeared full and flush in the joints, without cracks, or losing its original skin, or becoming crumbly; as often is the case with mortar of a tender kind, after having gone through two or three winters, or more: and in one place I remarked the foundation of a little bridge, that by some accident had been driven down; but the mortar, over which the current was making its way, I found, on trying it with my knife, to have acquired such a stony hardness, as, with a coat of moss, effectually defended it from the action of the water; yet it was considerably inferior, in hardness and firmness, to the balls I had made with lyas lime mixt either with *Tarras*, or *Puzzolana*.

190. ON my arrival at *Watchet*, I first examined the pier there, which, though but a rough piece of work, I found to be quite satisfactory, as to the mortar part; and learnt, that they made no scruple of mixing it up with *Sea* water.——On viewing the situation, in which the *Lyas Stone* lies here in its natural bed, I found, that the sea retreated from the shore to a considerable breadth, or distance, at low water; and in this inclining surface very many *Strata* of lyas stone, of different thicknesses, appear, chiefly from four or five to ten or eleven inches thick, but all apparently of the same quality; being indiscrimi-

nately taken by the lime-burners according as they find them most convenient to be come at.——These *Strata* are not much inclined to the horizon, but more so than the general inclination of the shore; and therefore, as they dip towards the low water mark, a vast number are exposed to view. The *Lyas* seems universally to lie in a bed of uncalcareous laminated blue matter, and which, when exposed to the weather, seems to turn to much of the same kind of looking clay, that I found by my experiments to be intimately mixed with the calcareous *Strata*.——The bed, or *Matrix* in which the Lyas lies, being of a softish perishable nature, it is found easy to detach the stone with an iron *Crow*; and therefore though there is plenty of the same kind of stone to be found in *Strata* within land; yet as there is no great demand for this kind of lime, the lime-burners can procure what they want in sufficient quantity from the shelving sea-shore just described, with more ease than by laying open the ground.

It perhaps will seem wonderful, that for a lime so excellent in quality there should be no great demand; for in reality I found but one small lime-kiln; and that not kept constantly at work: but considering the occasions of the neighbouring country for building-lime not to be great; and the charge, trouble, and difficulty attending the carrying it to a distance to be considerable; and that it does not suit the purposes of *Agriculture*, even upon the very spot where it is produced, the wonder will undoubtedly cease: and I was informed by the lime-burners themselves, that for the use of their own farm, they were obliged to get lime from the rocks of *St. Vincent* near the *Hot Wells* of *Bristol*; or of that quality, at the distance of more than 40 miles: for, they told me, were they to lay their own lime (though reduced to a fine powder) upon the land, the first shower of rain would turn it all to stone, without affording any sensible cultivation to the land: and as the rocks of *St. Vincent*, are somewhat like the *Plymouth* marble; this circumstance affords another proof, that the qualities of lime, for different uses, do not depend upon the *hardness*, but upon the *specific* qualities of the stone from whence it is burnt.

A question now arose, how I was to get supplied with lime in the quantity I wanted; as I found that the lime-burners were under a prohibition from the lord of the manor, to send away unburnt stone: and also that the difficulties of getting it on horseback across the country to *Exeter*, &c. were not exaggerated: but I was informed, that this lime, if burnt to a due degree, and quenched hot from the kiln, would fall to a powder as freely as any other kind of lime; and that to prevent its imbibing moisture from the air, they always mixed it up for use, as soon, or as *hot* (as they term it) as possible, and having so done, find it to set the stronger, when used for works under water. They also informed me, that, if kept *close* from the *Air*, it would preserve its virtue for a considerable length of time. Consequently nothing in this mode was to be depended on, but *Water tight* casks; the procuring of which without great expence and loss of time, appeared a considerable difficulty; as it was at first apprehended they must be brought from *Bristol*.——On enquiry however I found that much cyder was produced in this part of the country; and fortunately it was a time of the year, when many of the casks for this liquor were empty.——What quantity of *casking* would hold a given quantity of burnt lime was a matter untried; as this mode of sending it away was not in use with them.——I wished much to see the process of burning it, and quenching it when burnt; and therefore by way of investigating what quantity of casking would be wanted, I ordered a kiln of lime to be put on, and having procured some *Cyder* casks, and the lime to be quenched and sifted, immediately from the kiln; it slaked as I had been told, very freely, affording a very soft impalpable powder. We proceeded upon the package as follows.——I caused a quantity of their burnt lime, which they delivered for a *Hogshead* and half, to be weighed from the kiln, which was 4½ cwt. This being quenched, and sifted, the dry meal was the same weight as before: so that the water it had imbibed in quenching compensated for the waste in sifting: and in this state the produce from the hogshead and half, of *lime measure*, could be rammed into a cyder hogshead cask; so that in reality it was of less bulk and weight than it would have been if sent away *unslaked*, and of considerably less weight than it would have been if sent in the unburnt stone; which, in common with other limestones, is found to lose a considerable part of its weight in burning. The quantity therefore of 20 tons, which I proposed to procure, would be packed in 90 such hogsheads. I therefore employed a reputable merchant there to procure the casks, hire a vessel, and forward the lime; and 135 hogsheads of burnt lime, rammed into 80 caſks, containing in the whole 110 hogſheads wine meaſure, arrived at *Mill Bay* ſoon after my return*.

191. THE *blue Lyas* ſtone of *Watchet* is of a dead ſky blue†, of a very fine even froſted grain when broken, with few ſhining particles. There is alſo in ſeveral parts of that county another kind of limeſtone, which they call the *white Lyas*; which has the ſame kind of grain, with a ſmall quantity of ſhining particles, and has much the ſame appearance, the colour only excepted, as the blue; it alſo lies in *Strata* of nearly the ſame thickneſs; and though of a chalky whiteneſs, is quite as hard, or rather harder than the blue: yet it is held in no eſtimation for *Water Works*; and at which indeed when I had *analyzed* it, I did not wonder, as I found it almoſt wholly to diſſolve, and become ſuſpended in aqua fortis. The *Reſiduum*, which was very ſmall in quantity, was of a light reddiſh colour, and contained a few particles of tranſparent cryſtals.——In paſſing the cliffs upon the ſea coaſt between Minehead and Watchet, I found frequent veins of *Gypſum* or plaſter, interſperſed with *Strata* of limeſtone, of a kind having impreſſions of foſſil ſhells included in it; but obſerved no appearance of marks of foſſil ſhells in either the *blue Lyas* of Watchet, or the *white Lyas* of *Somerſetſhire*.

192. BEING now determined as to the compoſition of the mortar for the Edyſtone; I might here very properly put a period to this part of my ſubject: but my reader, after giving him the preceding account of its great utility, will not perhaps be diſpleaſed, if I communicate to him the principal obſervations that have occurred to me in a courſe of thirty years practice in water building.

As nothing could ſucceed better, or be more ſatisfactory, than the mortar I uſed, as will be further ſeen in the courſe of my proceedings; I wiſhed to examine all thoſe limes which diſcovered any degree of fitneſs for *Water Building*; and more eſpecially, if poſſible, to find out a ſubſtitute for *Tarras* and *Puzzolana* in this kingdom; that we might be in poſſeſſion of *all* the beſt materials for water building within ourſelves: and though I own I have not ſucceeded with reſpect to the latter, ſo far as my ardent wiſhes led me to hope; yet as I have ſince learnt how to compoſe water cement with a far leſs proportion of the foreign materials than I at firſt uſed, and upon the whole at a much leſs expence, I truſt this inveſtigation will be thought material and uſeful.

The Limes that I have ſince examined are as follows:

193. 1ſt. THAT of *Barrow* in *Leiceſterſhire*, of which we uſed conſiderable quantities in the *Calder Navigation*. I never was at the quarries, but having procured ſome of the unburnt ſtone, I found it had the appearance of blue Lyas, only ſomewhat of a more yellow tinge, and more of the ſlate kind: it burns to a buff coloured lime like that of Aberthaw and Watchet, and on diſſolution affords nearly [illegible]ths of its original weight, of blue clay, with a minute quantity of dirty grey ſand; ſo that I have no doubt of its being the true *Lyas*, though perhaps of a leſs perfect compoſition than that bordering on the *Briſtol Channel*. It contains more clay, can be carried further, and remains longer without injury‡; but in the actual uſe thereof as mortar, it does not appear to me to acquire quite ſo firm and ſtony a hardneſs, as the blue Lyas of *Somerſetſhire*. It makes however excellent water mortar, if properly treated, and will very well ſerve in thoſe parts of the kingdom that are more acceſſible to the *Trent* navigation, than that of the *Briſtol Channel*.——In fact, in travelling from *Glamorganſhire* through *Monmouthſhire*, *Glouceſterſhire*, and *Warwick-*

* This mode of conveyance was in reality ſo ſucceſsful, that ſeveral caſks of this very lime which remained, after the Lighthouſe was finiſhed, were afterwards carried into *Yorkſhire*, and uſed in the moſt critical part of the works of the River *Calder*, and remained perfectly good from the year 1757 to the laſt uſed in 1764: only, that as it had become ſomewhat lumpy, the fine powder was ſifted out, and the reſt by gentle bruiſing was reduced to powder, ſo that the whole paſſed through a fine wire ſieve.

† This was the deſcription of it at the time, but on breaking a ſpecimen of it that I have now by me, I ſhould rather ſay, it is of a dark lead colour, ſomewhat inclining to brown. I therefore ſuſpect it has altered its colour by keeping.

‡ The practice in ſending it away is, in the *burnt ſtone*, packed *unquenched* in caſks that have held ſugar and grocer's dry goods; but where the demand is conſiderable, I have practiced myſelf the getting the unburnt ſtone, and calcining it upon the place.

ſhire,

ſhire, into *Leiceſterſhire*, I found ſuch frequent inſtances of ordinary walls and cottages, built with ſtone that appeared to me to be blue *Lyas*, the mortar alſo being of the ſame hue, that I have not a doubt, but that the curious naturaliſt, in making this expreſsly an object of ſearch, would be able to trace it from *Aberthaw* and *Watchet* quite to *Barrow*; though probably with ſeveral breaks, as is uſual in the arrangement of the *Strata* of the earth. At *Bath* they pave the ſtreets with a ſpecies of Lyas; and to render the pavement more durable by keeping out the wet, they joint the paving with mortar of the ſame kind of ſtone.——The Bath *Free Stone* is of the pure calcareous kind; and it is remarked, that when it is walled with this kind of mortar, which is *frequently*, if not generally, uſed for the purpoſe, the joints are more permanent, and reſiſt the weather even better, than the ſtone itſelf: and it is this circumſtance, which gives that peculiar firmneſs to be obſerved in the light and thin walls of the buildings of that city.——From *Leiceſterſhire* it appears to paſs by the Vale of *Belvoir* into *Nottinghamſhire* and *Lincolnſhire*; for, a ſpecies of this kind of lime is uſed in ſome of the buildings about *Newark**; and the *Great North Road* is repaired with the blue Lyas ſtone for a conſiderable length in the poſt ſtage between *Newark* and *Grantham*: at *Long Bennington* (a village of *Lincolnſhire*, through which the road paſſes on that ſtage) there is a lime-kiln for burning it. I have not yet ſeen it farther north than this, nor any where north of the *Trent*. The limeſtone at Long Bennington contains $\frac{1}{5}$ blue clay.

194. 2d. PERHAPS nothing will better ſhew that the qualities of lime for water mortar do not depend on hardneſs or colour, than a compariſon of the white Lyas of *Somerſetſhire*, (which, though approaching to a flinty hardneſs, has yet a chalky appearance) with what is called near *Lewis* in *Suſſex*, the *Clunch Lime*; a kind of lime in great repute there for water works, and indeed deſervedly ſo. This is no other than a ſpecies of chalk, not found, like the Lyas, in thin *Strata*, but in thick maſſes, as chalk generally is: it is conſiderably harder than common chalk, but yet of the loweſt degree of what may be denominated a ſtony hardneſs; it is heavier than common chalk, and not near ſo white, inclining toward a yellowiſh aſh colour.——This ſtone, when analyzed, is found to contain $\frac{3}{20}$th parts of its weight of yellowiſh clay, with a ſmall quantity of ſand, ſeemingly of the cryſtal kind, not quite tranſparent, but intermixed with red ſpots. Hence the fitneſs of lime for water building ſeems neither to depend upon the hardneſs of the ſtone, the thickneſs of the *ſtratum*, nor the bed or matrix in which it is found, nor merely on the *quantity* of clay it contains: but, in burning and falling down into a powder of a *buff* coloured tinge, and in containing a conſiderable quantity of clay, I have found all the water limes to agree. Of this kind I eſteem the lime from *Darking* in *Surrey* to be; which is brought to London under the idea of its being burnt from a *Stone*, and in conſequence of that, of its being *ſtronger* than the chalk lime in common uſe there; though in fact it is a *chalk*, and not much harder than common chalk: it contains $\frac{1}{7}$ part of light coloured clay of a *yellowiſh* tinge.

195. 3d. THERE is in *Lancaſhire* a lime famous for water building, called *Sutton* lime: I have lately had an opportunity, by favour of JOHN GILBERT, Eſq. to get a ſpecimen of the ſtone in its natural ſtate. I had long ſince ſeen it in the Duke of BRIDGEWATER's works both in the burnt ſtone and ſlaked, made up for uſe, and in the water. I obſerved that it agreed with the Lyas in being of a *buff Caſt*. The ſtone itſelf is of a deep brown colour, and the piece I have is from a ſtratum about three inches thick, with a white clayey coat on each ſide. The goodneſs of the quality, as water lime, does not therefore conſiſt in the colour before it is burnt; for we have already ſeen *blue*, *whitiſh*, and now *brown*, to be all good for that purpoſe; but they all agree in the colour or hue, *after* they are burnt and quenched: and having analyzed the Sutton limeſtone, I find it to contain not only near $\frac{3}{8}$th parts of the original weight of the ſtone of brown or red clay, but alſo $\frac{1}{32}$dth of fine brown ſand; ſo that in reality I have ſeen no lime yet, proved to be good for water building, but what, on examination of the ſtone, contained clay: and though I am very far from laying this down as an abſolute *Criterion*, yet I have never found any limeſtone containing clay in a conſiderable quantity, but what was good for water building; and limes of this kind

* The lime quarries from whence *Newark* is ſupplied with this kind of lime is from the village of *Cuddington*, about 2½ miles S. E. from Newark, and betwixt the North Road and the *Trent*.

all

all agree in one more property, that of being of a dead frosted surface on breaking, without much appearance of shining particles.

106. SINCE the above was written, I have had the opportunity of examining others of the *Water-Limestones*. I find a species of lime has been used in some of the works about *Portsmouth*, and recommended as very good for water building, where the expence of *Tarras* mortar made with chalk lime could not be *afforded*. It is called *Grey Lime*, as having been burnt from a species of stone called *Grey Chalk*. This by inspection I observed to agree so nearly with the *Clunch* lime I had formerly observed near *Lewis* (and then analyzed) that in a consultation with His *Majesty's Engineers* concerning certain works at *Portsmouth*, I ventured to recommend it to be used in those works, in *preference of common Chalk Lime*, for forming a proper *Water-Cement*. This *Grey Lime* goes by land carriage from the parish of *Berryton* near *Petersfield* in *Hampshire* to *Portsmouth*. I visited the place, and observed that the country thereabouts was of this kind of chalk; and they call it here *Grey* lime, by way of distinction from common chalk or *white* lime: yet in its colour, hardness, and appearance both before burning and after, it is so like the *Sussex Clunch* before described, that I would not undertake by sight to distinguish them. Its appearance was also similar to that of the *Darking* lime before mentioned; and though the *Grey Lime* afforded, on dissolution, a less quantity of clay than *Sussex Clunch*, yet it yielded [illegible]th part of clay; which is a considerably greater proportion than the *Darking* lime affords; and yet I have proved this last in use to be a very competent *Water Lime*.

In my return from *Portsmouth* in April 1787, I recollected that about twenty-five years ago I was consulted about putting on foot the extension of the navigation of the river *Wey* from Guildford to *Godalmin*; and being then shewn the different chalk pits in the neighbourhood of Guildford, I recommended it to the *resident* surveyor to make use of one, in preference to the rest I saw, for building the locks, &c. merely because it had a *clayey look*; not imagining at that time (which was considerably antecedent to my acquaintance with the *Sussex Clunch*) that any *very* good water lime could be produced by any kind of *Chalk*. This induced me now to visit *Guildford Lock*; and in going thither, I found the *hawling* track for the navigation by horses, made good and covered with this very chalk stone broken small: and on examining the lock I found the mortar joints of the brick walling very compleat, especially where they were frequently immersed in water.——On bringing away a fragment with me for examination, I find it to contain [illegible]th parts of a dark coloured clay: the stone, however, is of a *yellowish* hue, much like all the chalks I have mentioned as containing clay.——Whether this lime has by these or any other means become known in the neighbourhood of *Guildford*, as peculiarly good for water works, I had not the means then of getting proper information: but whether so, or not, this may prove an useful hint to the London *Builders*, as these lime-stones may, by means of the water-carriage, be brought *raw* down to *London*, and burnt here; where coals are cheaper than at Guildford: and I am also led to think, that the curious naturalist will find some connection of this lime-stone to subsist through all this range of *Chalk Hills*, from Lewis to *Petersfield*; and probably from thence into *Surrey*, to Guildford and *Darking*.

In travelling the west road from *Bridport* in *Dorsetshire* to *Axminster*, the country puts on much the appearance of the *Blue Lyas*; and from a shard I broke off from a wall at *Axminster*, I have proved that it contains clay in considerable quantity; but was particularly happy in being informed from the ocular testimony of my highly respected friends the honourable Mr. CAVENDISH and Dr. BLAGDEN, the *blue Lyas* actually exists in quantity at *Lyme** in the same county; and is there burnt into lime for sale: which place being a small *Sea-port*, upon the strength of this information, I not only recommended it in 1787 to be used in the *King's Works* at *Plymouth*, instead of lime from their own marble, where water is concerned, but propose also to use it for the same kind of works at *Ramsgate* harbour. And I have not the least doubt, but that after it is known, *what to look for*, good water lime will be discovered in many

* *Lyme* being almost right across the *Isthmus*, and not above forty miles distant from *Watchet*, it is probable this *Stratum* is found at i[illegible] places.——Since the above was settled for the press I have been at LYME, and have had the opportunity of confirming the above from [illegible] ocular inspection. There is a small limekiln upon the pier, (or *Cobb* as called;) but what goes away by water, is [illegible] stone.

distant

distant parts of this kingdom, either of the *Lyas* or the *Chalk* species; which last, though seemingly very distinct, yet so nearly conduces to the same end, that (exclusive of my *original partiality*) I am almost at a loss which to prefer.

The following *Table* contains, in one view, the account of nine different *Water* limestones that I have already particularly mentioned to have analyzed.

N°	Species of Limestone.	Proportion of Clay.	Colour of the Clay.	Reduction of Weight by burning.	Colour of the Brick.
1	Aberthaw - - -	[illegible]	Lead colour	4 to 3	Grey stock brick.
2	Watchet - - -	[illegible]	The same	4 — 3	Light colour, reddish hue.
3	Barrow - - - -	$\frac{1}{18}$	The same	3 — 2	Grey stock brick.
4	Long Bennington -	[illegible]	The same	—	Dirty blue.
5	Sussex Clunch - -	$\frac{1}{20}$	Ash colour	3 — 2	Ash colour.
6	Darking - - -	$\frac{1}{17}$	The same		
7	Berryton Grey Lime -	$\frac{1}{15}$	The same		
8	Guildford - - -	$\frac{2}{19}$	The same		
9	Sutton - - - -	$\frac{1}{16}$	Brown		

197. UPON the subject of a *Succedaneum* for *Tarras* or *Puzzolana*, I have not seen any thing similar in appearance to *Tarras*, but what has been of the *calcareous* kind; but as the puzzolana was found to contain some iron, and I had seen masses of gravel strongly cemented (as it appeared to me) with nothing but pieces of malleable iron turned to rust, I had better expectations of success from the iron tribe. I therefore tried the scales that fall from the iron at a smith's anvil, which have long been known to be an excellent ingredient in making calcareous cement, and particularly where exposed to weather, or where water is concerned; and which being well powdered, and mixed with lime, in the same proportion, and treated in the same manner, as puzzolana, I found (so far as I could observe) to produce an *equal* effect.——A peck of smith's forge scales is easily collected occasionally, to do a small *Job*; but to procure four or five tons, would be far more expensive than to bring so much puzzolana from *Italy*. With a view therefore to works requiring large quantities, I tried *Iron Ore*, after it had passed the fire, and undergone what is commonly called calcination.——This being powdered, I found had a very good effect in water mortar, in causing it to set speedily, in preventing cracks, and finally, in hardening it. On this account it was used in the *Calder Navigation*, for the inside mortar of the best work, and for the *face work* of the subordinate parts: but its strength in hardening lime was far inferior to that of *Puzzolana* or of *Forge Scales*. What I used was the siftings of the iron stone, after calcination at the iron furnaces; which being deemed too small and light to go into the furnace, was thereby the better adapted to my use. I found that at the iron works it had been frequently made use of, to mix with lime in making mortar for the construction and repair of the water-building part of their *own* works; and the parts so sifted not being too large for the joints of their masonry, and having it in plenty at hand, they used it as it was; but after a land carriage of several miles, when brought to us, we ground it on a mill, to open its qualities and make it more effectual, as well as go further. This material, among the furnace men in these parts, is called *Minion**.

198. MINION, or iron stone burnt where it can be had in plenty, is a good *succedaneum* for puzzolana and tarras; and if it is made up with lyas, or other proper water lime, in equal quantities, will make a mortar more firm and hard than common lime, made up with the common quantity of tarras or

* *Minion* is supposed by Mr. MITCHELL to be what chiefly falls from the outside of the lumps of the iron stone, and therefore containing more clay.

puzzolana *: and hence we may be said to have materials within ourselves, to serve the general purposes of water works; but not so perfectly and compleatly, as by the use of either of the foreign materials above specified.

Wherever I have met with a reddish, or a brownish stone, I have generally made trial of it, but never yet found any thing to answer so well as forge scales; except once, that I picked up a kind of coarse deep brown sand stone, somewhat of a tender nature; which having burnt, powdered, sifted, and mixed with *slaked* lime, I made into a ball, and it proved of equal firmness with forge scales: but as it was a fragment found upon the surface of the earth, intermixed with others of different colour and kind, without the appearance of my being able to procure a quantity of it, I saw no probable use likely to result from this discovery, further than that of the reason for which I mention it; which is, that of demonstrating the existence in nature of the material we want, in this kingdom, if we could but tell where to find a quarry, or sufficient stratum of it; in which, though I have not succeeded myself, yet others may find a quantity either of this, or something equivalent to it †.

199. I COME now to shew the means I have used to make a given quantity of tarras, or puzzolana, produce a greater quantity of good *Water Mortar*, than either the common composition, where the dear material is sparingly used; or that I used at the Edystone, where nothing was spared that had the appearance of being of service.——And if upon this head, I should somewhat enlarge, I flatter myself, I shall be forgiven by a majority of my readers.——Limestone, as it is now generally known, loses about [illegible]ths its weight by burning, but shrinks an inconsiderable quantity in point of bulk ‡; but upon quenching it, when fully burnt, it falls freely, and will produce somewhat better than double the quantity of powder or *slaked lime*, in point of measure, that the burnt limestone consisted of; and this will be nearly the case, whether it is common lime or *water* lime. Supposing it common lime, if this is beat into a paste with a sufficient quantity of water, it will not in this state occupy quite half the space it did before in powder; but if to this paste from two measures of lime, we add one measure of tarras, which makes the ordinary composition of *Tarras Mortar*, the quantity will be enlarged, so as to produce about 1¼ measure of mortar; and then the bulk will be something greater than it was in either the burnt or unburnt stone §.

200. THE use of sand in mortar, so far as I have been able to observe, is twofold; 1st. To render the composition harder; and 2dly, To increase it in quantity, by a material, that in most situations is of far less expence, bulk for bulk, than lime. As there is no apparent change in the sand, by the admixture of the lime, the sand seems only to render the composition harder, by itself being a harder body; for the best sand, being small fragments of flint, crystal, *quartz*, &c. is much harder than any body we

* The following composition I directed to be used in building the first *Lock* upon the *River Calder*, in the year 1760; and which I lately transcribed from the *Memorandum* Book of Mr. JOSEPH NICKALLS, *Civil Engineer*, at that time *resident Surveyor* of the River Calder.

For *Face* Mortar, *Barrow* Lime	— — measures	4
Ground *Minion*	— — —	2
Coarse Sand	— — — —	2
Fine Sand	— — — —	2

And for the rubble backing; to the above composition, add eight measures of small gravel, or pebbles, the largest not larger than a horse-bean; which application of *Pebbles* was taken from what I observed at *Corf Castle*, §. 99.

† This stone was picked up in the high part of the country, in the beaten track of a moor, called *Wooley Edge*, not far west of the direct road between *Wakefield* and *Barnsley* in *Yorkshire*, and where a number of stones of the same kind may be found; but yet it would be attended with some trouble to gather a cart load of it.

‡ My experiments were upon *Water* limestones; but according to the experiments of the *Bishop* of LANDAFF, upon various kinds of common limestone, it did not appear with certainty to have shrunk at all. See WATSON's *Chemical Essays*, vol. ii. page 230.

§ Two measures of *Water Lime* in powder, will produce nearly one measure of paste; and this, with one measure of tarras or puzzolana, will produce nearly 1$\frac{1}{10}$ measure of mortar.

know

know of, that can be formed of lime only; and which, in paſte, is to be conſidered as a cement to the harder materials, and therefore compoſes a harder body; for the ſame reaſon that, if we had nothing naturally, but lime as a cement, and ſhould build a wall with flints, cryſtals, or rough ſtones cemented therewith, this wall would be far harder than if built with lime alone.

201. THE experience of ages has ſhewn, that a conſiderable quantity of ſand and other matter may be introduced with advantage in the making of mortar; but the proportion has never been agreed in: yet from common experience it appears, that there is ſcarcely any lime, but what, if well burnt and beaten, a load, or meaſure of lime, will take two loads or meaſures of ſand; that is, the quantity of ſand that can be introduced into its compoſition may be equal to the lime in powder: and conſequently if, as in tarras mortar, one meaſure of tarras is ſufficient to give to two meaſures of ſlaked lime a ſufficient *indurating* property, to make the compoſition acquire the propoſed degree of hardneſs under water; then if another meaſure of clean ſand is added, this will only give to the lime that quantity of the harder material that it would bear for building in the air; and this without hurting its cementing property in water; for as the ſand can hardly be ſuppoſed to act on either material, ſo as to alter their *chymical* action on one another; it will, at the ſame time that it increaſes the bulk of the whole to half as much more, be cemented together by the other ingredients, and make (for the ſame reaſons as in dry work) a *harder* compoſition.——Thus far we are warranted to proceed from the common practice; and as this increaſes the quantity, that would reſult from the common tarras compoſition, in proportion of 2 to 3, I was therefore willing to try this matter further. Thus,

A compoſition of this kind is further increaſed in bulk, by another meaſure of ſand, ſo that one cube foot or meaſure of the common tarras mortar compoſition will by this means become two, and quite as good in every reſpect.——Finding this idea ſo far to anſwer, not only in experiment, but my expectations ſatisfied in works at large, I was induced to try whether lime would not bear a ſtill greater addition of ſand; and I ſoon found that it would, with good beating, take in, for every two meaſures of ſlaked lime, one meaſure of tarras, and three of clean ſand; which would produce nearly 3½ meaſures of good water mortar, or full 2⅓ times the common quantity of mortar from the ſame quantity of tarras and lime; this being near upon four times the bulk in *ſolid mortar*, of the unquenched lime, or the unburnt ſtone.

202. STILL purſuing the ſame line of experiment, to ſee how far this matter could be carried, it appeared that even yet a greater proportion of ſand might be introduced; but to bring it to a proper conſiſtence and toughneſs, ſo as to be a good cement to large ſtones, I found it needed ſo much *more* beating, that the *labour* became, in moſt caſes, of more value than the ſaving of materials*.——Thus far I had proceeded

* This laſt proportion of lime to ſand (allowing for the tarras, which does not appear to me to make ſo great an increaſe of bulk as is made by common ſand) nearly agrees with the greateſt mixture of ſand with lime in the experiments of Dr. HIGGINS; ſee *Calcareous Cements*, page 48; wherein N° 5, contains a mixture of lime to ſand as 1 to 8; yet as this is expreſsly by *weight*, and as the weight of Thames ſand is nearly 4½ times the weight of ſuch common lime as I have tried, bulk for bulk, this will not amount to the full proportion of two meaſures of ſand to one of lime in powder: and though the *Doctor* ſays that this "Specimen was not ſufficiently plaſtic for common "uſe, or, as the workmen expreſs themſelves, it was *too ſhort*;" yet as his experiments ſeem, in a great meaſure, to turn upon the method of compounding calcareous cements for *dry work*; where they are continually in a *ſtate of moiſture*, this objection will not apply: beſides, it appears VITRUVIUS allowed two meaſures of ſea or river ſand to one of lime, and three of pit ſand to the ſame quantity of lime; and that he means *Lime in the Powder* is plain, becauſe he ſays expreſsly, the lime when *quenched* is mixed in the proportion of one to three of ſand, as judiciouſly pointed out to me by Mr. NEWTON, who has tranſlated that ancient author. That VITRUVIUS was not only a judicious, but a *practical* obſerver, as well in regard to *Mortar*, as other articles of building, appears from the diſtinction he makes betwixt *Sharp River* ſand, and *Pit Sand* which is generally ſoft; for of river ſand he allows but two to one of lime: and I have long ſince found the neceſſity of forming a compoſition of fine and coarſe ſand for mortar, unleſs the ſand is naturally ſo mixed; as appears by the firſt note on § 200; for, as the lime will receive the moſt ſand in that way, without loſing its plaſticity, it will of conſequence make the hardeſt and firmeſt mortar. My practice has uniformly been, if there was plenty of one ſort of ſand, and a ſcarcity of the other, to make the mixture, by allowing of the moſt plentiful ſort as far as the proportion of 2 to 1. Dr. HIGGINS not only recommends a mixture of fine and coarſe ſands, but attempts to fix the beſt proportion. *Calcareous Cements*, § 12. beginning page 78. See alſo VITRUVIUS, B. II. Ch. IV. V. and VI.

It may be of uſe, and not out of place, here to obſerve, that, ſo far as I know, it is a *peculiarity* of this gentleman to fix the proportion of proceeded in the reduction of the expence of *Face* mortar; but as common lime, burnt from a pure limeſtone, either hard or ſoft, with an admixture of ſand only, will never acquire a ſtony hardneſs under water, by any treatment I could give it*; and as this is what is generally made uſe of in the back part of the walls, even of works intended to be of the beſt ſort, I was very deſirous to provide a kind of mortar that might not be too expenſive, and yet might internally acquire a ſtony hardneſs. Inſtead therefore of *Tarras* or *Puzzolana*, I ſubſtituted an equal quantity of *Minion*; and as the back part of the walls (or *backing*, as it was called) of the *Calder* works was in general done with *Rubble*, (or rough ſtone from the quarries) where the interſtices were large and open, and required a good deal of matter to fill them them full, I uſed the compoſition already ſpecified, with *common* lime, taking care to ſcreen the pebbles clean from ſand and dirt†; ſo that the whole compoſition would be again increaſed in a greater proportion than that of one to two: we now therefore from every meaſure of unſlaked lime and a meaſure of minion, together with the ſand ſpecified, obtained five meaſures of backing, or (as we called it) *Pebble Mortar*.—— Where minion is not to be had, as a ſubſtitute, if one half, or even one third of its quantity, of tarras or puzzolana is given inſtead of it, it will anſwer nearly as good an end, as a whole meaſure of minion.

203. HAVING thus aſcertained the leading facts with reſpect to the making a compoſition of water mortar for various uſes, it remains a curious queſtion, which being myſelf unable to reſolve, I muſt leave to the learned *Naturaliſt* and *Chemiſt*, why an intimate mixture of clay in the compoſition of limeſtone of any kind, either hard or ſoft, ſhould render it capable of ſetting in water, in a manner that no *pure* lime I have yet ſeen from any kind of ſtone whatſoever, has been capable of doing. It is eaſy to add *Clay* in any proportion to a pure lime; but it produces no ſuch effect‡: it is eaſy to add *Brick-duſt*, either finely or coarſely powdered, to ſuch lime, in any proportion, alſo; but this ſeems unattended with any other effect than what ariſes from other bodies that by paſſing the fire become porous and ſpongy, and thereby abſorbents of water, as already hinted; and excepting what may reaſonably be attributed to the irony particles that *red* brickduſt may contain. In ſhort, I have as yet found no treatment of pure calcareous lime, that rendered it more fit to ſet in *Water* than it is by nature, except what is to be derived from the admixture of *Tarras*, *Puzzolana*, or ſome *ferruginous* ſubſtance of a ſimilar nature§.

204. NOTHING

of the ingredients for making mortar by *weight*. I doubt not, but it anſwered *his* end beſt, in point of accuracy in *Experiment*; as he had the management of the preparation of the lime himſelf; but I apprehend this mode will by no means fit the *practical* builder; for, as the Doctor has fully ſhewn, that limes not thoroughly burnt, are conſiderably the heavieſt; it will follow that, by weight, the workman when the lime was bad in quality, would alſo get the *leaſt* of it: and I have in reality known inſtances where the proportions given by Dr. HIGGINS (though clearly enough expreſſed to be *weights*) were applied as meaſures; compounding ſeven *buſhels* of ſand with one of lime!

* Having had the opportunity of taking up a large flat ſtone, of a cloſe grain, of about five feet ſquare, that had probably lain above a *Century* at the bottom of a malt ciſtern, I found it had been well bedded in mortar, which had become coagulated to the conſiſtence of cheeſe, but having never come to a perfect dryneſs, it ſo far retained its natural humidity, that I found it might, with ſome pains, be beaten up to mortar, without any addition of water; and afterwards, being ſuffered to dry in the air, it ſet to a ſtony hardneſs, and appeared as good mortar for dry work, as any which that part of the country produced.

† See the firſt note on § 200.

‡ In the year 1760, having ſome buildings to make for myſelf in a part of the country where the limeſtone is of the more pure kind, and the lime tender and light coloured, I reſolved to try an experiment upon a conſiderable ſcale. I diſſolved clay of the yellow kind (which, when burnt, makes a good hard red brick) in water, in ſuch proportion, as that this water being made uſe of in wetting the quick lime to make it into mortar, it would have ſomewhat leſs than the quantity I had generally found in the blue *Lyas* limes. I at firſt imagined I had made a valuable acquiſition, as the mortar, that from its ſituation was to become dry, ſet very well; but ſome of this clay mortar being uſed where it was likely to continue long in a humid ſtate, though not actually expoſed to water, I found it to ſet very tardily; inſomuch that at the end of three months, I could make an impreſſion upon it with my fingers: however, after a twelvemonth it was tolerably hard; but on examining the building ſo done in the year 1786, I found all the dry work not ſo hard as the mortar of the ſame lime without clay. Some parts of both had equally periſhed, and that in the humid place had acquired but a very moderate degree of hardneſs: it was not in reality, as I judge, near ſo hard as the ſame mortar would have been, if no clay had been introduced; but here no common mortar had been uſed to compare it with.

§ Some years ago M. LORIOT publiſhed a treatiſe upon the compoſition of *Ancient Cements*, with a view to improve the modern. He ſeems

204. NOTHING more directly conduces to the perfection of water mortar, than a means of doing the work with very moderate quantities of it. For these purposes, it is a first principle, that all must be *filled full*; but the more *stone* there is used in a cube yard of masonry, the less room there will be for mortar. I have already described the methods I made use of in *reducing* the *quantity* of the more valuable materials composing the mortar for the *Calder* navigation, where the *ashler* walls were backed, as is generally the practice, with rubble stone, or with bricks; but when we came to the upper part of that navigation, in the neighbourhood of *Cromwell Bottom* and *Elland Edge*, being there supplied with a species of stone that naturally rises in *flat beds*, or that can easily be split to any thickness from two feet to two inches; I found a great utility arise from the particular texture of this stone, not only in composing the *ashler* part, (which scarcely needed any hewing, except a little regulation of the faces and end joints) but also in the backing; for the stones intended for this use being sorted, and suited together, so as to form the internal or backing courses of an *uniform* thickness, we were enabled to lay the pieces together, in the manner of a promiscuous pavement; and these being laid down upon a bed of mortar, and the interstices afterwards made good with small rubble work, to bring to a level and compleat the courses; by these means we were enabled not only to preserve a firm bond throughout, but to use very little mortar in proportion to what we had been accustomed to do in common rubble.

205. MY mind had long dwelt upon this idea, without having afterwards an opportunity of putting it in practice; no quarries affording *flat bedded* stones having occurred in the proximity of any of my future works; the occasion was therefore reserved to my being joined in consultation with the Gentlemen *Engineers* at *Portsmouth*, as already mentioned; when those gentlemen observing the moderate price at which they obtained not only *flat backing*, but *Purbeck* ashler in rough courses, from those quarries, the application in the way above mentioned immediately presented itself; and those gentlemen being very attentive to all improvements in the building art, we soon found by proper estimation, that walls might be built with this kind of stone upon this principle, and especially with the use of a mortar also investigated for that purpose, as already mentioned, not only at a less price than walls backed with common brick and tarras, but of superior bond and solidity * to any thing that has yet been done, except with block stone hewn within and without.

I need not acquaint the ingenious artist, that more or less mortar will be consumed, in proportion as the flat pieces which compose the backing are larger, and brought more closely together in the first instance: but it may be agreeable to him to be informed, that if the stones are tolerably bedded, a little work of the hammer will bring them so close together, that four cube feet of mortar will be sufficient to compleat a cube yard of backing.

seems to suppose the *grand secret* that has been *lost*, to consist in the admixture of a certain quantity of the burnt limestone unslaked, and *ground* to a powder, with lime wetted up in large heaps for use, as in the common method for large buildings.——I have made trial of this method, both in small and in large; for, however little of likelihood of advantage a proposition may contain, yet when this concerns a *physical* process, nothing can be safely concluded, but from actual trial. And I must candidly own, that the effect was better than I had expected; for I found the composition not only *set* more readily than mortar, as commonly made up, but much less liable to crack; and consequently, if this cement was made use of in water building, it was less apt to re-dissolve, because, it would more *speedily* get set to a firmer consistence, and so as more ably to resist the water from entering its pores; but when the water was brought upon it, in whatever state of hardness it was at the time, it at best but remained in that state, without any further induration, while the water remained upon it; and, as I expect, would so remain, till it had had some opportunity of acquiring hardness by further drying.——M. Loriot, I perceive, strongly recommends, where *water is concerned*, the use of *smiths forge scales*, and the *refuse of iron* to be joined with his composition; but this I apprehend is no *new* discovery of M. Loriot's, as these substances have been long known to produce a good effect upon all kinds of lime for water building. But after all the experiments I have made, it yet remains a doubt with me, whether, be it for dry works or water works, the use of *fresh* slaked lime, of whatever kind, as recommended by Dr. Higgins, is not preferable to the *same* kind of lime treated in M. Loriot's way. This I am sure of, that the method of the former gentleman is attended with less trouble and expence, as not requiring any part of the materials to be *ground* in a mill, or otherwise pulverized.——*Water Lime*, ever since I found out the distinction, I have always used as *fresh* as possible, as I was instructed at *Watchet*; but in the use of common lime, especially for dry works, I had nearly fallen into the common method of wetting it up, till I read M. Loriot and Dr. Higgins.

* Report of Colonel Pipps, Lieutenant Colonel Moncrief, Captain Twiss of His Majesty's *Corps* of *Engineers*, and John Smeaton, *Civil Engineer*.

226. BY way of recapitulation and sum of what I have said upon the article of *Water Cement*, I here subjoin a *Table*, containing a specimen of twenty different compositions, most of which I have used in different situations, and for different purposes.

A TABLE containing Twenty Compositions of Water Mortar, suited to different Situations and Circumstances.

N°	*Water Lime* with *Puzzolana*.	Lime Powder.	Puzzo-lana.	Common Sand.	N° of Cube Feet.	Expence per Cube Foot.
		Bushels.	Bushels.	Bushels.		s. d.
1	Edystone Mortar — — — —	2	2	—	2.32	3 8
2	Stone Mortar — — — — —	2	1	1	2.68	2 1½
3	——— 2d Sort — — —	2	1	2	3.57	1 7½
4	Face Mortar — — — — —	2	1	3	4.67	1 4
5	——— 2d Sort — — —	2	0½	3	4.17	1 1
6	Backing Mortar — — — —	2	0½	3	4.04	0 11
	Water Lime with *Minion*.		Minion.			
7	Face Mortar — — — —	2	2	1	3.22	1 5½
8	——— Calder Composition — —	2	1	2	3.57	1 1
9	Backing Mortar — — — —	2	0½	3	4.17	0 10
10	——— 2d Sort — — —	2	0½	3	4.04	0 9½
	Common Lime with *Tarras*.		Tarras.			
11	Tarras Mortar — — — —	2	1	—	1.67	4 0
12	——— increased — — —	2	1	1	2.50	2 9
13	——— further — —	2	1	2	3.45	2 0½
14	——— still further — —	2	1	3	4.35	1 8
15	Tarras Backing Mortar — — —	2	0½	3	3.50	1 2½
16	——— 2d Sort — —	2	0½	3	3.37	0 11½
	Common Lime with *Minion*.		Minion.			
17	Ordinary Face Mortar — — —	2	2	2	2.75	1 5½
18	——— 2d Sort — —	2	1	3	4.34	0 8½
19	Ordinary Backing Mortar — — —	2	0½	3	4.05	0 8
20	——— 2d Sort — —	2	0½	3	3.92	0 7½

Observations on the preceding Table.

1st. Those that would make mortar according to the preceding Table, should know, that the materials are all supposed to be in a *dry* state when measured.

2d. That the lime is supposed to be thrown into the measure with a shovel, with some *degree* of force; for if put in as light as possible, in the way to make the most measure of it, there will be a want of the real quantity; and if pressed down, the measure will contain considerably more than what can be expected in *purchasing* the material: and the same may be said of the puzzolana, the tarras, and the minion.

3d. Respecting

3d. Refpecting fand, it is particularly to be noted, that if in a moift ftate, the real quantity is confiderably lefs under the fame meafure, than if dry, and that in an *uncertain* degree: and as moift fand is moft frequently brought for ufe, it is advifable that the operator fhould take a means of finding the difference of the proportion, and allowing accordingly in meafure.

4th. I would alfo obferve, that, if the fand is not naturally a compofition of *fine* and *courfe*, it fhould be rendered fo by an admixture of different forts; the proportion of *one* to the *other* need not be much ftudied; what I have already faid in note * on § 202. will be a fufficient direction.

5th. The due beating of the mortar is however of *great* confequence; and, without going into that repetition of beating, which has been always looked on as effential to the making the common *tarras* mortar, fuch as N° 11, a degree of beating fufficient to give it all *poffible* confiftence and toughnefs, before it is ufed, is in reality *indifpenfible*: and the method that I have found to anfwer the end in the moft fatiffactory way is, to mix the due proportion of the lime and the *puzzolana*, the *tarras*, or the *minion*, together in the dry powder; and it will alfo be well, to have at leaft one third of the *fand* (either fine or coarfe) likewife dry: put as much water to the lime, as that with a fhovel or beater you can bring it to a pafte of a moderate confiftence, but rather more wet than to be properly ufed as mortar in that ftate; then by degrees beat in the moift fand, and afterwards the dry, bringing it to a confiftence by beating after every addition. The dry fand is intended to take up the fuperfluous moifture, fo as to render the mortar immediately fit for ufe; and if this has not brought it to a fufficient ftiffnefs, you may let it lie till it inclines to fet, and then beat it up to the due confiftence; or, if immediately wanted, you may beat in a little dry lime powder to drink up the fuperfluous moifture; always, however, *faithfully* remembering not to terminate the beating, till the mafs has got *all* the toughnefs that you find it will acquire by beating. This method fully anfwers where *Water Lime* is concerned.

6th. The cuftomary allowance for tarras mortar beating, firft and laft, is a day's work of a man for every bufhel of tarras; that is, for two bufhels of lime powder with one bufhel of tarras; fo that, by N° 11, if a labourer's day's work (as at London) is rated at 2*s.* then (the bufhel of tarras being valued at 4*s.*) the beating will be half the price of the tarras; and the mortar produced being only 1⅔ cube feet, the *beating* of the mortar will therefore amount to 14⅖*d.* per cube foot: whereas, in the way I have juft mentioned, a man in *half* a day will beat to a very good confiftence the whole produce that can be made, in any of the articles, from two bufhels of *Lime*; fo that the beating of the beft face mortar, as N° 4, being 4⅔ cube feet, will be done for lefs than 2¾*d.* at the fame rate of labour.

7th. In regard to the column of prices, they can only be confidered as *comparative*: the articles of carriage, dearnefs of particular materials and labour, will greatly vary in different fituations; but the prices being given as under, at which the different ingredients are rated in the preceding table, the ingenious artift will be at no lofs either to compare the different compofitions with one another; or find the value of them in his own fituation; or vary them to fuit his price and purpofe *.

	s.	*d.*
Water lime per bufhel in the dry powder — — —	0	9
Common lime ditto — — —	0	4
Puzzolana in powder, prepared — — — —	3	0
Tarras ditto — — — —	4	0
Minion ditto — — — —	1	0
Coarfe or fine fand, or mixed — — — —	0	2
† The labour of beating two bufhels of common lime to *tarras mortar*, is fuppofed	2	0
The labour of beating two bufhels of water lime for thofe articles —	1	0

* There are many cuftomary meafures and ways of meafuring amongft workmen, as well as in different counties: when I fpeak of a *Bufhel*, I would be underftood to mean the *Winchefter Corn Bufhel ftriked*, or the contents reduced to a level with the border.

I alfo fuppofe the forge fcales of iron (when equally powdered, and fifted clean from dirt and glaffy flagg) to be equivalent to as much puzzolana or tarras: ruft of iron, or iron ore burnt, powdered, and fifted, to be equivalent to minion; and each of thefe to about half the quantity of puzzolana or tarras: but as the materials themfelves may differ, I would advife the curious artift to be attentive to the refult of his *own* trials.——N. B. I fuppofe N° 5 equal in firmnefs and validity to N° 11; and N° 10 to N° 15.

† This article of labour is only applied in N° 11, 12, 13, and 14.

BOOK

B O O K IV.

An Account of Proceedings in the CONSTRUCTION *of the* STONE-*Work, &c. upon the* ROCK, *from the Beginning to the Finishing of the Building. With after Occurrences.*

C H A P. I.

Containing an Account of the FIRST YEAR's BUILDING *upon the* ROCK.

207. BY the end of May 1757, we had got every thing in readiness to carry out the *Neptune Buss* and begin the Work; it was however the 3d of June before wind and weather suited for our getting under way. On that day, being accompanied by Mr. JESSOP, eight seamen, the mould-maker, two moorstone masons, and six tinners, we sailed out of Plymouth Sound; but it falling calm, we came to an anchor about a league from the rock; and the next morning proving favourable, at six we laid hold of the ring of the buoy. We proceeded to heave up the moorings by means of our great tackle blocks, and could we have proceeded at the rate we began, we should have had them up in an hour; but the links of the buoy chain having been made each six inches in length, by way of getting faster forward with the work in making, we found, when these links came to a considerable strain upon the *davit* roll, which was of cast iron, and (as mentioned § 127.) not above nine or ten inches in diameter) they began to bend upon the convexity of the roll; and as I was apprehensive of the ill consequence that might attend their breaking, the following remedy occurred to me: I ordered the carpenter to cut some trenails into short pieces, of about three inches long, and to split each length into two; and those pieces being applied betwixt the chain and the roll at the flexure of each link, as it came to a bearing, prevented the middle part of each link from touching the roll, and therefore its streightness and figure could no way be changed by the strain in passing over the roll; and the pieces delivering themselves as the chain cleared the roll, they would serve the same purpose many times over.

The appearance of caution, begets an idea of danger to those who otherwise never would have had any apprehension of it; and though the risk of failure was lessened in a great degree by the proposed application, as was confessed by the whole company, yet it was observed, that if the chain *should* break any where between the roll and the tackle, the person that applied the pieces of wood would be in danger of being cut in two by the chain, or carried overboard along with it. This being the sense of my ship-mates, and as I always made it a rule not to put another upon doing what I was afraid to do myself, the *Post of Honour* naturally devolved on me; I therefore attended the getting in of the remainder of the eleven fathoms of chain, link by link, till we came to the great swivel of the bridle chain: and though this of course took some time, and left room for serious pause, yet the consideration of having previously tried the chain by a far greater strain than it was ever destined to bear, (see § 140.) prevented these reflections from being uneasy.——This business having been successfully executed, and our addition of five fathoms of large chain applied to the bridle, (see § 167.) at twelve o'clock this day, the 4th of June, we found ourselves once more riding as safely and securely at our moorings as we did the last season.

208. THE

208. THE weather did not admit of our landing that afternoon; but the next morning at eleven we landed, and immediately proceeded with fixing the *Fender Piles* on the eaſt ſide of the rock, which were intended to prevent the boats from rubbing againſt it, according to the idea given thereof, § 83. and as ſhewn in the elevation of the eaſt ſide of the rock in Plate N° 14. We alſo proceeded in fixing up the ſhears and the windlaſs, as ſhewn in the ſame plate; and though we made a conſiderable progreſs the ſame tide, which laſted till four o'clock, yet from the uſual uncertainty of weather, even in the beſt of every ſeaſon, it was the 10th of June before thoſe neceſſary matters were diſpatched; incluſive of the mooring the *Tranſport Buoy*, at eighty fathoms north of the landing-place*, in fourteen fathom water†.——By way of ſeeing that all our tackle acted properly, and as ſome trial of its ſufficiency, we hoiſted the Sea-Horſe yawl, a ſtrong heavy ſhip's long-boat, with ſeveral people in it, upon the top of the rock; and finding every thing to act properly and to be ſufficiently manageable, we were now ready for receiving the ſtone; and the whole company returned home in the yawl, except ſuch hands as were neceſſarily left to take care of the buſs.

209. ON Saturday the 11th of June the firſt courſe of ſtone was put on board the Edyſtone boat, (ſee Plate N° 10. Fig. 1.) with all the neceſſary ſtores, tools, and utenſils; and having appointed Mr. JESSOP, at his own requeſt, to be a foreman in the place of HILL, diſcharged, I took on this occaſion both the foremen, Meſſrs. JESSOP and RICHARDSON, along with me, as alſo the neceſſary hands. We landed at eight on Sunday morning the 12th of June, and before noon had got the firſt ſtone into its place, being that upon which the date of the year 1757 is inſcribed in deep characters‡; and the tide coming upon us, we ſecured it with chains to the old ſtancheons, and then quitted the rock till the evening tide, when it was fitted, bedded in mortar, trenailed down, and compleatly fixed; and all the outward joints coated over with *Plaſter of Paris*, to prevent the immediate waſh of the ſea upon the mortar, (ſee § 174). This ſtone, according to its dimenſions, weighed 2½ tons.——The weather ſerving at intervals, it was at the evening of Monday the 13th that the firſt courſe, conſiſting of four ſtones, was finiſhed; and which, as they all preſented ſome part of their faces to the ſea, were all of *Moorſtone*.

210. THE next day, Tueſday the 14th, the ſecond courſe, ſee Plate N° 10. *Fig.* 2. arrived; and ſome of it was immediately landed, proceeded with, and in part *ſet* the ſame tide: the looſe pieces being chained together by ſtrong chains, made on purpoſe for this uſe, and thoſe ultimately to the ſtancheons; or to Lewiſes in the holes of the work of Courſe I. that had already been fixed.——The ſea was uncommonly ſmooth when we got upon the rock, this evening's tide; but while we were proceeding with our work, within the ſpace of an hour and half, the wind ſprung up at N. E. and blew ſo freſh, that the *Weſton*, lying to deliver the remainder of her cargo, had ſome difficulty in getting out of the Gut; and had it not been for the tranſport buoy, to which ſhe had a faſtening by a rope, it would probably have proved impracticable to have got her out again. And we ſoon ſaw it was neceſſary to get every thing in the beſt poſture, time and circumſtances would admit, in order to quit the rock, with ſafety to ourſelves, and ſecurity to what we muſt neceſſarily leave behind us.

The pieces that were fixed and trenailed down, were ſuppoſed to be proof againſt whatever might happen; but the looſe pieces, and thoſe that were ſimply lowered down into their dove-tail receſſes, were conſidered as needing ſome additional ſecurity to prevent their being carried away by the violence of the ſea. Of the thirteen pieces of which Courſe II. conſiſted, five only were landed: N° 1. was compleatly ſet; N° 2 and 3 were lowered into their places, and ſecured by chains; and 4 and 5, which lay at the top of the rock, were chained together, and alſo to the ſlide-ladder, which was very ſtrongly laſhed down

* This was the great buoy that had rode at the moorings during the winter, and was moored by the ſame chain to which it had been faſtened during that ſeaſon: but for this ſervice it had been ſent home and repaired, and was attached to an old anchor of 12 cwt.

† See § 86, and Plate N° 3.

‡ To facilitate the work of getting down the ſtones, after they were landed upon the top of the rock, a kind of frame, ſomething in form of a ladder, was laſhed upon its inclining ſurface, upon which we ſlid the ſtones to their reſpective places.

to eye-bolts, purposely fixed on the rock for that intent.——Every moment the wind and sea so increased, that it was with the utmost difficulty our two yawls could be prevented from being staved upon the rock; and while we were endeavouring to get our tackle-blocks, mortar-buckets, and a great variety of loose materials and tools, on board the yawls, and to preserve our utensils and stores; we were risking the chance, whether we ourselves should not be left behind to be washed off the rock. Our light *setting Triangle* *, by which we hoisted and lowered the pieces of stone into their places, as being our greatest incumbrance, was also lashed to the slide-ladder.——Having at last got into our yawls, the wind and sea were so increased from the N. E. quarter, that we found it quite impracticable to make head against it, so as to row out of the Gut to the northward; we therefore had no alternative, but, compelled by necessity, we risked our passage through the rocks to the southward, aiming at the interval betwixt the Sugar Loaf and the House Reef, (see Plate N° 3.) and both boats providentially got through unhurt. We then, having doubled the south point of the House Reef, had to make our way to the north, by the west side thereof; which, as it was not quite low water at the rocks, afforded us some tolerable shelter, and gave us time to consult what to do: for, as the current of the channel tide was then setting strongly to the westward, and as our buss lay to the N. E. of the rocks, and of course right to windward, there seemed a necessity for our utmost exertions to recover the buss. We therefore agreed that the light yawl should row the headmost, taking the other in *tow*; by which means our united strength could be equally exerted for the benefit of the whole.——Accordingly, when by rowing north we had cleared the House Reef, we soon got into so much wind, sea, and current of tide, that we found, notwithstanding our joint efforts to get to the eastward, we were gradually carried to the west; and, after a struggle of an hour and an half in this way, we found it quite impracticable for *both* boats to get on board the buss. Each boat rowed with four oars; Messrs. SMEATON and JESSOP, with two seamen, and four other hands, were in the light yawl, and Mr. RICHARDSON, one of our best seamen, and eight other hands were in the Sea-Horse; which was to make her way westward to the *floating Light*, that lay to leeward (see § 122): and we in the light yawl determined to endeavour to gain the buss; and if that could not be effected, also to bear away towards the other vessel.

After labouring at our oars for an hour and an half more, we recovered the buss, (which lay not much more than 200 fathoms from the place where we parted with the Sea-Horse) to the great joy of ourselves, and anxiety for our associates, it then blowing a hard gale of wind, which continued increasing all night.

About four the next morning the wind shifted to the S. E. which produced so troublesome a sea, that the Weston, which had rode at the transport buoy all night, made signals of distress; and was therefore ordered to *slip* and make her best port. In the afternoon the wind coming to S. with the tide of flood, the Sea-Horse returned to the buss with all hands in safety, with grateful hearts for the kind treatment they had received on board the floating light, and for their deliverance; having found the utmost difficulty and danger in getting aboard the floating light, on account of the sea's running so high.

211. IN the evening we made a short tide upon the rock, and had the satisfaction to find that no material damage had happened to any thing; we therefore proceeded with our work, and compleatly fixed N° 2. of Course II: and next morning, Thursday June the 16th, the Weston returning from Plymouth, came to the transport buoy. We then proceeded both morning and evening tides, though they were not very favourable; and this day sent home Mr. JESSOP, to prepare himself and company to relieve Mr. RICHARDSON's; and for a supply of lime and other necessaries, of which we were in want. On the morning of Friday the 17th, we again landed for a short time; and, notwithstanding we did not meet with any thing amiss on our return to the rock on Wednesday evening after the hard gale of wind, yet this morning we found a part of the rock in the border of our work, that secured a corner of N° 3. was gone: we therefore, to secure that stone to its neighbour, applied an iron cramp, of which we had some in readiness in case of accident.——We were prevented landing in the evening by a fresh of wind

* This Triangle is represented as standing upon the wall of the building, supposed to be raised above the vaulted covering of the store-room, Plate N° 14.

and

and rain at N. W. but landed again on Saturday morning's tide, the 18th. However, we had not been long there before a great ſwell aroſe from the S. W.; and, though there had been no wind apparently to occaſion it, yet it came upon us ſo faſt, that we were obliged to quit the rock before we could get our work into ſo ſatisfactory a poſture of defence as I wiſhed. It was, however, as follows, N° 1, 2, 3, 4, and 5, were compleatly fixed as intended; N° 6 and 7 were fitted, and lowered upon their mortar beds; N° 8 was ſimply got into its place, with a weight of lead of five cwt. upon it*; which, in all ſuch trials as had hitherto been made thereof, had lain quietly. Not having time to get the ſtone, N° 9, into its place, we chained it upon the top of the rock to the ſlide-ladder, as we had done before on Tueſday. In this condition we left the rock, having ſtaid till we were all wet from head to foot.——The ſwell continued the remainder of the day, and the wind freſhening at S. W. in the night, at five o'clock on Sunday morning J. Bowden made the ſignal of diſtreſs, and was therefore ordered to *ſlip* and go into port.

In the afternoon, on tide of flood, the ſea frequently broke in a large denſe body over the head of the ſhears, which were twenty-four feet in height above the top of rock, and the ſeas running very *ſhort* where we lay, the bowſprit of the buſs ſometimes dipped in the water.——We could plainly ſee the ſtone on the top of the rock till towards the evening, at about high water, when we obſerved ſomething of timber to have broke looſe, and to lie in a wrong ſituation; ſoon after which it diſappeared, as alſo the ſtone; ſo we concluded it was the ſlide-ladder and the ſtone that had gone together.——The next morning, Monday the 20th, the wind was rather increaſed than abated; but no further alteration was apparent on the rock ſince the laſt night.——Towards evening the wind veered to the ſouth, and blew a ſtorm till three o'clock on Tueſday morning, when it began to abate. About nine o'clock it became more moderate; and finding that bread was running ſhort among the workmen, as we were not likely very ſoon to get to work again, I diſpatched the greateſt part of them home in the Sea-Horſe yawl: and about twelve o'clock the wind and ſea having become ſtill more moderate, I judged it practicable to row a-head againſt it, ſo as to get to the weſtward of the rock, and reconnoitre our damages: accordingly, taking four oars in the light yawl, it being then near low water, I obſerved, when the ſea fell away from the rocks, (every ſea then breaking bodily over it) that N° 9, and the ſlide-ladder to which it was chained, were both gone; that the two pieces of moorſtone N° 5 and 6, which had only been let down upon their mortar beds without further faſtening, were alſo gone; that N° 3 had broke its cramp and was gone; and that the 5 cwt. that had been laid upon the moſt projecting part of the piece N° 8, had, by the force of the ſea acting edgewiſe upon it, been driven to the eaſtward till it was ſtopped by the riſe of the third ſtep, againſt which it ſeemed abutted; ſo that having thereby quitted the piece N° 8, upon which it was laid, that was gone alſo: we therefore, as it appeared, had loſt five pieces of ſtone; the loſs of which was in the firſt inſtance alleviated, by finding that the firſt courſe appeared ſo thoroughly united with the rock, that its ſurface begun to look black with dark-coloured moſs fixing upon it, and giving it the ſame hue as the rock itſelf: alſo, that our ſhears and windlaſs were all ſtanding without the leaſt derangement.

I did not wait for the ſubſiding of the winds and ſeas, ſo as to enable us to land, and look out whether or no we could recover any of the loſt pieces; I immediately *made* for Plymouth in the light yawl, and landed at Mill Bay at five o'clock on Tueſday evening the 21ſt; and, having collected the moulds of the ſtones we had loſt, and choſen proper ſpare blocks, I ſet a couple of men to work upon each piece of ſtone, day and night, till finiſhed.——This diſaſter, though it furniſhed a few reflections, yet they were not of the unpleaſant kind; for, as every part of the ſtone-work, that was *compleated* according to its original intention, appeared to have remained *fixed*, it demonſtrated the practicability of the method choſen; and at the ſame time ſhewed the preference of wedging to cramping, as the cramp had failed: and alſo the utility of trenails† as a ſecurity till the mortar was become hard.

* This weight, which was in the ſhape of the ſegment of a ſphere, I had got prepared, as a means of holding down ſuch ſtones as were ſimply lowered into their receſſes, and which for want of time could not be got fixed in a more effectual manner; for, from the figure thereof, its baſe or flat ſide being laid upon the flat ſurface of the ſtone, the action of the ſea could have very little hold upon it, being all a ſmooth ſurface, the ring excepted.

† The method of trenailing and wedging will be fully deſcribed in its due place.

In

In lefs than two days the five pieces of ftone were compleated; and on Thurfday the 23d in the evening I went on board the Wefton with the ftones, carrying alfo Mr. JESSOP and company; but there being little wind, we were obliged to row all night; and when, by this labour, we had got within a league of the bufs, it began to blow fo hard at E. that we thought it advifable to bear away for fome weftern port. Accordingly at feven in the morning we came to an anchor in Fowey harbour; and that day took the opportunity of viewing the progrefs of our moorftone works at *Lanlivery*. The wind continued frefh at E. the next day; and as the day after, being Saturday the 25th, it again became RICHARDSON's turn to go out, I ordered BOWDEN to beat to windward, if poffible, and get to his moorings at the tranfport buoy, as foon as he could; and with Mr. JESSOP and his company, returned over land to Plymouth.

212. AT four o'clock on Monday morning the 27th, the weather ferving, I went out with RICHARDSON and company, in the Edyftone boat; we got to the bufs at ten, and found the Wefton at the tranfport buoy, but could not land till the afternoon's tide, being a compleat week fince we had been laft upon the rock. We firft replaced the ladder, and afterwards proceeded, without more than ufual interruptions, till the 30th in the evening, when we clofed and compleated the Courfe N° II. and began upon Courfe III.——The execution of thefe two courfes had taken us up from the 12th to the 30th inclufive, and though they confifted of no more than feventeen pieces of ftone in the whole, yet I found myfelf no ways *difheartened*; for, in eftablifhing thefe two courfes, I confidered the moft difficult and arduous part of the work to be already accomplifhed, as thefe two courfes brought us up to the fame level where my predeceffor Mr. RUDYERD had begun.

While the new ftones of Courfe II. were making, I received intelligence from the bufs, that the feamen there, during our abfence, had been into the Gut, and had obferved fome of the pieces we had loft to be lying in the bottom of it: I therefore, befides forming new pieces, ordered an utenfil to be made, by means of which it feemed likely I might get fome of thefe pieces up again: and though all the new ftones were landed and fet in their places before I had an opportunity of trying the tool; yet I was willing to convince myfelf, how far it might be ufeful upon any future fimilar occafion.——Accordingly, between the tides of the 30th, (the water falling away fo as to leave only ten feet depth in the Gut) I made a trial of the inftrument*, wherewith I fucceeded in getting up one of the ftones, which proved to be N° 9, that was chained to the ladder at the top of the rock; and I might have got up two others that lay there, had they been wanted; but the mere recovery of ftones, after a fufficient experiment had been made, was fcarcely worth the time.

The next day, Friday July the 1ft, we were able to land; but as the wind blew frefh at S. W. I judged it unfafe to bring the Edyftone boat into the Gut to deliver any ftone. I obferved, that during the laft tide, the fwell had wafhed fome of the pointing out of the exterior joints, and alfo fome of the grouting out of the upright joints; but as a heavy fea feemed likely to come on with the tide of flood, I judged it to be to no purpofe to repair the cement while a *violent* fwell continued; I therefore employed the company in cutting off the iron ftancheons belonging to the former building, as they now began to be in our way, and as the *hold* we got of them ceafed to be of ufe, in proportion as we got more faftening from the lewis holes of our own work.——It was not long before the mafter of the Edyftone boat gave warning, he could lie no longer at the tranfport buoy; I therefore took my paffage on board of it to Plymouth, and landed in the afternoon.

213. THE weather having become more favourable, on Sunday morning the 3d of July, I went on board, accompanied by Mr. JESSOP, and his party, to whom, as they had never had the opportunity of fetting a ftone, it behoved me to attend. We however not only met with a repulfe this day, but could not make any further attempt to go out till Tuefday the 5th; and then the wind, though gentle, being contrary, had not the company on board the bufs come with their two yawls and towed us thither, in all probability the day would have been fpent in fruitlefs attempts. Our difficulty was confiderably increafed by the

* See the explanation of this inftrument, amongft the tools and utenfils contrived or adapted to the Edyftone works, in Plate N° 18.

coming

coming on of so thick a fog, that all our efforts united, we had much ado to regain the buss.—— RICHARDSON told me they had had such bad weather, that the slide-ladder had again broke its lashings and driven away; that they had however got all the irons cut off close to the rock; but that the last tide, though there was only a breeze at S. W. the swell was so great, and came on so suddenly, as to put them in great danger of being washed off from the top of the rock, before they could quit it.

At two o'clock this day we landed, and JESSOP's company set six pieces of stone, and effectually repaired the cement; and next day a proportionable dispatch was made, though the weather was not very mild.——In the night, betwixt eleven and twelve o'clock, the watch upon deck espied a sail upon the rocks; whereupon we immediately sent one of our yawls to her relief; which soon returned with the whole crew, several of whom were in their shirts, and in great distress. They informed us that the vessel was the *Charming Sally* of *Biddeford*, a snow of 130 tons burthen. They had been at *Dartmouth*, from whence they were returning in ballast; and as there was no stress of weather at that time to drive them upon the rocks, we could not but wonder how they had contrived to get *thither*: we were informed, that not knowing exactly where they were, they took the rocks to be so many fishing-boats, till it was too late to clear them; and that on the vessel's striking, she filled so quick that the boat floated upon the deck before they could get into it. In steering westward, she had cleared the south point of the south-east reef, and fell upon the south reef near the highest part. See Plate N° 3.——The vessel sat almost upright upon the rocks, and the masts remained standing the whole of the day; but in the night following she was wholly beaten to pieces.——Her crew, consisting of seven hands, having been refreshed on board the buss, the next day rowed off in their boat to *Looe*; and as we had not landed since the 8th, nor now more likely, I took the opportunity of returning to Plymouth in a Cawsand fisherman, who came with an intent to pick up something from the wreck; in which however he was disappointed.

214. ON Monday the 11th I again went out with RICHARDSON and company; Course III. consisting of twenty-five pieces, was closed on the following day, and Course IV. begun.——The tide of the 13th in the evening was remarkably quiet, and allowed us to go on with our work uninterruptedly; but just after we had got on board the buss, a sudden squall of wind arose from the S. W. which at once threatened a most dreadful storm; and it blew so hard, that we expected the mast to go by the board; but before the necessary orders could be given, by way of preparation, it became a perfect calm; the squall not having continued more than a minute, as it seemed to us. This was followed with a breeze from the east, and frequent flashes of lightning till the tide of ebb.

Thursday the 14th of July the company pursued the work of Course IV; and now both companies being fully instructed in the method of setting the basement courses, I returned to Plymouth; from whence I proposed to visit each company as often as should seem expedient, but always once in each company's *turn*, if wind and weather should permit.

215. I WENT out with JESSOP's company on Monday the 18th; but we were repulsed by bad weather, which continued to the 23d. The 21st, RICHARDSON's company having almost exhausted their provisions, and not being likely to get any supplies, came home in the Sea-Horse yawl: and gave account, that a few days before they came home, in hoisting one of the stones out of the vessel upon the rock, by neglecting to belay the tackle-fall of the *out-hawler Guy*, the shears came down flat upon the rock in the midst of the men, but providentially without doing any harm to either men or shears. He also acquainted me that they had had the greatest swell from the south they ever experienced, and that the 500 lb. weight had been washed from the work, but that they had found it entangled in the rocks above low water mark.

About this time I had intelligence from Portland, that two vessels laden with stone for the Edystone, waiting a favourable opportunity to sail for Plymouth, had all their hands pressed by the lieutenant of a tender stationed there; notwithstanding the service they were upon, and their having on that account Admiralty protections. This circumstance would have proved very distressing, had not the Lords of the

 Admiralty,

Admiralty, on application, sent immediate orders, by express, for discharging the men: and it is a great satisfaction to me when I say, that on this, as well as on every other occasion, we found the *Admiralty* Board was ready and disposed to give all the furtherance to our work in their power; though we did not always find that countenance from their servants.

216. CONTRARY winds, ground swells, and heavy seas for several days, interrupted the regularity of our proceedings; however, taking such opportunities as we could, the Course N° IV. consisting of twenty-three pieces of stone, was closed, in the morning's tide of the 31st of July, (see Plate N° 10): and in the evening's tide five pieces of Course V. were set.——Our work went on regularly for some days together; and on visiting the work upon the 5th of August, I found the Course N° V. containing twenty-six pieces, closed in, (see Plate N° 10); but that by some inadvertency in proceeding with the interior part, the masons had been obliged to set two of the outside pieces so as to be further out than they should have been by an inch each. However, as I found the work was sound and firm, I thought it better to cut off the superfluous stone from the outside, than to disturb the work by the violence that must have been used in unsetting the pieces; I therefore determined to let them stand as they were, till the cement was become so hard as to support the edges of the stone while the faces were working afresh; and which, from the mortar of our first and second course, we found was likely to be the case before the close of the season. ——One of the dovetails had also given way in driving a trenail, owing to a flaw in the stone; for the remedying whereof we applied a cramp.

This day our additional boat, that had for some time been fitting out, called the *Assistant*, and of which I appointed SAMUEL MEDLING to be master, brought out and landed at the rock her first cargo of stone, containing a part of Course VI. some of which were proceeded with and set: the Edystone boat also arrived with another cargo of lime and puzzolana, as well as stone, and came to the transport buoy; but the wind beginning to blow hard, she was obliged to look out for a harbour.——At this time we were in greater want of lime and *Puzzolana*, than of stone; and as nothing could proceed without these necessary materials, and it being uncertain when the boat might return, I contrived as follows to get a cask of each on board the buss before she left us.——The sea was so hollow and tumultuous, that though it was practicable for the light yawl to row near enough to throw a small rope on board the boat, yet it was impracticable for the yawl to receive any thing of weight over her side without danger of filling. I therefore ordered W. SMART, the master of the boat, to lash a cask of each to the shrouds with *Spun Yarn*; so that when the lashing was cut, either of the casks might instantly go overboard. A small rope from the buss having been fixed to each, and the lashings successively cut at a favourable moment, the casks immediately fell into the sea, and were easily towed on board the buss, the materials not suffering any material injury by being wet with sea water: and this expedient proved of the more value, as by this means we proceeded with the work of Course VI. several tides sooner than otherwise we could.

217. THE 8th of August at noon, the weather being exceeding fine, with a low neap tide, I took the opportunity of drawing a *meridian* line upon the platform of Course VI. the sea never going over the work during the whole tide, which was the first time it had not washed *over all*, since we began to build: we therefore took this favourable opportunity of carefully making good all our *pointings* and *groutings*, wherever the water had washed during the bad weather that had succeeded the last departure of the Edystone boat; and which was the case with it in places where it had not had time, to set before a rough tide came on; but I observed with much satisfaction, that whatever, not only of the original work, but of the repaired pointing, had once stood a *rough* tide, without giving way, the same place never after failed. ——I also observed, that as in mending the pointings we had in some places made trial of Dutch tarras as well as puzzolana, interchangeably, the puzzolana, for hard service, was evidently superior to the tarras: and some particular joints had proved so difficult, that I was obliged to try other expedients; the best of which was to chop *Oakum* very small, and beat it up along with the mortar. This was our *last* resource, and it never failed us.

218. ON

218. ON landing at Mill Bay, the 9th of Auguſt, I had the ſatisfaction to find four veſſels arrived from Portland with ſome pieces of ſtone, which their detention had cauſed us to be much in want of. Upon the 11th I again went out in the veſſel that contained the remaining pieces of Courſe VI; thoſe I ſaw fixed; and that courſe, conſiſting of thirty-two pieces, cloſed in, the ſame evening. See Plate N° 10.—— This compleating our ſix baſement courſes, brought our work upon the ſame level to which we had, the preceding ſeaſon, reduced the top of the rock; and upon this, as a common baſe, the reſt of the ſtructure was to be raiſed by regular entire courſes.——The time this part of the work (conſiſting of 123 pieces of ſtone) had taken up, was from the 12th of June to the 11th of Auguſt incluſive, being a ſpace of ſixty-one days. We now conſidered our greateſt difficulties to be ſucceſsfully ſurmounted, as every ſucceeding courſe had given us more and more time, as well as more and more room; and this will appear from our proceedings; for it has already been noticed that the firſt two courſes, conſiſting of nineteen pieces of ſtone only, had coſt us ſeventeen days.

219. HAVING now got the work to this deſirable ſituation, I apprehend it will be agreeable to my reader, to be more particularly acquainted with the method in which the ſtones were ſet and fixed. ——I have intimated § 151, that when each ſeparate piece, of which a courſe was to conſiſt, was ſeparately wrought, they were all to be brought to their exact places with reſpect to each other upon the platform in the work-yard, and ſo marked, that after being numbered and taken to pieces, they could again be reſtored to the ſame relative poſition. This was done upon the compleat circular courſes by drawing lines from the center to the circumference, paſſing through the middle of each ſet of ſtones; and likewiſe concentric circles through the middle of each tier or circle of ſtones, ſo as to indicate to the eye their relative poſition to each other: but to render the marks not eaſily delible, where thoſe lines croſſed the joints, a *nick* was cut and ſunk into the ſurface of the two adjacent ſtones; for doing which, a piece of thin plate iron was employed, with ſand, upon the principle that ſtones are ſawn; ſo that not only the ſight, but feeling, could be employed in bringing them together again exactly; for the ſame or a ſimilar plate being applied to the nick, the leaſt irregularity of its poſition would be diſcoverable.——In a ſimilar manner the ſtones of the *Baſe Courſes* were marked by lines drawn parallel to the length of the ſteps, and others perpendicular to the ſame, the croſſings being ſawn in as before deſcribed. There was, however, a nicety in this part of the work that required particular attention, and that was in forming a proviſion for ſetting the four *radical* ſtones, that occupy the four *radical* dovetails into which each ſtep was formed, as may be obſerved in the ſeveral figures of Plate N° 10.——Thoſe ſtones were formed, from the work of the rock's being actually moulded off, as mentioned § 159: and from the manner already deſcribed of bringing thoſe moulds to agree after they were brought home from the rock, § 160, thoſe ſtones were laid upon the platform thereby, and then marked with lines upon their own ſubſtance, in the manner juſt mentioned: and as the diſtances of each of thoſe ſtones were then aſcertained by gauge-rods of white fir-wood, while upon the platform; it muſt be expected, as each ſtep was reduced to a level plain, as the platform was, that when laid upon the rock in their due poſitions and diſtances, by the gauge-rods, they would nearly fit the dovetails that had been cut in the rock to receive them; and where there was the leaſt want of fitneſs, as might poſſibly happen with bodies of ſo rigid a nature, either the ſtone or the rock was cut, till each ſtone would come into its exact relative poſition, and then all the reſt would follow one another by their marks, in the ſame manner as they had done upon the platform.

220. IT is neceſſary to be noticed, that the waiſt of each piece of ſtone had two grooves cut, from the top to the bottom of the courſe, of an inch in depth, and three inches in width: applicable to thoſe grooves, were prepared a number of oak wedges, ſomewhat leſs than three inches in breadth, than one inch thick at the head, nearly [illegible]ths thick at the point, and ſix inches long. The diſpoſition of theſe grooves is ſhewn in the courſes of Plate N° 10, where the little black parallelogram figures, placed along the lines deſcribing the joints of the courſes, repreſent the tops of the grooves, and their place on the right hand or left of the joint line, ſhew in which ſtone the groove is cut. It is alſo to be noted, that where the flank ſide of a ſtone

a stone was not more in length than a foot or fourteen inches, one groove was generally deemed sufficient; but those of eighteen inches or upwards had generally, in themselves or the adjoining stone, a couple of grooves.

221. THE mortar, which was compounded as shewn in § 188*, was prepared for use by being beat in a very strong wooden bucket made for the purpose; each mortar-beater had his own bucket, which he placed upon any level part of the work, and with a kind of rammer or wooden pestle†, first beat the lime alone, about a quarter of a peck at a time, to which, when formed into a compleat, but rather thin paste with sea-water, he then gradually added the other ingredient, keeping it constantly in a degree of toughness by continuance of beating.——When a stone had been fitted and ready for setting, he whose mortar had been longest in beating came first, and the rest in order: the mason took the mortar out of the bucket; and if any was spared, he still kept on beating; if the whole was exhausted, he began upon a fresh *Batch*. ——The stones were first tried, and heaved into and out of their recesses, by a light moveable triangle, which being furnished with a light double tackle‡, the greatest number of all the pieces could be purchased by the simple application of the hand; and this made our stones to be readily manageable by such machinery as could commodiously be *moved* and carried backward and forward in the yawls every tide. To the first stone, and some few others, we took the great tackle, that we might hoist and lower them with certainty and ease; but there were not in the whole above a dozen of stones that required it.

222. THE stone to be set being hung in the tackle, and its bed of mortar spread, was then lowered into its place, and beat down with a heavy wooden maul, and levelled with a spirit level‖: and the stone being brought accurately to its marks, it was then considered as set in its place. The business now was to *retain* it exactly in that position, notwithstanding the utmost violence of the sea might come upon it before the mortar was hard enough to resist it.——The carpenter now dropped into each groove two of the wedges already described, one upon its *Head*, and the other with its point downward, so that the two wedges in each groove would then lie *Heads and Points*. With a bar of iron of about 2½ inches broad, ½ of an inch thick, and 2½ feet long, the ends being square, he could easily (as with a rammer) drive down one wedge upon the other, very gently at first, so that the opposite pairs of wedges being equally tightened, they would equally resist each other, and the stone would therefore keep its place; and in this manner those wedges might be driven even more tight than there was occasion for; as the wood being dry, it would by swelling become tighter; and it was possible that by too much driving, and the swelling of the wedges, the stones might be broken: and further, that a moderate fastening might be effectual, a couple of wedges were also, in like manner, pitched at the *top* of each groove, the dormant wedge or that with the point upward, being held in the hand, while the drift wedge or that with its point downward, was driven with a hammer; the whole of what remained above the upper surface of the stone was then cut off with a saw or chissel; and generally, a couple of *thin* wedges were driven very moderately at the but-end of the stone; whose tendency being to force it out of its dovetail, they would, by moderate driving, only tend to preserve the whole mass steady together; in opposition to the violent agitation that might arise from the sea.

223. AFTER a stone was *thus* fixed, we never in fact had an instance of its having been stirred by any action of the sea whatever; but considering the unmeasured violence thereof, the further security by trenails, suggested § 163, and now prepared, will not seem altogether unnecessary, when we reflect, that after a stone was thus fixed in its place by wedges, a great sea coming upon it, often in less than half

* See a b No 1. of the Table in § 205.

† See description of tools and utensils, Plate No 18.

‡ See also description, Plate No 17.

‖ These were provided on purpose, being such as were used § 81. and saved much loss of time that would otherwise have attended the use of levels with *Plumbets*, which, (as far as I know) were the only ones then used in masonry.

an

an hour) was capable of washing out all the mortar from the bed underneath it, notwithstanding every defence we could give it by plaster or otherwise; and that when the bed of mortar was destroyed, the sea acting edgewise upon the joint would exert the same power to lift it up, that the same sea would exert to overset it, in case its broad base was turned upright to oppose it; and as the wedges only fixed and secured the several pieces of which each course consisted to each other, and had no tendency to keep the whole course from lifting together, in case the whole should lose its mortar bed; it seemed therefore highly necessary to have some means of preventing the lifting the whole of a course together, till the solidity and continuity of the mortar should totally take away that tendency.——Adverting now to what was said § 163, that a couple of holes, to receive oak trenails of an inch and [illegible] in diameter, were bored in the work-yard through the external or projecting end of every piece of stone; we must now suppose these stones set in their places and fixed by wedges; then one of the tinners with a *Jumper* began to continue the hole into the stone of the course below, and bored it to about eight or nine inches deep; but this hole was bored of a less size, by [illegible] of an inch in diameter, than the hole through the stone above*; in consequence, the trenails having been previously dressed with a plane till they would drive somewhat freely through the upper hole, would drive stiffly into the under one, and generally would become so fast as to drive no further before their leading end got down to the bottom; and if so, they were sufficiently fast: but as they sometimes happened to drive more freely than at others, the following method was used to render them fast, for a certainty, when they got to the bottom.——The leading end of every trenail was split with a saw for about a couple of inches, and into this split was introduced a wedge about [illegible] of an inch less in breadth than the diameter of the trenail; it was a full quarter of an inch in thickness at the head, and sharpened to an edge: when therefore the head of the wedge touched the bottom of the hole, the trenail being forcibly driven thereupon, would enter upon it, till the whole substance was jambed so fast, that the trenail would drive no further; and as the wood would afterwards swell in the hole, and fill the little irregularities of boreing by the jumper, it became so fast that, as it seems, they could sooner be pulled in two than the trenails be drawn out again†. The trenail (originally made somewhat too long) being then cut off even with the top of the stone, its upper end was wedged cross and cross.——There being generally two trenails to each piece of stone, no assignable power, less than what would by main stress pull these trenails in two, could lift one of these stones from their beds when so fixed, exclusive of their natural weight, as all agitation was prevented by the lateral wedges.——The stone being thus fixed, a proper quantity of the beat mortar was liquefied, as mentioned § 183, and the joints having been carefully pointed up to the upper surface, the *Grout* so prepared was run in with iron

* The jumpers were kept to the same gauge by means of two brass rings turned to the proper size; so that when the jumpers by wearing became too little, they were sent to the smith to be made to their full size, by the hammer, according to the gauge ring referred to.

† It probably may be a satisfaction to the practical reader, as this mode of fixing by trenails may be useful on many occasions, to have some sort of proof of what is here advanced. He will remember the case of the *stemming* a hole for *blasting* rocks with gunpowder, that, after the proper quantity of powder is in, the ramming the hole, for five or six inches above the powder, with dry clay, or even the very powder of the stone that has been cleared out of the hole in boring, will, on firing the powder, produce so compleat a resistance, that the rock will sooner be split in another direction than the stemming will be driven out of the mouth of the hole. Now this does not happen because the stemming is of more solid or tenacious matter than the rock itself, but because the power to drive it out can act only upon the *end* of it, equal to the area of the circle of the hole; whereas the *hold* by which the stemming (or *wad*) is retained in the hole takes place in every point of the surface of the cylinder that it occupies. As for instance, suppose the hole to be 1⅛ inch diameter, then the area of it is nearly one square inch; and suppose the length of the cylinder occupied by the wad to be 6 inches, then the circumference of a circle, whose area is one square inch, being 3½ inches nearly, the circumference of the whole cylinder so engaged will be 21 square inches; so that it would require a force 21 times greater than that whereby the matter of the *Wad coheres* to the solid, to dislodge it from the hole lengthwise.——I do not find an instance in my Journal, nor does my memory furnish me with one, wherein the necessity occurred of getting any trenail out again after it had been driven; had that happened, it must have been bored out again, as I know of no force that could have been applied, which would have drawn it out.

Having mentioned the affair of blasting, it perhaps may not be amiss here to add, that the efficacy of the gunpowder to split the stone, rather than to drive out the stemming or wad, is greatly owing to a further circumstance. The force of the powder to drive out the wad is only in proportion to the area of the hole; whereas its power to divide the stone in a direction parallel to the hole, is as the area of a parallelogram formed by the diameter of the hole, multiplied by the length that the charge occupies; that is, the diameter of a hole whose area is one square inch, being 1⅛ nearly, if the length is 6 inches, the product will be 6¾; and so many times is the force that the same charge of powder exerts to split the stone, more than that to drive out the wad. Besides, every force exerted to drive the wad out of the hole, probably tends to make it take the stronger hold, in consequence of the parts of it being jambed harder together, as the force is greater.

 ladles,

ladles, and was brought to ſuch a conſiſtency as to occupy every void ſpace; and though a conſiderable part of this was water, yet that being abſorbed by the dry ſtones, and the more conſiſtent parts ſettled to the bottom, the vacuity being at the top, this was repeatedly refilled till all remained ſolid: the top was then pointed, and, when neceſſary, defended by a coat of plaſter.

The ſeveral courſes repreſented in Plate N° 10, are ſhewn as they would appear, when compleated with the whole of their wedges and trenails: and beſides theſe, there being alſo generally two *Lewis* holes upon the upper ſurface of each ſtone, thoſe ſerved as temporary fixtures for the work of the ſucceeding courſe.

224. IT was the ſame evening's tide of the 11th of Auguſt, that the baſement was compleated and the center ſtone of Courſe VII. was landed.——Of the preceding courſes, each was begun by the ſtones that engrafted in the dovetail receſſes cut in the rock; theſe ſtones therefore being immoveable by any aſſignable force acting horizontally, rendered thoſe ſo likewiſe that depended upon them; but having now brought the whole upon a level, we could not have this advantage any longer; it therefore became neceſſary to attain a ſimilar advantage by *artificial* means.——For this purpoſe the upper ſurface of Courſe VI. (ſee Plate N° 10. Fig. 6.) had a hole of one foot ſquare cut through the ſtone that occupied the center; and alſo eight depreſſions of one foot ſquare, ſunk into that courſe ſix inches deep, which were diſpoſed at regular diſtances round the center, as is ſhewn in that figure: theſe cavities were for the reception of eight cubes of marble, in maſonry called *Joggles**.——As a preparation for ſetting the center ſtone of Courſe VII. a *parallelopiped* (which for ſhortneſs ſake I will call the *Plug)* of ſtrong hard marble from the rocks near Plymouth, of one foot ſquare and twenty-two inches in length, was ſet with mortar in the central cavity, and therein firmly fixed with thin wedges. Courſe VI. being thirteen inches in height, this marble plug, which reached through, would riſe nine inches above it; upon this, the center ſtone (ſee Plate N° 11. Courſe VII.) having a hole through its center of a foot ſquare, was introduced upon the prominence of the plug, and being bedded in mortar, was in like manner wedged (with wedges on each ſide the plug) and every remaining cavity filled with grout. By this means no force of the ſea acting horizontally upon the center ſtone, leſs than what was capable of cutting the marble plug in two, was able to move it from its place: and to prevent the ſtone more effectually from being *lifted*, in caſe its bed of mortar happened to be deſtroyed, it was fixed down in the manner above deſcribed, by *four* trenails; which being placed near to the corners of the large ſquare of that ſtone, they not only effectually prevented the ſtone from lifting, but aided the center plug in preventing the ſtone from moving angularly or *twiſting*, which it might otherwiſe have done, notwithſtanding its weight, which was two tons nearly†.

225. WHILE the center plug of this courſe was preparing to be fixed, an accident happened, which, without ſome preſent reſolution, might have prevented my ſeeing the firſt ſtone placed. The level platform we then had obtained being ſomething of a novelty, I was enjoying it by walking to and fro upon it; by ſome inattention I made a falſe ſtep into one of the eight cavities for the *Joggles*, and not being able to recover myſelf, tumbled over the brink of the work down among the rocks on the weſt ſide; but the tide being then retreated, I preſently recovered my former ſtation, at firſt ſuppoſing myſelf but little hurt; but ſoon finding a very great and unuſual numbneſs in one of my thumbs, on looking upon it, I perceived, from its irregular direction, it was put out of joint. I reflected that I was at leaſt fourteen miles from a ſurgeon, and as far back again, and both ways ſubject to the uncertainty of winds and ſeas; I therefore laid faſt hold of it with the other hand and gave it a violent *pull*, upon which it ſnapped into its place; and I immediately proceeded to fix the plug. I had not much pain or uneaſineſs from it the firſt tide; but it was above ſix months after this accident, before I could make free uſe of it.

* When a ſmaller piece of ſtone, of any ſhape or kind, is let in between two larger ſtones, and partly into one, and partly into the other, ſo as to prevent their ſhifting place with reſpect to each other, thoſe pieces of ſtone are termed *Joggles*.

† An Edyſtone ſilver medal (ſee Plate N° 18.) was laid under the center ſtone, together with ſeveral pieces of money.

226. AFTER

226. AFTER fetting the firft center ftone of Courfe VII. we immediately proceeded to fet the four ftones that furround it, and which were united thereto by four dovetails, projecting from the four fides of the center ftone. Thefe ftones being fixed in their dovetails by a *pair* of wedges on each fide, at bottom and top, as has already been mentioned, and held down by a couple of trenails to each furrounding ftone, and ftill further ftcadied by joint wedges at the head of the dovetails, and alfo in the *mitre* or *diagonal* joints betwixt each furrounding piece; the whole formed a circular kind of ftone of ten feet diameter and above feven tons weight: and which being held down by a center plug and twelve trenails, became in effect one fingle ftone; whofe circumference was fufficient to admit of eight dovetail receffes to be formed therein, fo as to be capable of retaining in their places a circle of eight pieces of ftone of about 12 cwt. each, in the fame manner and upon the fame principle, that the *radical* pieces of ftone were engrafted into the dovetail receffes of the rock; and which being in like manner wedged and trenailed, we proceeded with circular *Tiers* of ftone, in the manner fhewn in Plate N° 11. Fig. 1.——It is however to be remarked, that the mode of applying the wedges and trenails being fufficiently explained in the feveral figures of Plate N° 10. and alfo in Plate N° 11. Fig. 1. to avoid a repetition of fmall work, the feveral fucceeding figures fimply fhew the general fhapes and difpofition of the different pieces compofing a courfe, and other incidental larger matters, wholly omitting the particular application of the wedges and trenails; yet it is to be obferved that they were every where equally applied, till we got to the *top* of the *Solid*.

227. WE went forward with Courfe VII. without any thing but common interruption for fome days.——It was remarked that upon the 12th of Auguft, the wind being eaftwardly, and moderate, there was the greateft fwell in the Gut that we ever had experienced, when we attempted to land ftones; the boat rofe and fell full four feet perpendicular, which rendered the management of it, and landing of the pieces extremely difficult; and had not our *purchafes* been very fpeedy in their action as well as forcible, we could not have done it at fuch a time; for after a ftone was raifed from the floor of the boat, the boat would rife under the ftone fo as fometimes to unhook it from the tackle, yet happily the boat fuftained no damage: and having now feen the five ftones of the center compleatly eftablifhed, I left RICHARDSON and company, after fetting the firft of the third tier, to compleat and go on with the reft in the fame manner.

228. MY much efteemed mafter and friend Mr. WESTON, who came from London to be witnefs of our proceedings, arrived at Plymouth during this interval. I went off with him early on Wednefday morning the 17th, attended by Mr. JESSOP and his company, and landed upon the rock at ten; RICHARDSON and company were then about to begin to fet the fifth tier, or circle of ftones which was to contain the eight cubes before defcribed.——Thefe cubes were fo difpofed upon the furface of Courfe VI. that the cavities cut on the under fide of Courfe VII. to take the upper half of each cube, fhould conftantly fall in the broad part of the ftones of the fifth circle; which will appear plain by confidering the dotted lines relative to Courfe VII. upon the furface of Courfe VI. (fee Plate N° 10. Fig. 6.) There could confequently be no application of wedges in the upper courfe to the faftening of the circle of ftones (N° 5.) upon their refpective cubes: when therefore the ftones refpectively came upon them, we put as much mortar upon the top of the cube, as would in part make good the joint betwixt it and its cavity, but not enough quite to fill it; becaufe if too full there was no ready way for the fuperfluous mortar to efcape; but a hole, of the fize of thofe for the trenails, being previoufly bored through each of thefe pieces, anfwerable to the middle of each cube; when the ftone was fet, wedged and trenailed, then it was very practicable, by *dreffing* a trenail fo as to become a *Ram-rod*, to drive as much mortar down the hole as would compleatly fill every vacancy betwixt the ftone and its cube; infomuch that we foon perceived, that if this was attempted before the ftone was compleatly trenailed down, that it would very eafily raife the ftone from its bed, as might indeed be expected from the principles of *Hydroftatics*: but being done after fuch completion, it brought the whole to the moft folid bearing that could be wifhed; and when the cement was *hardened* anfwered the end quite as effectually as if they had been wedged.

It may here be very properly faid, that fince thofe cubes could be of little ufe in keeping the work firmly together before the mortar was *hardened*; and after that had taken place, they could be of no

uf

uſe; becauſe the number of 108 trenails, of which one of theſe courſes conſiſted when compleat, being ſuppoſed ſufficient to keep it from liſting and moving out of its place; as the mortar hardened, and every additional courſe was an addition of its own weight upon the former, if thoſe cubes could have been diſpenſed with in the firſt inſtance, they might have been ſo ever after.——This reaſoning I can very well admit to be true; yet, when we have to do with, and to endeavour to controul, thoſe powers of nature that are ſubject to *no calculation*, I truſt it will be deemed prudent not to omit, in ſuch a caſe, any thing that can without difficulty be applied, and that would be likely to add to the ſecurity.——It may further be remarked, that as this building was intended to be a maſs of ſtone held together by the natural and artificial union of its parts, it would have been out of character, that when compleated, it ſhould be beholden to certain parts of *Wood* for its *Conſolidation**.

229. I HAVE mentioned, § 67. that I originally conceived more than one way of preventing the courſes from ſhifting place upon one another. My firſt conceptions were to form a riſe (or a depreſſion) of three inches, bounded by a circle ſomewhat about the diameter of that in which the joggles are placed; which ſtep or depreſſion would have formed a ſocket, whereby the courſes would have been mutually engrafted, not much different from what nature has pointed out in the *baſaltine* columns of the *Giant's Cauſeway:* but conſidering how much unneceſſary trouble and intricacy would be hereby introduced, by one part of the bed of the *ſame* ſtone being liable to be three inches higher than the other, I judged that the end would be very ſufficiently anſwered by the much more plain, eaſy, and ſimple method of joggles; eſpecially as, for this purpoſe, the firmeſt and tougheſt kind of ſtone might be choſen, and the number multiplied at pleaſure. One *plug* in the middle, of a foot ſquare, and eight *joggles* of a foot cube each, of the hardeſt marble, diſpoſed in the manner deſcribed, ſeemed to me, along with the additional ſtrength and ſecurity ariſing from the trenails; as alſo from the infinite number of little indentures upon the ſurface of the courſes, as well as the Lewis Holes, each being filled with an extuberance of mortar, which, when hard, would in effect become a *ſteady pin*; from the *coheſion* of the mortar as a ſolid, promiſing to be no leſs than that of the ſtone; together with the incumbent weight of every part of the building above; every joint thus ſeparately conſidered, ſeemed in point of firmneſs ſo ſatisfactory to my mind, that if the whole of this proved too little, it was out of my power to conceive what would be enough.

230. WHILE I am upon this part of my ſubject, I will take an opportunity of obſerving that it was a part of my problem, which I will not take upon me to ſay that I have accurately ſolved; but I have endeavoured to do it, ſo far as my *feelings*, rather than *calculations*, would bear me out: That the building ſhould be a column of *equal ſtrength*, proportionate in every part to the ſtreſs it was likely to bear, (regard being alſo had to its *uſe*,) was a view of the ſubject I was naturally and forcibly led to, as I found it eternally rung in my ears from all quarters, that *a Building of* STONE *upon the Edyſtone would certainly be overſet.* I therefore endeavoured to form it, and put it together ſo, that while a ſimilarity of uſe permitted a ſimilar conſtruction, no man ſhould be able to tell me at *what* joint it would overſet; for, if at any given height the uppermoſt courſe was, when compleated, ſafe, it became more ſafe by another courſe being laid upon it; and that upper courſe, though ſomewhat leſs in weight, and in the total coheſion of its parts, than the former; yet every courſe, from the firſt foundation, was leſs and leſs ſubject to the heavy ſtroke of the ſea.

231. IN the morning and evening's tide of the 17th we ſet the whole of the fifth tier, and conſequently the whole of the eight cubes were then inlaid. The morning of the 18th we again landed; but Mr. WESTON, after expreſſing his entire approbation of our proceedings, returned to Plymouth in the Aſſiſtant; I ſtaid in hopes of ſeeing the whole courſe cloſed. In this morning and evening's tide, though rough, we had got ſet five pieces of Circle 6. and had landed the remaining three; as alſo one of the

* Indeed the application of theſe cubic joggles ſo well accords with my feelings in reſpect to ſtability, that I ſhould even now have regretted it if they had been omitted, and ſhould be ſorry to have them *now* removed, if it was poſſible.

largeſt

largest pieces of moorstone for the east side, (see Plate N° 11. Fig. 1.) This evening's tide we worked with links, and it began to blow so fresh that we had much ado to keep them in, being obliged to make a fire of them upon the surface of the work. We were under the necessity at last to quit the rock with some precipitation, and were very glad to get into our yawls; things being left in the following posture. Two of the pieces, Tier 6. were simply dropped into their places on the north-west side, while the third piece, being about a ton, and the piece of moorstone near upon two tons, were chained together, and to the work of Course VII. that was already set; these two loose pieces being upon the top of that course near the east side: the triangles were lashed down upon the floor of the work, as we had practised several times before.—— The sea became so rough in the night, that the Weston at the transport buoy was obliged to *slip* and make for an harbour. Next day the wind increased, so that the sea broke over the shear-heads at low water. I waited in hopes of an alteration of weather till the 22d, when I returned to Plymouth in the yawl, the wind being S. W.——Upon the 25th, though the weather continued still bad, the Assistant carried out RICHARDSON and company, and brought home Mr. JESSOP and company, who left every thing well upon the rock, as far as they could discover from the buss, but had shared their last pound of bread. The bad weather still continued to increase till the 28th, when there was a violent storm at S. W. so that the *Antelope* man of war in the *Sound*, of fifty guns, dragged her anchors, and was in great danger of driving upon the rocks.

The 29th I perceived with my telescope, from the *Hoa*, the buss to ride safe, but could not see the shears, or indeed any thing else upon the rock distinctly, except the breakers. The day following being more clear, and the sea somewhat subsided, I distinctly saw the buss and the rock; but the shears not being visible, I immediately went on board the Edystone boat to reconnoitre the state of things, and left orders with Mr. JESSOP in the mean time to prepare new shears.——The wind being N. W. I passed the rock several times under sail, but there was no possibility of landing.——I observed that not only all the work which had been compleatly set was entire, but that the two stones mentioned to have been simply lowered into their places also remained therein, and that the 5 cwt. still rested upon the stone whereon it was left. The west face of the building had got so compleat a coat of sea weed that it was only distinguishable from the rock by its form: but the shears and triangles were entirely gone; the two pieces of stone that had been chained together and to the work, were also gone; the windlass frame broken and much damaged, and the roll gone; the fender piles and the transport buoy however remained in their places.——The buss I was told had rode it out very well, but not without frequently alarming the company on board, with an apprehension of her breaking loose, she having shipped many heavy seas on deck, and one so great they expected the deck to have been staved in; they had veered out seven fathoms of bridle cable, but were afraid to ease out more, lest it should touch the rocks.——This was in reality the greatest storm we had ever experienced while out at the rock; yet we were less chagrined for the damages done, than thankful that they were not greater.

232. THE 1st of September JESSOP and company went out to shift RICHARDSON; who sent me a letter, informing me they had caught an opportunity of reconnoitring the Gut, and found the two stones washed off from the rock to be lying therein, and which, as he apprehended they could be weighed, there would be no need to proceed with new pieces on shore. It was the 3d of September before this company could make a landing to do any thing upon the rock; so that since the 18th ult. there had been an interval of fifteen days in which we had been totally interrupted by bad weather in the very prime part of the season. However, every thing having been expedited on shore to get refitted for work, this day I went out therewith, and began to set up our new shears, windlass, &c. and with the shears got up the piece of Portland of Circle 6. which was set, as also the others that had been left loose in their dovetails; but the tide of flood coming on, had deepened the water too much before we could try to get up the other.

The getting up of the piece of Portland stone was effected by means of the same utensil wherewith we got up that mentioned § 212; and though it lay the wrong side upward, yet as the trenail holes always reached through the stone, into which the instrument was introduced, (see its description,) this difference of circumstance was at present of no consequence; but when the next day we introduced it into one of the trenail holes of the piece of moorstone, that lying also the wrong side upwards, (for the holes being bored from the upper side, were therefore naturally a little taper), this circumstance prevented the pin from going in so far as it otherwise would have done; the holes being also nearer the corner, and the stone double the weight of the former, when the stone was got up to the surface of the water, it then becoming heavier by losing its buoyancy, the pin became bent, and thereby the hold of the tool upon the stone releasing, it dropped down again to the bottom; it however fortunately fell upon its end, and in this position we found means to get a chain round its waist.——To one of the strong chains, which were about ten feet long, wherewith we used to chain our loose pieces of stone upon the work when we left them, we fastened a rope to each end, and lowering the chain in a loop beyond it, we could then, by bringing the two ropes together, bring the chain round the waist of the stone; but the difficulty was to confine the two parts together so close to the stone, as to prevent its turning out of the chain when we came to heave upon it: for this purpose I bethought me of putting an iron ring over the double rope, the weight of which might draw the two parts together; but that not proving to do it sufficiently, while expedients were concerting, JOHN BOWDEN, whose invention was ever ready, cried out, "*Twist the ropes*, master;" and by this simple expedient, the parts being drawn so close that the ring went home, it was impossible for the stone to slip, and therefore, not long before it was relanded upon the rock*.——The depth of the water was twelve feet.——The three parts of the *Lewis* by which this stone had been chained, were found in the hole, but the bolt and shackle were gone. The like parts of the lewis were left in the work to which the same chain was hooked, but the bolt was gone, and half of the shackle found in one of the cube holes. We also remarked that the surface of the work upon which the stones had lain, that had been chained, was brought almost to a polish, as well as the under bed of the Portland piece that was driven into the Gut. ——As the shears were fastened at the top as well as the bottom, it is difficult to suppose they could at once leave the rock; most probably therefore it was the legs of the shears that broke the windlass after one or both had got loose at bottom; otherwise it is not easy to imagine that the water could lay such hold of its frame as to break it in the manner it was broken, being wholly of iron. (See Plate Nº 14. Fig. 1.)

233. SEPTEMBER the 5th the seventh circle was finished and the eighth begun; and this day the wind being variable from N. E. to N. W. and very moderate, was remarkable, as being the first time of the people having worked, till they were obliged to quit the rock for refreshment: and now every thing being reinstated, it was some time before we met with any but the ordinary interruptions.——On the 7th I had notice from Mr. JESSOP of his expecting to compleat Course VII. that day, being the first circular course: I therefore went, accompanied by Messrs. WESTON and RICHARDSON, on board the Edystone boat, which was loaded with the center, and its surrounding stones, of Course VIII. We arrived at the buss in the night, and were informed by Mr. JESSOP, that the weather had been so calm that the top of the work had not been wet for three days; that therefore they had worked from light in the morning to dark in the evening, but not in the nights. That Course VII. was compleatly closed, pointed and grouted; and that the top of the work, where it needed, had been levelled, and every irregularity in the face of the work rectified.——In the morning of September the 8th, we landed at break of day, and the Edystone boat having been unloaded, we proceeded to set her cargo: and, besides the satisfaction that Mr. WESTON enjoyed in setting the center plug of Course VIII. which was managed in all respects as already described of Course VII.† he was entertained with the appearance of a fleet around us, consisting of a convoy of

* On this occasion it may not be amiss to observe the great advantage that arises, in the greater operations of mechanics, from the having commodious tackles and utensils. We had not compleated the setting up of the windlass, when we found it necessary to heave up the two stones before mentioned; we therefore (applying a sufficient number of men to the main tackle) heaved them up *by hand*: and though there was no *difficulty* in this, yet I could not help remarking the vast difference there was in the *Time* and *Power*, between the application of men's strength in this way and by the windlass. I therefore afterwards purposely noted the minutes they were in heaving up one of the large moorstone pieces of Circle 7. by hand from the boat; and by the time this was done the windlass was compleated; and then, by a few trials therewith, found that four men at the windlass hoisted a stone in *half* the time that it took twelve men to do in *heaving by hand*, though the *Tackle* remained the same to both.

† It may be necessary to say, that this center plug was four inches shorter than the *first*; because Course VI. being thirteen inches thick, was four inches more than half the *medium* thickness, of the courses above, which were eighteen inches at an average.

above

above a hundred ſail of *Weſt India* and *Mediterranean* merchant ſhips; to whoſe future ſafety, we had the ſatisfaction to ſuppoſe ourſelves contributing.——After ſetting the plug and the center ſtone, Mr. WESTON returned to Plymouth.

The fineneſs of the ſeaſon now continued to favour the expediting of our works, inſomuch that Courſe VIII. which was begun upon the 8th, was executed in five days, being entirely compleated on the 13th at the ſame hour. Every thing went regularly on till the 20th; ſo that in return for our continued interruption from the ſtormy weather for fifteen days, our works had an uninterrupted progreſſion for eighteen days, when Courſe IX. was advanced to the fifth circle: but at this time, notwithſtanding the wind had been moderate at E. for a week paſt, yet there came on ſo great a ground ſwell from the ſouth-weſt, that though both the companies had uſed their joint endeavours to get the Edyſtone boat into the Gut, they had not been able to effect it.

234. THE greateſt hinderance we had met with during the laſt fine ſeaſon aroſe from the uncommon *lowneſs* of the tides, which were ſo much ſo, that our ſtone veſſels were liable to be catched by the keel in going out from the Jetty Head in Mill Bay. This inconvenience was in a great meaſure remedied by a thought of Mr. JESSOP's, who contrived to borrow a *Punt* or flat ſquare veſſel, which, being loaded at the Jetty Head, was then hauled out into deep water, where her cargo could be ſhifted into the boats of paſſage, at any time of the tide.——An incident however happened, reſpecting our uſe of this punt, that demonſtrates the extreme degree of malevolence which *ſometimes* poſſeſſes the breaſt of man. She was loaded on Monday the 12th in the evening, and hauled out as uſual; and the next morning (the night having proved uncommonly calm) the punt was found, on hauling up her moorings, to be ſwinging by a ſingle yarn, the reſt having been cut with a *knife*, at three fathoms under water; doubtleſs that it might not be diſcovered, otherwiſe than by the effect of the veſſel's being driven upon the rocks, and there ſunk with her cargo, to our no ſmall diſappointment in the progreſs of the work: a circumſtance, that as it could not contribute to any man's advantage or pleaſure, indicated a degree of *turpitude*, at which, were it not for ſuch inſtances as theſe, it could hardly be ſuppoſed the human mind was capable of arriving.

235. IT was not till the 25th that any of the boats could keep the ſea; for when they attempted to go out, they were as often obliged to return with their cargoes: however, the Weſton's cargo being firſt wanted; J. BOWDEN, always deſirous to promote the ſervice to the utmoſt of his power, went out this day to the tranſport buoy, with a reſolution to ride it out there if poſſible, and which, with great difficulty and ſome hazard, he did; and in the evening of the 26th his cargo was landed, which enabled the work to go on again as intervals offered. I went out on the 27th, and was witneſs to the great difficulty there was in preſerving the boats from being wrecked in the gut; the eaſterly wind having raiſed ſo great a ſwell on that ſide of the rocks, that two of them ſucceſſively broke their faſtenings, and were in the utmoſt peril of being ſtaved; yet ſteadily endeavouring to uſe our *beſt efforts* to expedite the work, no material damage in reality happened; though the boats rolled to that degree, that every moment one would have expected the maſt of the veſſel and the ſhears to have got entangled together ſo as to carry one or both away.

236. THE 29th of September all the remaining pieces belonging to Courſe IX. were happily landed from the Weſton, and the veſſel got clear of the Gut.——We found the beſt method of a boat's going into the Gut was; when ſhe arrived at the tranſport buoy, for one of the yawls to carry her a rope to the landing-place, as alſo one to the principal rocks on each ſide, entering the Gut; thoſe on board then heaving upon whichever of theſe three ſeemed moſt requiſite, alſo veering out a ſufficient rope *double* from her bows, and paſſing through the ring of the tranſport buoy, ſhe goes into the Gut *ſtern foremoſt*; and by theſe means has a faſtening head and ſtern, as alſo one on each ſide.——When going out of the Gut, ſhe heaves by the double rope towards the tranſport buoy, and when clear of the rocks ſhe can either go to the buoy, or, by the rope's being double, ſhe can ſlip her hold of it, and get under ſail. ——A ground ſwell coming from S. W. ſoon after, obliged us to quit the rock; but the next day we landed, and ſet the remaining ſtones, which compleated Courſe IX; and the maſons proceeded to rectify the face

face of the work, where it was in any degree wanting thereof, that there might be no need hereafter to disturb any part of the coat of weed, which was likely to fix upon it during the winter.

237. BEING now arrived at the eve of October, I maturely considered our situation; and finding that we had been eighteen days in compleating the last course, whereas the former one (Course VIII.) was begun and finished in five; though the weather, both on shore and above-head, had remained to all appearance much the same; I from thence concluded it to be very probable, we might not get another course compleated in the compass of the month of October; so that when I reflected on the many disasters we had suffered last year, by continuing out till the month of November, and how little work we in reality did after *this* time, it appeared to me very problematical whether we might be able, with every possible exertion, to get another course finished this *Season:* and considering how very ineligible it was to have a course lie open during the winter, in this stage of the work; and that we had now got three compleat courses established above the top of the rock, the sum of whose heights was four feet six inches; and that we could not leave the work in a more defensible state, whether as relative to the natural violence of the sea, or the possibility of *external* injuries; from these considerations, it appeared to me highly proper to put a period to the out-work of the present season; and this opinion was heartily concurred in by Messrs. Jessop and Richardson.

We therefore proceeded to take down the shears and windlass, and to weigh the transport buoy chain and anchor, which we successfully did, by applying all hands thereto on board the Weston; but in effecting this we providentially escaped what, if it had taken place, would have proved in all probability a very unfortunate disaster.——The anchor, as mentioned § 208. being of 12 cwt. was a heavy one in proportion to the size of our *Craft*; and it was weighed by means of its buoy rope, and got close to the bows of the Weston. The chain of the transport buoy then hung down in a loop from the ring of the anchor, the other end being supported by that buoy; which, that the whole might float together, was confined to the side of the Weston by a small *luff*-tackle which laid hold of it.——We then proceeded to hoist the transport buoy into the Weston by her runner and tackle, from the mast-head; but the hook being too small to encompass the ring of the buoy; it was fixed by means of a salvagee: and this small circumstance saved us; for by the time the buoy was hoisted out of the water, observing that its weight and appendant chain a good deal *heeled* the Weston, and was in consequence making a strong effort to quit the vessel's side, I ordered the tinners to *hold fast* the *luff-tackle*, which they unfortunately mistook for an order to *let go* the luff-tackle; on this the buoy immediately quitted the vessel's side: I happened to be with others in the yawl on the outside of the buoy, where we had been fastening the salvagee; and seeing the buoy separating from the vessel, and driving us outward, and that the weight of the buoy and chain was gaining more and more purchase upon the mast, as it heeled more outward; in consequence, there being nothing to prevent the further separation of the vessel and the buoy, this advantage must have become every moment greater, till the vessel had overset, filled, and sunk: in this dilemma it occurred to me to make use of my *Pocket Knife* to cut the salvagee; which being instantly done, the Weston immediately righted, and the buoy was soon after got on board in the manner it was first intended.

238. THE 1st of October we proceeded to heave in the bridle cable of the buss, and instead of it to fix to the great swivel of the moorings (which we found unhurt) a new buoy chain that we had received from London, to be applied instead of the other; which being made with short links, would relieve us in future from the anxiety we had in heaving up the bridle chain and swivel the beginning of this season. (See § 207.) This was put down, and the great buoy and chain affixed upon the top of it, which had rode the whole of last winter, and had served us as a transport buoy during the season we were then about concluding. The buss was now rode by this buoy till the wind should come fair to carry her into harbour; the whole being ready to cast off at a moment's warning.——This business being compleated, and a good opportunity of landing on the rock offering itself, I again went upon it with Mr. Jessop and the masons; and having compleatly rectified the outside, and finished every thing to my mind, we went on board the Weston and Assistant with the company, leaving the buss to the care of the seamen, who were all

all on board, except the two masters of the boats, BOWDEN and MEDLING, in their respective vessels, and landed at Plymouth the same evening.——The next day, Sunday October the 2d, BOWDEN and MEDLING went out to assist SMART and the other seamen in bringing in the buss as soon as the wind came fair.——They sailed with the buss on Monday the 3d at four P. M. but it was not till the next day at noon that she arrived at Mill Bay: she was hauled up upon the beach the same evening, and I took leave of the work-yard for that season; exhorting the men to diligence and unanimity, and leaving every thing about the work up to the entry door ready to go to sea, which was intended to be pitched upon the fourteenth course, I set forward from Plymouth for London the 5th of October*.

* Besides what precedes, in relation of the incidents of the last season, I have omitted one in its proper place, that may indeed be esteemed more of a ludicrous than a serious nature; and, as it was not set down in my Journal at the time, depends now altogether upon my memory; as however the thought might, in like case, have its utility, I will give it a place in this note.——I think it was after we had got the shears refitted, after the storm § 232. I was desirous to shew the people the advantage that might be had from the construction of the shears, in enabling us to get off from the rock, in case any of us should be left there, when the yawls could not possibly go alongside to take us off in the usual way: and, to introduce the affair the more readily, I set about to give them an example. From Plate N° 14. it will appear that the shears were kept upright, and were managed, by two strong *guy* (or guide) ropes, one passing from the head of the shears over the area of the house, which was fastened to the rocks, above low water, on the west side of the rock; the other, counter-acting it, passed over the Gut, and was fixed to one of the rocks in the south reef on the *east side* of the Gut. This last rope therefore wholly crossed the Gut, obliquely from the top of the shears, down nearly to low water mark. I mounted to the head of the shears, and clung upon the guy rope, and, as the descent was with a considerable declivity, it was easy to work myself downwards, which I did without difficulty, till I approached somewhat near the surface of the water; I then ordered the yawl to come underneath me, to take me in, and when I found my feet in the boat, I concluded I had nothing to do but quit hold with my hands; but the very moment in which I quitted hold, the boat took a sudden *yaw* or *sheer*, which canted me overboard, head-long into the sea. No ill consequence however happened, except a thorough wetting to myself; but failing of ultimate success, though by means of a *collateral* circumstance not necessarily connected with the operation, no one ever repeated the trial; that is to say, we were never put to the real *want* of it, though every one present was convinced of the practicability of the *manœuvre*, in case necessity should in future call for it.

C H A P. II.

Comprehending the Account of Transactions from my leaving Plymouth in October, 1757, to the Conclusion of the Working Season of 1758.

239. THE interval between the conclusion of the outwork of the year 1757, and the commencement of that in 1758, furnished some memorable events.——The first that happened was of an untoward nature. In the beginning of December there happened a violent storm, so great as to drive the floating light from her moorings, and oblige her to go into Plymouth; and from whose master we learnt, that in passing by the Edystone all then appeared to be well. From this time the weather continued so tempestuous that it was the month of March before any of our boats could venture out to reconnoitre, when I received a letter from Mr. JESSOP, containing the disagreeable news, that the great buoy of the moorings was gone, as also the buoys of the anchors; but that the seamen were at work *sweeping* for the anchors, and though they had not been so lucky as to find them, yet when the weather became more favourable, they did not doubt of success.——This was a matter that required the fullest attention; and, on a consultation with the proprietors, it was determined not to rest the matter solely upon the efforts of our seamen, but, to spur the whole body of fishermen, &c. upon the coast to exertion, a reward of £ 50 was offered to whoever should recover the moorings. At the same time it was further determined not entirely to trust to our hopes of finding them, and therefore, without loss of time, a new set of chains was bespoke of Mr. WILSON of *Blackwall*, who had made those already described; so that these might be going on while endeavours were used to find the former; and if found, there would be no other loss, than that we should have so much

much ſpare chain upon hand as ſhould be made at the time; and which, as what *had happened* might happen again, there poſſibly would be occaſion for in future. This matter being therefore now in a proper train, I ſhall proceed to an event of a more pleaſing kind.

240. THE proprietors of the Edyſtone acquainted the Corporation of TRINITY HOUSE that their engineer being now in town, and, having made a conſiderable progreſs with the work upon the rock, was, together with themſelves, deſirous of giving them full information of the proceedings; and that nothing would be more ſatisfactory to the public, as well as to themſelves, than to merit their approbation. This was the 21ſt of March, and on the 22d they received an anſwer from Mr. SHUTTLEWOOD, Secretary to the Corporation, appointing the Saturday ſe'nnight following.

In this interview I had the pleaſing ſatisfaction of fully explaining to that honourable Board, not only what I had done, by means of the models and drawings I had laid before the Board of Admiralty, but alſo what I propoſed further to do; obſerving, that what was already executed would *equally ſerve* as a very firm foundation and baſement for a *Timber* ſtructure, in caſe it ſhould be their opinion that ſuch a one would be preferable to that of ſtone propoſed: but, after a full inveſtigation, they were pleaſed to honour the propoſition with their decided opinion, that nothing could anſwer ſo well as the building propoſed; which opinion was ſtill the more acceptable, as it was that of the *moſt competent* judges.

The Board, after many enquiries concerning the place and manner of our moorings, were pleaſed to offer me a ſet of mooring chains, they had at Falmouth, in caſe we ſhould need them, which though neither new nor ſo heavy as thoſe prepared, by their directions, for the Neptune buſs, yet might ſerve on occaſion, as we did not expect to continue out in the *worſt* of the ſeaſon. The corporation were alſo pleaſed to deſire me to give them at times an account of my proceedings and progreſs, from Plymouth; by their doing which, I eſteemed myſelf much honoured, as well as obliged by the offer of the chains.

241. AFTER this the accounts from Plymouth continuing conſtantly the ſame; that every thing was going on briſkly in the yard; that the ſeaſon was but little favourable to the ſweeping for the recovery of the moorings; and that the attempts which had already been made, proved abortive; I took a reſolution of going down to Plymouth, though not by way of proceeding with the building, till the ſeaſon arrived when the weather was more likely to continue ſettled, as well as fine; yet, as I had frequently found difficulties to be ſurmounted when I was preſent, that continued obſtacles when I was abſent; and though the operation of *ſweeping** was not a thing to which I had been accuſtomed, I notwithſtanding found myſelf much inclined to be preſent, in order to expedite the buſineſs as far as in my power.

242. I ARRIVED at Plymouth on Sunday the 16th of April, and found every thing at Mill Bay to my ſatisfaction; the laſt cargo of ſtone from Portland having been delivered in December, and Courſe XXXI. was in hand working, being that whereon the windows of the ſecond room were to be placed. The ſolid part of the houſe was entirely compleated and off the platform, ſo that had our moorings been in readineſs, I might have been tempted to have carried out the buſs.——But I was ſcarcely arrived at Plymouth before an expreſs came after me, upon a difficulty that had ariſen in the progreſs of the *Calder Navigation* Bill, and I was wanted to attend a committee of the *Houſe* of *Commons* upon the 24th inſtant: I therefore was obliged to content myſelf with a conſultation with our ſeamen and Mr. JESSOP; and it was their opinion, that as, from the roughneſs of the rocks at the bottom, the anchors would natu-

* The operation of *ſweeping* for an anchor is as follows. A couple of boats of a proper ſize are manned; and, as near as they can judge of the place where the anchor lies, they, at a competent diſtance from each other, row or ſail abreaſt, having a hawſer or ſmall cable paſſing from one boat to the other, and of ſuch a length that a conſiderable part of it may drag upon the ground. This, on a plain bottom, will naturally hang upon the arm of the anchor ſtanding obliquely upward; provided the ſhank of the anchor lies eaſtward, that the tide runs weſt at the time of taking the ſweep, and the boats are moving *with* the tide; for it is evident, if the hawſer hooks upon the anchor, that the two boats will tend to come together, and, the two parts being brought into one boat, if ſhe heaves upon them till ſhe approaches nearly over the anchor, as the cable will be prevented by the broad part or *Flake* from ſlipping off the arm, a proper purchaſe being then applied, the anchor may be weighed.

rally

rally get into the hollow places, the ſweep ropes had conſtantly gone over without touching them; and therefore they adviſed to ſweep with a ſmall rope, not ſufficient to weigh the anchor; but firſt to hook it, and then to ſweep with a larger rope with weights upon it, ſo as to ſink it into the hollows, and thereby catch the anchor alſo.

243. IN this ſituation I left our ſeamen to make the trial, the promiſed reward not having as yet excited any others to the attempt. I attended upon the 24th at the Houſe of Commons, and upon the 30th was back again at Plymouth; when, on my arrival I was told by the ſeamen, that by the ſcheme concerted before I left them, they had the preceding day the good fortune to hook one of the anchors, which they weighed off the ground; but were unable to bring it to the ſurface, on account of the heavineſs of the chain to which it was fixed, and the ſmallneſs of our veſſels; however, they had ſecured the ſweep rope by letting drop a *Runner-Ring*, as mentioned § 232, and had fixed a buoy thereon.——It happened that the tides ran ſo remarkably ſhort at this time, that our buſs did not float at high water. We therefore procured the uſe of a ſloop that lay in the harbour, which the very next day was fitted out with a roll proper for heaving up the anchor and chains; and, at three in the morning the 2d of May, I went on board with Mr. JESSOP, all our ſeamen, and eight or nine hands from our yard; the *Aſſiſtant* accompanying us. We arrived at the moorings at eight; at firſt we could not ſee any thing of the buoy the ſeamen had fixed, but when the tide was fallen away we got ſight of it, and ſoon weighed the mooring anchor; but by the time we had got it above water the wind began to freſhen at eaſt, and raiſed ſuch a ſwell that we durſt not attempt to get it upon deck, ſo as to haul in the chain and come at the bridle; and therefore were obliged to be contented with ſecuring our temporary buoy rope upon the anchor, lowering it down again to the bottom, and then return to Plymouth.

The weather remained unfavourable till the 11th of May, when we went out with the buſs; and, having conſidered the numberleſs diſappointments which we had experienced, chiefly as it ſhould ſeem, from the ſtiffneſs of the ropes and unevenneſs of the bottom, I had determined to get a ſix inch cable *laid* of a ſufficient length for ſuch purpoſes, and the yarns to be ſo looſely twiſted together that it might be conſidered as of the nature of a *Salvagee:* carrying this along with us, and finding the place of the anchor by means of the buoy we had fixed upon it, we laid effectual hold of the anchor with it, which was in twenty fathoms water, and ſoon got it up to the bows; but when we began to heave in our ground chain, we found it to come in much heavier than we expected. We thereupon fixed our great tackle to it in addition, and hove all *taught*, but without procuring any more of the chain. We therefore made all faſt, and, it being nine P. M. concluded to let all ſtand till the next morning. The wind then beginning to freſhen at E. the buſs got ſome motion, and while we were refreſhing ourſelves there came on a ſudden rumbling of the chains, which put the buſs into ſo great a tremor, that we concluded the chains were gone overboard to the bottom; we ran upon deck, and, to our great ſurprize, found all ſtanding as we left it: after this two or three more rumblings enſued, but gradually leſs; ſo that it would ſeem the chains had by degrees diſentangled themſelves from the rocks, as after this the buſs rode without any particular ſtrain upon the tackle; and the wind continuing freſh, we did not reſume our work till day-break on the 12th.——The ground chain now came in kindly, and about ten o'clock we came to and got in the bridle and ſwivel, the buoy chain being faſt thereto; as alſo the under buoy and the upper chain; which, as it appeared to me, had ſunk the under buoy to the bottom, it being much water ſoaken. In fact, we recovered the whole of our moorings, except the upper or great buoy, and the bolt by which it had been fixed; ſo that from the appearance we concluded the failure had been in the *Forelock** of the bolt; but whether it had gradually worked itſelf looſe by the continual motion, or by ſome violent jerk of the ſea, or blow from ſome veſſel's having run upon it, we could not determine.——By three o'clock we got the chains and the anchor lowered, and the buſs as compleatly moored, in our own opinion, as ſhe ever had been in either of the former ſeaſons; which, conſidering the number of diſappointments we had experienced, muſt be ſuppoſed to have been attended with unuſual joy and ſatisfaction.

* A *Forelock*, in ſhipwrights terms, is the key or wedge by which a bolt is drawn tight, or prevented from ſlipping out.

244. DURING

244. DURING the time I was out upon this business, I took an opportunity at pinch of low water to view the works upon the rock. It was with no small difficulty that I landed; but I was much surprized, notwithstanding what had been reported of the soundness of the work, to find it so perfectly entire; for, except a small spawl which had been washed from the rock itself, the whole did not seem to have suffered a diminution of so much as a grain of sand since I left it on the 1st of October: on the contrary, the cement, and even the grouted part, appeared to be as hard as the Portland stone itself; the whole having become one *solid mass*; and indeed it had that appearance, as it was then entirely covered with the same coat of sea-weed as the rock, the top of the work excepted, which was washed so clean and white, that the lines thereon appeared more distinct than they had done upon the platform in the work-yard; no weed having fixed upon the upper surface except in the cube-holes and lewis-holes, which constantly holding water, were grown over with green weed like the outside. The fender piles were indeed all gone, but this was a trifling disaster, as they could soon be renewed; and we thought ourselves happy in the prospect of getting to work upon the rock so early in the season.

245. SATURDAY the 14th of May the whole of the Portland stone work being compleated in the work-yard, the stone-cutters in that branch were dismissed: and upon the 16th the fender piles at the rock were restored; contenting ourselves now with two, fixed as is shewn in Plate N° 14. The shears, the windlass, and all the rock tackle, with the transport buoy, being compleatly fixed*, our boats were now loaded with stone, and the first sailed to the transport buoy; but though the weather was not favourable for delivering their cargoes, yet it being seasonable, I determined they should keep out from Mill Bay, that they might take the earliest opportunity, and no time be lost. And now, what could hinder our progress? Yet such however is the uncertainty of human affairs, and particularly of those that depend upon the state of the winds and waves, that, from this time till the 2d of July, instead of prosecuting the work, our thoughts and attention were wholly employed to remedy disasters.

246. HAVING employed the 16th of May in writing an account of our late proceedings to the TRINITY BOARD, I went out to the buss to take the first opportunity of landing the center stone of Course X. the vessel that had it on board riding at the transport buoy; thus every thing continued fair and promising, and we expected every hour that the ground swell would subside sufficiently to give us leave to get the vessel into the Gut. In this state we were obliged to wait from day to day till the 23d, when, about three o'clock in the morning, the watch upon deck came down to acquaint me that the buss had dragged her eastern anchor, for that she had got a considerable distance from the buoy; whereupon we all hastened upon deck, and found that we had really got out of the accustomed place; however in a little time the buss came apparently into her former situation, and finding the bridle *taught*, we concluded she had taken some extraordinary swing, and that all was come right again. After waiting awhile for the approach of day, we could not discern our buoy, and we observed that we were removed further from the rock, so that, on applying to the bridle a second time, we found that the chain was dragging upon the rocks: but how it had been separated, as the buss had not rode with any extraordinary strain since she was last placed at her moorings, we could by no means guess; and finding that we still continued driving from the rock, we concluded to drop an anchor as soon as we got into clean ground. The spring-tide of flood however came on so strong, that though the wind blew a fresh gale at E. we were carried so fast to the eastward that we concluded it unsafe to anchor, and therefore advisable, for the present, to *bend* our sails (which had indeed been all unbent and stowed down in the *hold* for the summer) and try to gain *Plymouth Sound*; which being done with as much dexterity and readiness as could be expected from three seamen, assisted by masons and tinners, we got under way, and proceeded to heave in our bridle cable, at the end of which was the great swivel with the five fathoms of chain that had been added at the end of the last season, but no-

* During this interval upon the rock the masons were employed in reducing the whole area of the work to a strict level; and it was very remarkable to observe, that the *strokes* of the mallet and tool were equally compleat and perfect in *driving a fair chissel draft* across the joints, as upon the entire stone; which was a proof of the firm coherence of the component matter.

thing

thing farther; and finding that even the swivel had struck against the rocks, we concluded that the bolt and shackle, joining this chain to the former, by some accidental stroke had got its forelock broken or beat out*, and then, by the continual working of the sea, it could not be long before the shackle became unbolted, and in consequence the vessel set adrift: but having carefully placed a buoy upon our western anchor, we were not apprehensive of any other ill consequence from this accident than the hindrance which the repetition of the same operation that was performed upon the 11th and 12th instant must necessarily occasion.——At ten o'clock on the 23d we came to an anchor in the Sound; from whence the winds and seas prevented our stirring for several days.

247. THE 3d of June, at two A. M. I went with Mr. Jessop and company on board the buss, and go out near the rocks at nine; but how great was our surprize and mortification to find that the buoy, which we had taken great precaution to secure upon the anchor, was gone. We therefore came to an anchor about a mile to the N. W. of the rock, which we judged to be in clean ground, and I went in a yawl with Mr. Jessop to make enquiries at the floating light.——The master informed us, that on Wednesday the 24th ult. he went on shore in his boat; but it being then thick weather, it was thought advisable to make the rock in their way to Plymouth, that they might more readily hit the Sound; and he then observed the buoy floating, and that two *Polparra* fishing boats were in sight.

On our return to our station about twelve we began to sweep for our moorings as before, but without success; this we repeated at six, when the tide became again favourable; next morning we tried again, and laid hold of something which we judged to be the under buoy of the western anchor; but the tide running too strongly, prevented us from using our salvagee rope: we therefore went upon the rock, where we fixed the chains and rings for steadying the boats in the Gut; and after clearing away the weeds from the cube holes, we set the center plug ready for fixing the center stone of Course X; which done, we returned to our sweeping work, not doubting but that we should be able to hook the under buoy with the salvagee rope, and we accordingly constantly met with it; but the weather being untoward, the short sea raised thereby occasioned so great a motion of the yawls, as to cause the sweep rope to disengage itself from its hold: and soon after there came on so great a sea as to prevent all further trial at present, and made it prudent for us to weigh the buss's anchor; so that in the evening we arrived with her in Mill Bay, through a rough sea, fresh wind, thick fog, and rain.

248. WHAT we had been told by the master of the floating light could not fail to give us some suspicion of the *Polparra Fishermen*, as having cut away the buoy for the sake of the *cork*; a jealousy I should not have given way to, if I had not recollected the cutting the moorings of the punt the last year, and several other instances of villainy of like nature, which in such cases it would be always worth while to endeavour to detect and punish. With this view I accepted the offer of a friend in the Custom House, that I could depend upon, to go to Polparra; and, under colour of searching for run liquors, to try to discover the buoy; which was accordingly done, though without further success than a confirmation of our *suspicions*: for they learnt that three boats had been out the very day the master of the floating light saw the buoy in his way to Plymouth, and that they had brought home a large parcel of fish of a kind peculiar to these rocks; so that they might easily have disengaged the layers of cork composing the buoy, and cut them to pieces for their *Crab-pots* and *Seines*, while at sea, to prevent discovery.

249. FROM this time we were always prepared to go out in search of our moorings, and frequently attempted it, but were obliged as often to return. On Friday the 23d, the Weston and Assistant having unloaded their cargoes of stone, our men went out with a declaration that they would not return till they had found the moorings. They did not come back in some days; and, as I was not able to see any of the boats with my telescope from the *Hoe*, the Cawsand fishermen also reporting that they had not

* As this bolt and shackle would necessarily be in review on getting in the bridle, as mentioned § 243. the cause of this derangement must have happened after that.

feen them at fea, and it had blown very frefh all the time, we began to be uneafy for them; imagining they had fhared the fame fate as a fifhing boat, which about three weeks before had been picked up by the *French* for the fake of intelligence: but upon the 28th of June in the evening they returned to Plymouth, having, by diftrefs of weather during the interval they were out, been obliged to take refuge in *Yealm* harbour, where they lay two days and nights, and afterwards returned to fweep for the moorings; in which trials they ftill laid hold of fomething with their fweep rope, but never had the good luck to lay hold of it with the falvagee rope; however they continued their trials till wind and weather drove them in.

250. DURING this time we received a parcel of chain from the fmith in London; for, as he had continued very diligently at work upon the new chains, that were ordered upon the firft difcovery of the lofs of our buoy, and had proceeded with them till we had got (as we thought) compleatly moored upon the 13th of May; the quantity of chain then made, amounting to forty fathoms, was, by way of *precaution*, immediately put on board a veffel that was about to fail for Plymouth, and was now fortunately in our poffeffion. We had moreover received the Corporation's chain from *Falmouth*, amounting to twenty-feven fathoms, and had ready two mooring anchors, which had been purchafed when the new chain was befpoke.——In this ftate of things, as the feafon was approaching that we might expect fuitable opportunities upon the rock, and lofs of *time* being the greateft lofs that could happen to us; on a confultation, we judged it proper to fpend no more now, in fweeping for the moorings, but to carry out the bufs and moor her in the beft manner we could with the chains we had; becaufe this would not prevent a proper endeavour to recover the moorings, when time and feafon was lefs precious: and though the Corporation's chain of twenty-feven fathoms was not above half the weight of an equal length of our own, yet we judged it might be very fufficient for our *Eaftern* anchor; and the new chain was of fufficient length to allow thirty-five fathoms for the weftern anchor, and five fathoms to turn up for a bridle; which, together with the five fathoms of bridle, and the fwivel, which we had left, would be very fufficient for our purpofes. Our feamen therefore were ordered to go out the next day, if the weather fuited, to make *one* more trial at *dead of neap*, when the tides run lefs rapid; and if unfuccefsful, to return in the evening to affift in carrying out the bufs: this indeed once more proved to be the cafe; fo that every thing being ready, we went on board her the 1ft of July in the evening, and weighed. The wind being then at north, was very fair for carrying us out; but before we cleared the Sound it began to frefhen to a ftiff gale, it therefore became neceffary to confider, as our veffel would not turn to windward, how we were to get back, in cafe we fhould by any accident be prevented from mooring. We therefore came to an anchor in *Cawfand Bay*; and as in the evening it became very moderate, though from the fame quarter, we weighed and made eafy fail, having the whole night before us; and by three next morning we got out the length of the Edyftone. As the tide had overhauled us, and driven us to the eaftward of our proper mooring-place, we let go an anchor and warped the bufs to her proper *birth*: but before we could *ground* our weftern anchor, the tide of ebb fet fo ftrong as to carry us too much to the weft; we therefore defifted for the prefent, till the ebb abated, and landed on the rock, unloaded the Edyftone boat of her cargo, and fet a part of it. We returned to the bufs about noon to get down our moorings, which we happily compleated by four P. M. much in the fame manner we had originally done § 126; our eaftern anchor lying amongft the rough rocks in fourteen fathoms, and our weftern in fixteen fathoms water; the houfe bearing by the compafs S. W. by W. diftance about 200 fathoms.——And here I muft obferve, that one misfortune frequently becomes a confolation for another; for if none of thofe accidents had befallen us, if our bufs had kept its ftation and all our effentials had duly performed their duties, we could have reaped little advantage from them; for we had repeatedly experienced that the progrefs of the work was by no means proportioned to the length of time that the bufs continued at her moorings; fo that, from the time of our firft going out with the bufs to this day, winds, ground fwells, and feas, had afforded fo few opportunities of forwarding the conftruction, to any material purpofe, that in fact we had loft little or no time; and our principal fufferings were from that vexation and trouble of mind, which fuch difafters are apt to produce.

251. FROM

251. FROM the 2d to the 5th inclufive we began and finifhed the Xth Courfe; and by noon on the 6th we had fet the center, and two of the furrounding ftones of Courfe XI; I therefore left Mr. RICHARDSON and company to proceed; and, as the method was the fame as has been particularly defcribed in the courfe of laft year's work, there will be little further occafion to trouble my reader with any account of the building work; except to mark its progrefs, with the incidents attending, and fuch *alterations* in the method, as were neceffarily occafioned by the different modes of conftruction, which the different purpofes naturally required.——Our prefent run of fine weather was not lafting, for though we compleated the Xth Courfe in four days, it was not till the 18th (twelve days longer) that the XIth Courfe was finifhed. However, the feamen that were relieved upon the 16th brought word that the bufs had rode it out very well, without being under the neceffity of veering out any more cable.

252. ON the 17th at midnight I went out, and found RICHARDSON and company at work delivering the Affiftant's cargo, that had been on board ten days; and by the 24th the XIIth Courfe was finifhed; as was the XIIIth the 5th of Auguft; and on the 8th of that month the XIVth was compleated, and therewith the *Fundamental Solid.*——From hence begins that part of the building, alfo called *the Solid*, which includes the paffage from the Entry-Door to the *Well-Hole* for the ftairs. The Plates N° 11. Fig. 2, 3, and 4; together with the Section N° 9, will explain, by infpection, the conftruction and proportion of thefe parts much better than words; I fhall therefore think it fufficient to fay, that as, for the fake of the well-hole, we muft neceffarily lofe our *Center Stone*, the four ftones furrounding it that in the former courfes were by four dovetails united to the center ftone, were, as now prepared, to be united to each other by *Hook-Scarf-Joints*, fo as to compofe, in effect, one ftone: and as, in confequence, we had alfo loft our center cubes, it became expedient, that the work might have an uniform texture and ftrength, that thofe four ftones, making a compleat circle for the ftair-cafe, fhould be provided with cubes to prevent their being fhifted by any fhock applied horizontally, (fee Fig. 4.) as well as with trenails to hinder them from lifting. By this means the *principle* of confolidation would be effectually preferved: but as the top of the XIVth or Entry-door Courfe, was twelve feet above the top of the rock, that is, twenty feet four inches above the bafe of the Ift Courfe, the ftroke of the fea muft here become lefs violent, and therefore a lefs degree of refiftance would be equally fufficient. And as the large cubes would too much cut the work, which was here of confiderably lefs *area*; and as feveral cubes would be requifite for the *Well-Hole Stones*, I had determined, above the Entry-door Courfe, to increafe the number of cubes from eight to fixteen, and to diminifh their fize from twelve to fix inches; but ftill to be of folid grey marble, and two of them to be introduced into each of the four well-hole ftones.

253. UPON the 9th of Auguft at two A.M. I landed on the rock, and marked out the Entry and Stair-cafe; and having unloaded the Edyftone boat, which was loaded with the firft pieces of Courfe XV. we immediately proceeded with it; and from this time were bleffed with fuch an uninterrupted continuance of fine weather, that upon the 20th day of Auguft the XVIIIth Courfe was compleated, which reunites the building into a compleat circle by covering the paffage to the ftair-cafe: the external face of the ftone of that courfe, which makes the cover or *head* of the entry door, having the figures 1758, denoting the year in which this part of the work was accomplifhed, cut, in deep characters, upon it. During this fine feafon we had however one accident, that might have proved of bad confequence, if Providence had not interpofed. Upon the 15th, while all the people were at work upon the building, and the yawls attending in the Gut, by fome accident the hook by which the *in-hauler* guy of the fhears was attached, became undone; and in confequence the fhears came forward, overfet into the Gut, and falling upon one of the yawls confiderably damaged it, and hurt two of the workmen, fo that they were obliged to be fent home to the care of a furgeon; but they were foon recovered, and returned to their work with their company the next turn.

254. ON the 24th of Auguft the fine weather, and in confequence the works, were interrupted, the XXth Courfe being then in hand; and it was not till the 24th of September that, with every poffible exertion,

exertion, the XXIVth Course was finished; which compleated *the Solid*, and composed the floor of the *Store-Room*.——During this month of froward weather, it happened upon the 30th that the men, who went in the yawls to help the Assistant out of the Gut, after so doing, the wind becoming fresh at E. with a strong tide of ebb, were not able either to get on board the buss, or land upon the rock; so that those remaining upon the rock could not get on board the yawls: those in the yawls were therefore under the necessity of lying upon their oars all night, in the wind and rain, to the leeward of the building; those upon the rock amused themselves with their work; which, having their lanterns and candles, they were enabled to do. On the morning of the 31st the wind abated, and they got happily off without any other harm, than that there was not a dry thread amongst the whole company. This was the first and only time that either company were ever detained upon the rock: and, considering the number of escapes we had had, it was rather surprizing that this had not happened oftener.

On Wednesday the 6th of September it blew a storm, and when I landed on the 8th I found the forelock, which fastened the foot of the south leg of the shears, broken, and the two legs driven together: but the house being now almost as high as the top of the shears, the in-hauler guy tackle had been hooked to a lewis in the floor of the top of the building, which supported the shears from falling, otherwise they must have been destroyed, as happened before about the same time last year. (See § 232.) No other part of the tackle however had received any injury.

255. IT being, as said, the 24th of September when we finished the solid, had nothing been further in view than the completion of the building the *next* year, I certainly should have been very well contented now to have put a period to this year's work; but, conceiving it would be of great utility to the public, I had been for some time past meditating upon the practicability of exhibiting a light from the house during the ensuing winter, provided we could get the *Store Room* compleated; of which I thought there was little doubt, when I considered how much less of solid stone was necessary to raise one room with its vaulted stone cover, than was necessary to finish as much in height of the solid; and that for the execution of this, every thing was ready in the yard for putting together.——Accordingly, upon the 28th of September I wrote to the proprietors; and also gave an account of the advancement of our works to the Board of *Trinity House*; intimating the practicability thereof, in case I could get the *Store-Room* compleated: and also the probability of doing it, as it certainly could be effected in eight or ten days of working weather. I also set forth the general outlines of the method, by which I proposed to do it; which was, that besides making good the stone floor above the store-room, a strong platform of timber was to be laid over all, and that covered with a *Tarpaulin* well secured down. Upon the middle of this platform I proposed to set up our triangle, wherewith we hoisted and set our stone; the legs to be well lashed down, and to suspend the *Lantern* thereon that was made for the *Neptune Buss*: and, as nothing would project beyond the circumference of the area of the top of the building, the lantern being in the center would be effectually screened from the stroke of the sea; and every thing would be sufficiently strong to resist the falling *broken water*, which would immediately shoot off from the platform: and as I meant to lay three floors in the well-hole, I could convert the whole of that cavity, as well as the passage, into store-rooms, so as to make sufficient conveniency for *two* men, which appeared to be all that was *absolutely* necessary for the keeping a light.——As I doubted not but this proposal would be approved, and there was no time to lose, I went on with it in the same manner as if I had received an order for that purpose; and I not only got prepared the wooden platform and tarpaulin, but fixed with two of my hardiest workmen to keep the light for the winter; which for *double* their constant wages they agreed to undertake: and as, under these circumstances, our platform would be full forty feet above the base of the building, and every thing very substantial, I did not doubt but that my two men would fare much better in the year 1758, than Mr. WINSTANLEY's did in 1698; and quite as well as Mr. RUDYERD's could do in the year 1708*.

256. THE 25th and 26th of September Course XXV. being the first course of the superstructure, was successfully compleated in its place; but as the mode of construction now became entirely different

* See Mr. Winstanley's account § 20 and 21; and Mr. Rudyerd's § 34 and 50.

from

from the former, it becomes neceſſary to give an account thereof, as alſo of the reaſons for the change. The building was carried up ſolid, as high as there was any reaſon to ſuppoſe it expoſed to the heavy ſtroke of the ſea, that is to thirty-five feet four inches above its baſe, and twenty-ſeven feet above the top of the rock, or common ſpring-tide high-water mark. At this height, as it was reduced to ſixteen feet eight inches in diameter, it became neceſſary to make the *beſt uſe* of this ſpace, and make all the room and convenience therein that was poſſible, conſiſtent with the ſtill neceſſary ſtrength.——The rooms being made of twelve feet four inches diameter, this would leave twenty-ſix inches for the thickneſs of the walls. Theſe being made with ſingle blocks in the thickneſs, ſo that ſixteen pieces might compoſe the circle, would, from its figure, compoſe a ſtout wall; yet moorſtone, as has been obſerved, being a tender kind of ſtone in reſpect to the union of its component parts; any method of dovetailing the blocks together at this thickneſs, appeared to me impracticable to any *good* purpoſe. What ſeemed to be the moſt effectual method of bonding the work together, was that of *cramping* with iron, which would confine each ſingle piece to its neighbouring piece in the ſame circle: and if to this be added, that every piece ſhould, at *each end* of it, lay hold of an *inlaid* piece, or *Joggle*, in the ſame nature as the cubes, then not only all the pieces in the ſame courſe would be united to each other by the cramps, but ſteadied from moving upon the under courſe by the joggles, and of conſequence would be faſtened at thirty-two points; for, in each courſe there being ſixteen joggle ſtones, as each end of each principal piece, at its baſe, took hold of half a joggle, there would be thirty-two points of confinement in the circle above; that is, the joggles being made to occupy the middle of the upper bed of each block, in that ſituation they would croſs the joints of the courſe above. Theſe joggles, as well as the reſt, were of ſawn marble, and made eight inches long, four inches broad, and three inches thick: each end of each block therefore would occupy four inches in length, four in breadth, and 1½ inch in the height of each joggle; and this I judged quite ſufficient to keep every courſe in its place, at the height that this kind of work was begun, and ſo as to conſtitute a piece of ſolid maſonry. There was however another matter, that it ſeemed quite material alſo to attend to; and that was, to render the habitable rooms contained within thoſe ſhells of walls, perfectly *dry* and comfortable in all weathers; and this was a matter that ſeemed to merit very particular attention; for the ſeas that are ſaid to riſe up againſt, and in a manner to *bury* the houſe in time of ſtorms, (ſee § 21.) would make effectual trial of every joint.

The level joints being preſſed together by the incumbent weight of the building, would keep firm and ſound that coheſion of parts produced by the mortar; ſo that being once made *water-tight*, there was no doubt but they would ſo remain: but with reſpect to the upright joints, the *leaſt* degree of ſhrinking, either of the ſtone or of the mortar between, tended to open the joint, ſo that it might always remain leaky in a greater or a leſs degree; for we know of no degree of ſeparation of parts, however minute, ſhort of abſolute contact, which will ſtop or prevent the percolation of water. For this purpoſe I conceived, that if flat ſtones were introduced into each upright joint, ſo as to be lodged partly in one ſtone, and partly in its neighbour; much upon the ſame idea, that *Dutch* laths were formerly introduced into the joints of chamber floors, to hinder the paſſage of wet; the water might be prevented from making its way through the upright joints of the walls.

The manner in which it was executed was as follows, (ſee Plate N° 11. Fig. 6.) At each end of each piece of ſtone, anſwerable to the middle between the inſide of the wall and the outſide, was ſunk a groove 2½ inches wide and three deep, running from the top to the bottom: when therefore two contiguous pieces of ſtone were put together in their places, the two grooves being applied to each other, they would form a *Rhomb* of ſix inches in length, and 2½ inches in breadth, which in this ſtate would be an unoccupied cavity from the top to the bottom of each courſe; the reſt of the joint, where the ſurfaces of the two ſtones applied to each other, was made good with mortar in the ordinary way, and brought together by the *gentle* blows of a beetle. For the groove mentioned, a ſolid *Rhomb* was prepared, of about two inches thick by five inches broad, and in length a little leſs than the depth of the cavity, which generally was eighteen or twenty inches; and for the ſake of firmneſs of thoſe ſlender pieces of ſtone, I made choice of the flat paving ſtones from *Purbeck*, which, as mentioned § 100, is a laminated marble of great ſtrength and ſolidity. The *Joint Stones* (which was the name we gave thoſe *Rhombs*) thus prepared, would readily go down the cavities; but to fix them ſolid, a quantity of well-tempered mortar was prepared, made more soft than ordinary, by the addition of a little water; a competent quantity being put down to the bottom of the hole, the joint stone was put down upon it; and, by the simple pressure of the hand, was forced down to the bottom, causing the semifluid mortar to rise up to the top, and compleatly fill the cavity: and when forced down in the way described, having in this state a small quantity of superfluous moisture about it, a few *very* gentle blows or raps were given upon the top of it by the handle of a mason's trowel, which producing a small degree of agitation, while the dry stones were absorbing the moisture, contributed (like the beating of mortar) to bring all the parts into their most *friendly* state of contact, and in consequence, to their firmest state of union; and this happened in the course of a few minutes, so that no further agitation could be of any service.

As the cramps, that were to bind the contiguous pieces together, must cross the joints upon their upper surface, they were of course to be applied *after* the joint stones were settled in their places. Precaution was therefore necessary not to apply too much exertion in forcing down the joint stones: for, however gentle the operation may appear, according as it has been described, yet it was found advisable not to put in the joint stones till an additional piece had been got down upon its joggles, and plain jointed, at each side of the two pieces, whose joint stone was to be put in; for by this means there were the united efforts of all the joggles, and adhesion of the beds, of two stones on each side of that where the effort was applied. Without an attention to this, the lateral force arising from merely pressing down a joint stone, was capable of breaking the adhesion of the joint where it was applied.

257. THE cramping was applied the last thing. The top or *flat bars* of the cramps were about thirteen inches long, two inches broad, and [illegible] of an inch thick, and were turned down at each end about three inches in length; forming a cylinder of 1[illegible] inch diameter. Jumper holes were previously bored when upon the platform, and the cramps fitted to their places; the surface of the stone under each cramp being sunk [illegible] of an inch, so that the two stones together would compleatly receive, or rather bury, the cramps: the joint stones, as said above, being made so much shorter than the height of the course, as not to interrupt the bedding of the cramp. The places for the cramps being properly fitted and cleared (as we now were not liable to be driven off the work in a moment, as had formerly been the case) we took the opportunity, whenever time allowed it, of fixing the cramps of a whole course together. There was no danger of the cramps not fitting; as, besides that all the cramps were forged to fit a gauge-bar having a couple of holes at the assigned distance, they were also fitted and marked to their particular places at Mill Bay, while upon the platform.——Every cramp being now ultimately tried to its place, it was then put into a kettle of lead made red hot; and the cramp continued there till it was also reddish. About a spoonful of oil was poured into the two cramp-holes, and the cramp being put into its place, the ebullition of the oil caused by the heat of the iron, quickly gave a compleat oily surface, not only to the whole cramp, but to the whole unoccupied cavity in the stone; then the hot lead being poured upon it, the unctuous matter caused the metal to run into and occupy the most minute cavity unfilled, and compleatly to cover each cramp; and they became by this means defended from the salts of the sea, even had they remained *uncovered*, upon Mr. RUDYERD's principle*: but as every cramp, from construction, would be covered by the middle of the base of the stone in the next course above, it became defended from moisture in the most effectual manner possible; and thus by cramping in general a whole course together, the contraction of the iron in *cooling* would greatly add to the tightness wherewith every stone was bound to its fellow.——Thus, according to this mode of fixing, (besides the union of the parts by the mortar itself) to resist all violence and derangement whilst it was doing, and before the induration of the mortar, every course was retained in its place by sixteen joggles, and each single stone by two half joggles at its lower bed; they were further steadied to each other by the joint stones, and lastly by the cramps, which compleatly prevented a separation: and this method proved so effectual, that we were not only free from all derangement of the stones, when in their places, but I did not find a leaky joint, except one, in the whole building. By a due consideration

* § 27.——It is there said that instead of *Lead* Mr. RUDYERD had used coarse *Pewter*. The lead we used was *Pig Lead*, which is harder and stiffer than Pew[illegible] lead: and as we used no cramps, as an *essential* part of the building, till above the store-room floor, I judged pewter, merely for the sake of stiffness, *there* to be unnecessary.

of

of Plate N° 11. with the particular references to it, the whole of this procefs will become perfectly intelligible.

258. ON Saturday the 30th of September, Courfe XXVIII. was compleatly fet; and being the firft courfe, upon which was refted the vaulted floor, which made the cieling of the ftore-room and floor of the *upper* ftore-room; and, as here again occurred a difference in the mode of fixture, in this, as in all like cafes, I attended the performance of the work: and that was the *leading* in of the firft *circular chain*, that was lodged in a groove cut round the middle of the upper furface of this courfe; which this day was fatisfactorily performed; and the next day, Sunday October the 1ft, Courfe XXIX. was fet, and its circular chain leaded in alfo; which operation, with the reafon thereof, it will be proper here to defcribe.

The ordinary way of fixing the feveral courfes by joggles and joint ftones; and alfo the bonding them together by cramps, has already been defcribed; but thofe courfes, upon which the floors refted and depended, feemed to demand every *poffible* fecurity.——It will be feen in the general fection, Plate N° 9, that each floor *defignedly* refted upon two courfes: it will alfo appear, by infpection, that the circumference of the floors was not made to reft upon the floping abutments of an arch, in lines tending towards the center of the fphere, of which the under fide of the floor was a portion, but it refted upon a triple ledge going circularly round the two fupporting courfes. In confequence of this, had each floor been compofed of a *fingle* ftone, this lying upon the horizontal bearings furnifhed by thefe ledges, would, while it remained entire, have no lateral preffure or tendency to thruft out the fides of the encompaffing walls*: and that, in effect, the feveral pieces, of which the floors were really compofed, might have the fame property as *whole* ftones; the center ftone was made large enough to admit of an opening, from floor to floor, or *Man-Hole*, to be made through it; and being furnifhed with dovetails on its four fides, like thofe of the entire folid, it became the means by which all the ftones in each floor were connected together; and confequently, the whole would lie upon the ledges like a fingle ftone, without any tendency to fpread the walls. But, if by the accident of a heavy body falling, or otherwife, any of thofe ftones fhould be broken, though this might not deftroy its ufe as a floor, or its properties as an arch; yet the parts would then exert their *lateral preffure* againft the walls: and therefore, as a fecurity againft this, it became neceffary that the circle of the inclofing walls fhould be bound together, and the building, as it were, *hooped*.

This would be in a great meafure brought about, by the cramps tying the neighbouring ftones together, as already defcribed for the ordinary courfes; but yet this was no abfolute fecurity, becaufe the outfide ftones might break and feparate, between cramp and cramp: and I fuppofe it was for reafons of this kind, that Sir CHRISTOPHER WREN, in the conftruction of the *Cupola* of *St. Paul's*, did not chufe to depend upon cramping the ftones together, of the courfe that ferved as a common bafe to the infide dome, and the cone for fupporting the lantern; but chofe to furround the whole with continued chains of iron†.——Upon this principle, an *endlefs* chain was provided for each of the two floor courfes, fee Plate N° 11. Fig. 7. The bars compofing the links being 1½ inch *fquare*; that the moft iron might be included in a given fpace, the corners only were a little canted off; and the double parts being brought near together, the whole was comprehended in a groove, of fomewhat lefs than four inches wide, and as much in depth; into which the chains being introduced and brought to a ftretch, the reft of the cavity was filled with lead; of which each took about 11 cwt.

Had the author of the *Parentalia* informed us particularly how this was done, it would have been ufeful to me to have known it. It is obvious that it muft be in a manner impracticable to heat chains of fuch a length as even ours, in the manner I treated the cramps; or that the whole of the circle could be run at once: becaufe if fo attempted, the metal firft poured in would have fo *far* to run, that one ladle-

* This method of abutting by ledges alfo prevented the fhell of the walls from being unneceffarily thinned by a longer continuance of floping lines.

† "Although the dome wants no butment, yet for greater caution it is hooped with iron in this manner. A channel is cut in the bandage of Portland ftone, in which is laid a *double* chain of iron ftrongly linked together at every ten feet, and the whole channel filled up with lead." WREN's *Parentalia*, p. 294.

full

full would cool and set, before another could be put down upon it; so that the mass of lead, instead of enveloping the iron of the chain, as one solid piece, and thereby excluding all moisture, would in many places be composed of *Laminæ* without any firm cohesion.——In our work, it was performed in the following method. The chains were oiled all over before they came from the shore; and the circumference of the groove was divided into four parts by stops, or dams of clay; to prevent the lead from flowing further than one quarter at a time. A couple of iron kettles were provided, capable of melting commodiously, when full, six cwt. of lead each; and that quantity was brought in each to a *full* red; that is, somewhat hotter than we used for the cramps, as the iron of the chain as well as the stone were cold. The whole quantity of lead being brought to a heat that we judged proper, and the quarter groove being supplied with oil sufficient to besmear the whole surface, two persons with each a ladle, as briskly as they could, poured the melted metal into the same quarter of the groove; and as soon as it was full, and the lead began to set, one of the clay dams was removed, and the melted hot metal was poured upon the end of the former mass, till it was perceived to re-melt and unite with the fresh metal. This done, the dam at the *other* end of the first run mass was taken down, to prevent its cooling more than was necessary, and the third quarter was treated like the former; the end of the mass rendered solid by cooling, being re-melted by the fresh hot metal: lastly, both the remaining dams being taken down, and the metal at each end having a considerable heat, it was found practicable to dissolve both the ends of the former masses; first applying both ladles to that which had had the greater time to cool, and afterwards to the less: by this means the whole was brought to a solid consistence, and the chain entirely buried in the lead.——It is however to be remarked, that to preserve proper impressions in the lead, for the joggles of the course above, those impressions were made by confining down bricks in proper places, which when removed, the proper marble joggles were set with mortar in their places.——Thus the floor courses were in effect *keyed*; and the hoops securely protected from moisture and rust; first by a coat of oil together with a body of lead; and secondly by the whole being lodged in the middle of the wall.

Some may perhaps think this extreme precaution of the chain courses, and the forming of the *floors* upon a system of dovetails, might have been dispensed with; and probably it might, if the whole of this work must have been executed upon the *Edystone Rock*; but it is to be remembered that the iron chains were executed on *shore*, at so much per cwt.; were fitted to their places in the work-yard at *Mill Bay*; and the *extra* work in the jointing of the floors was the produce of so many days work of a stone-cutter in the same place: so that little extra expence attended the fixing at the rock, except a little more *Lead*, and a little more *Fire*.

259. MONDAY October the 2d we proceeded to set up the centre, composed of sixteen ribs, (see Plate N° 18. Fig. 3.) for putting the floor together upon; but I must here note, that having the evening before had the opportunity of landing the five large stones composing the middle of the floor; those were, previous to the setting up the centre, got up upon the top of the wall; for all the rest could be got up through the man-hole left in the middle of the centre, answerable to that of the centre stone; and this afternoon we landed all the remaining pieces belonging to the floor, being in the whole thirty-seven; which we lodged in the well-hole for the stairs, and in the store-room under the centre. This I was not a little anxious to get done; for we had now got into the building every piece of stone that I had it in view to set this year, as necessary for the establishment of a light; but this solicitude had nearly cost us our boat the *Weston*; for though the past week had been the finest this season, yet before the boat could be got out of the Gut, it began suddenly to blow so fresh at E. that it was not without the greatest difficulty and exertion, that she was got out of it without damage.——Being myself wanted at Mill Bay, to forward our equipment for rendering the house habitable, I returned in her to Plymouth; and, as rough weather came on, I got that work well advanced. I went out again on Thursday the 5th, and saw the two first stones of the floor set in their places in the outward circle *; but after doing this, we had some risque and difficulty

* I first set the Pieces we began with, the outward circle of stones, because at all adventures they were to fit the outside shell of the building, and if set last they would not have gone into their places.

culty

culty in getting aboard our yawls. The company before my arrival had employed themselves in getting down the windlass and shears, as having no further occasion for them this season.

The weather continued broken till Saturday the 7th, on which day the Edystone boat came out, having on board the roof or platform, for covering the building, and protecting it, as mentioned, from the entrance of the downfall spray; together with the doors, iron-work and timber for fitting up the same for habitation; *Coals, Water*, &c. and the carpenters for fixing those temporary works. This afternoon we landed, and went on with the setting of the outward circle of floor stones, made the holes in the wall for fixing the hinges of the entry and store-room doors; and did not doubt but that *one* favourable day, would enable us to compleat this floor; and then we proposed to begin directly to lay on the *Platform* roof; which would be perfected in two or three hours: and as this being done would render the building water-tight; we then intended immediately to make a *lodgement* therein, and go on to the entire completion of this temporary part of the work; however, towards evening, while we were proceeding, a ground swell began to come on, and to such a degree as reminded us of the necessity of retiring, though two stones were wanted to compleat the outward circle, (see Plate N° 11. Fig. 7.); and as the sky began to look *foul-weather-like*, I endeavoured to see every thing put into the *best* posture for receiving a storm. In particular, I caused the middle stone to be laid upon the *centre*, by way of weight, to keep it steady. Three of the four stones that were to connect with the centre stone were laid upon the top of the wall on the N. E. side; and the fourth I caused to be hoisted and suspended upon the triangle, in the posture that is shewn Plate N° 14. at Stage 2nd. So that the triangle, which was all of it compleatly within the area of the top of the building, would be kept down by the weight of this stone, which was between seven and eight cwt. ——The other three that lay upon the wall, I caused to be carefully drawn within the circumference thereof, so that there might not be the least projecting part for the water to strike against in flying upwards; which I judged quite necessary, though the walls were then upwards of forty-three feet above the foundation stone, and near thirty-five feet above the top of the rock. After righting all matters to our satisfaction, we had again an escape in getting into our yawls.

In the night the wind came to S. W. and S. and in the morning the swell was so great as to oblige the Edystone boat to quit the moorings: and as I wanted to be at Plymouth to expedite and finish our intended equipment and stores, which I had greatly at heart, and we were not likely to proceed soon to business, I left orders with Mr. Jessop for the compleating of the floor, and took my passage home in the boat.——The evening of this day, Sunday October the 8th, it blew a storm, the men of war in the Sound frequently firing guns of distress. About break of day on Monday morning the wind suddenly veered to N. W. but it still blew very hard.

260. THIS morning, October the 9th, I went up to the *Hoa* to look out with my glass; I could just discover the house, and the sea breaking over it, so as at intervals entirely to bury it, but could discover nothing of the *Buss*; however, the air being very hazy, the hull of that vessel being low, and its mast a small object, I judged that to be the reason I could not see her.——In the afternoon, the air being somewhat less hazy, I looked out again; the sea was breaking over the house as before, but still no buss was to be seen, which created some apprehension for her and the people.

Tuesday October the 10th I again went up to the *Hoa*, and though the wind had remained fresh at N. W. now above twenty-four hours, yet the sea was still breaking over the house, rising up in the form of a white pillar, considerably higher than the building, and of such magnitude as at times to intercept every part of it from view: but the air being now more clear, in the intervals of its retreat, I could distinctly perceive the triangle standing upon the house, and the stone suspended thereon; but to my great mortification, found that the buss was really gone from her moorings, and no where to be seen.——This, in reality, turned out a day of thorough regret; for, besides the uncertainty of the fate of the *Neptune Buss*, it brought me the resolution of a *General Court* of the *Corporation* of Trinity House, upon my proposal of the 28th of September, for the exhibition of a light upon the house during the winter; which more effectually put a stop to all further attempts to proceed this year, than the parting of the buss from her moorings. Their answer was to this purport: that having taken into consideration the proposals

 (mentioned

mentioned § 255.) "on reading the acts of parliament, the application from the merchants and owners "of ships, the patent for the floating light, and the inclosed *Narrative* of the first light-house erected "there *, they are of opinion, that a light cannot be exhibited on the Edystone rock till the light-house is "re-built."——This rebuff, I own, mortified me much, not only that I should in *appearance* fall short of the expedition which my predecessors Mr. WINSTANLEY and Mr. RUDYERD had shewn, to procure the public a temporary light in the course of the *third* season; but that my exertions on this head were frustrated †.

261. THIS evening at ten Mr. JESSOP returned to Plymouth, and, to my no small joy and satisfaction, brought me an account that the buss was safe at anchor in *Dartmouth Harbour*.——He further informed me, that on Sunday, about two hours after I left them, it began to blow a storm at S. S. W. and that in consequence thereof he ordered the decks to be cleared, and every thing put in order; but did not *hand* the main-sail, because, by holding wind, it might be the occasion of their breaking loose. Towards night however the storm increased, and the sea frequently intercepted from them all sight of the building, as the broken column of water rose considerably higher than the top of the triangle: that at night the storm still increased, and about eleven o'clock the cable parted at the *Bows*.——Upon this they hoisted their fore-sail and mizen, and endeavoured to stand in for the land; but the sea proved so tempestuous, that with the little quantity of sail they had, they could not keep a proper steerage; and it being also excessively rainy and dark, they were afraid of running on shore before they could see it: they therefore determined to lay her *to*, with her head to the S. E. that they might have daylight before they drove to the land. About two o'clock the wind came to the W. and at break of day they found themselves about three leagues from, and abreast of the *Start*. They then bent their main-sail, hoisted their *Jib*, and stood in for the land with the wind at N. N. W. (see the Chart N° 1.); but the Neptune buss was so slow a sailer, that it was four P. M. before they got off *Dartmouth*: they then, by the help of a pilot, came to an anchor in the *Road*, and the next morning warped into the harbour; and after seeing the vessel safely moored, Mr. JESSOP and part of the workmen made the best of their way to Plymouth.

Wednesday October the 11th JOHN BOWDEN was sent with one of the seamen over land to Dartmouth; the former to take charge of, and the latter to assist in bringing the buss round to Plymouth, as soon as the wind should prove fair.——This day the wind continuing at N. W. and having become so moderate as to produce smooth water in Plymouth Sound; though I now laid aside all further idea of carrying out the buss to her moorings again this year, we prepared every thing on board the Edystone boat and Assistant to go out with a competent set of workmen the next morning, to do whatever might appear necessary upon the building, after such a trying storm; and at least, if possible, to set the two remaining pieces of stone, that were wanted in the outward circle of the vaulted floor; for that being done, the *centre* might be taken down, as every circle of stones would support itself: and I was desirous, if it should be found practicable, to do something to secure the *Moorings*; there being only one buoy, upon one of the anchors. ——Every thing was thus prepared, but early next morning there came on a fresh of wind at E. which rendered it to no purpose to attempt to go out.

The wind continued fresh at E. for several days running, and brought home the buss, which was moored in Mill Bay on Friday evening: and on Sunday came on a storm at E. and a continuance of bad weather from the same quarter.——Nothing therefore being *necessary* further to be attempted, and every thing going on well in the yard under the care of Mr. TYRRELL, I left the necessary orders what to do, in case of favourable weather, and every thing to the care of Mr. JESSOP; and took my departure for London on the 25th of October: after which, no further events, of consequence to this business, happened in the remainder of this year.

* The narrative referred to was an extract from that of WINSTANLEY, recited § 17 to 27 inclusive.

† It is very possible I might not at that time have reflected, that we heard nothing of any *floating* light being *then* maintained; so that till a *temporary* light was erected *upon the Building* itself, the public were not served with *any* light.

C H A P. III.

Containing an Account of the Transactions of the FOURTH *and* LAST YEAR'*s Work, to the finishing of the Building in the Year* 1759.

262. DURING my stay in London, in the early part of the year 1759, I received regular accounts of the proceedings at Mill Bay, which were carried on with all the dispatch I could wish, while I was myself forming and making out the necessary designs for the iron rails of the balcony, the cast iron, the wrought iron, and the copper works for the lantern; which, together with the plate glass work, were all done in London. The weather having continued unfavourable to visiting the works at the Edystone during the winter, I got no report thereon till I received Mr. JESSOP's letter dated the 27th of March, wherein he informed me that on the 21st of that month, being the first opportunity he could catch after the violent storm which had happened on the 9th preceding, and which had done very great damage to the ships, houses, and buildings at Plymouth; they put to sea, and at a distance observed the triangle standing, with the stone hanging upon it, as it was left at the conclusion of the last season's work; so that when they had got by the Edystone, and doubted not but to have laid hold of the *Transport Buoy*, they found it was gone! whereupon they came to an anchor; and getting into the small boats, went into the Gut and landed. They found not only the solid but the hollow work perfectly found and firm; all the mortar having become quite hard; and in short every part of the work in the situation in which it was left by the workmen in October: the only derangement was, that the sea had carried away the south fender pile from the rock; and also, from the top of the wall, one of the three stones that I had taken care to draw within the verge of the circumference of the wall, as mentioned § 259. That they had found the fourteen pieces of stone set in the circumference of the floor, stuck quite firm to the wall, though two of the pieces requisite to complete the circle were left unset; and that, finding the *centre* itself quite tight and firm underneath them, they had lowered down the stone suspended on the triangle upon it, and removed from the wall the other two remaining stones to lie upon the centre; and lastly, that they took down the triangle and stowed it away in the well-hole for the stairs: but, on further search, nothing of the buoy that was left upon the mooring chains was to be seen. Mr. JESSOP also informed me, that he had put in hand a new transport buoy, and was preparing a south pile; that he had given the necessary orders for fitting out the buss to sweep for the moorings; and that the XLVth Course was then upon the platform*.

After this the seamen went frequently out, and often swept for the moorings, but without success; although the proprietors had offered £. 10 as a bounty to the seamen in case they recovered one set of the moorings, and £. 20 in case they recovered both sets.——I then proposed the sweeping with a cord, every yard of which to have a lead upon it like those used for nets, which by sinking into the hollows of the rocks might lay hold of the *fluke* of an anchor; and thereby ascertain its place, which would facilitate the laying hold of it with a proper pliant sweep rope, as mentioned in the operations of last year (see § 242.) This Mr. JESSOP made trial of, and informed me that after a considerable time spent, it had proved ineffectual; so that now, looking upon the recovery of our moorings as hazardous, I thought it time to set about the providing a new set. Accordingly, the 29th of May I ordered forty fathoms of new chain to be made at *Blackwall*, intending to send it down by land; and this, with some old chain purchased in

* This course makes the chain course for springing the arch of the balcony floor, and forms the cove on the outside.

Wapping

Wapping laſt year, which we had then at Plymouth, and was thought ſufficient for our eaſtern chain if occaſion required; I judged would ſerve our purpoſe for the preſent year, in caſe we could not recover any of the others: and Mr. Jessop was alſo directed to look out for a couple of anchors ſuitable to our purpoſe.

263. THE caſting the corner pillars for the lantern being attended with ſome difficulties, to which the ordinary workmen in the caſt iron foundery *at that time* were not equal, I was recommended to Mr. Prickett, then of *Farthing-Fields*, Wapping, whom I found equally intelligent and ingenious, and who executed my buſineſs to perfect ſatisfaction*.——The caſting of ſaſh frames of copper, each in one piece, was a difficulty I was deſirous to ſee accompliſhed before I ſet out for Plymouth. The inſpection of Plates Nº 12 and 15, will give my reader an idea of this buſineſs as well as the former, eſpecially if he alſo conſults the technical deſcription of thoſe plates.——Thoſe copper frames, conſiſting of nine panes each, being ſixteen in number, were ſucceſsfully caſt by Mr. Kinman of *Shoe Lane*; a work which did him credit.——The fitting together of the whole work of the lantern with wrought iron framing, as alſo the balcony rails, I ſaw in good forwardneſs, and left in the hands of Mr. Broadbent, an *Engine*-maker, in *Piccadilly*; of which work he acquitted himſelf to full ſatisfaction.

264. DURING this ſtay in London, I had more than once the honour of attending the *Board* of *Trinity House* by their deſire, and they were pleaſed to approve of our methods and proceedings. The latter time, which was upon the 2d of June, was to give my opinion upon a propoſal that had been made, and ſtrongly recommended to them by an *Optician* in London, who propoſed to grind all the panes of glaſs for the lantern of the Edyſtone to circular ſegments; ſo that the whole together ſhould form a ſphere of fifteen feet diameter: to this I obſerved, that it was in reality a method of making an *eaſy* thing *difficult* and expenſive, without the leaſt ſolid advantage. For, the propoſer ſeemed to imagine it needful that the rays of light ſhould proceed from the lantern in right lines in every *poſſible* direction; whereas thoſe rays that proceed in an horizontal direction out of the lantern are thoſe *alone* that are ſeen from the ſurface of the ſea by diſtant obſervers; all the reſt either going over their heads into the air, or falling down into the water before they reach them: and as, for the ſufficient ſpreading of the lights, ſo as not to interfere with each other, it had been found needful to place them in *Rings*, at two *different* heights; it would be only that ring of lights which was even with the centre of the ſphere, whoſe rays could proceed perpendicularly through the globular panes; the others above or below, muſt paſs through with a proportional obliquity: whereas the rays proceeding horizontally would paſs through the *upright* ſides of the lantern in a direction equally near the perpendicular, whether the light exhibited was high or low. And for this explanation, which fully convinced the Board of the inutility of the ſcheme, I received the thanks of the *Deputy Maſter*, in the name of the body.

265. HAVING left all neceſſary orders for the works going on in town, I arrived at Plymouth the 22d of June, where I found all the ſtone-work hewn out, the two courſes compoſing the cove and balcony floor upon the platform, with the balcony rails, and the baſe or plinth courſe of the lantern thereon; and every thing in all the forwardneſs I could expect.——I found that on the 13th inſtant ſo violent a ſtorm had happened at Plymouth, that the leaves of the trees and buſhes, on the windward ſide, had been blaſted, to the extent of four and five miles from the ſea; as I ſuppoſed, by the ſalts thereof being impetuouſly driven againſt them. In this ſtorm the Neptune buſs had received ſome damage, but had been got thoroughly repaired, and was then out with the ſeamen, ſtill in ſearch of the moorings.——Five of our beſt hands being grown ſelf-important, demanded an increaſe of wages, without which they would not go

* The ingenious Mr. Prickett, to whom the *Iron Foundery* of this kingdom owes much, is ſtill living, and is now maſter of the *Falcon* Iron Foundery, near *Blackfriars* Bridge; which is the very ſpot where the famous Mr. Jones, commonly called Gun Jones, had his foundery, and where caſt the ſmaller work of the railing that incloſes *St. Paul's*, London; for which he had the contract: but the larger parts of that work were caſt by Mr. Prickett's father, a relation of Mr. Jones, who had his foundery at the *Foreſt of Dean*, in *Glouceſterſhire*.

any

any more off to the Edystone. I now judged that as the want of earning a sufficiency of money could be no *just* cause, the shortest way to restore peace, unanimity, and preserve our original system, was to discharge them; which I accordingly did*.

Mr. Jessop and the seamen having now found by experience, the great advantage in point of strength which ropes of all kinds preserved by not being hard twisted; and conceiving that the circumstance of too hard twisting, had been the occasion of the parting of our bridle cable the last season; petitioned that we might have thirty fathoms made on purpose for us, and laid quite pliant; in consequence of which we might also increase its strength by a number of yarns, and yet diminish its stiffness. This I readily agreed to, and accordingly a bridle cable was *laid* perfectly pliant, though it was 12½ inches in circumference, that is 2½ inches more than the former.

The old chain before mentioned, which upon the strictest examination was found very sound and good in general, and every link of it, that appeared to have suffered any material waste, having been cut out and replaced with new, was now found to contain thirty-two fathoms compleat: a couple of suitable mooring anchors, as also a proper transport buoy, chain and anchor having been provided; all these were put on board the buss; and we now did not want any thing but the new chain from London, which coming by land, we could have the greater certainty of its arrival, which was upon the 2d of July, and it was put on board the buss the same evening†.

266. ON Monday morning July the 3d, at four, I attended the party out with the buss; but, owing to the usual uncertainty of calms, wind, and tides, and the still inherent property of our vessel as a slow sailer; it was not till eight the next morning that we came to an anchor at our mooring ground; yet at three P. M. we had compleated this business in the way already described § 126. the west anchor lying in sixteen fathoms water, and the east in fifteen, the rock bearing W. S. W. by the compass, distance by estimation three hundred fathoms. The new chain was our western chain, and the eastern joined it at ten fathoms from the swivel; in consequence so much could act as a bridle in either direction; and to this was *bent* our new pliant bridle cable.——We then proceeded to lay down our transport buoy; but the wind freshened, and obliged us to desist.

Thursday the 5th of July the wind being at N. W. and moderate; we this morning laid down the transport buoy in ten fathoms water; the rock bearing S. W. by S. by the compass, distance eighty fathoms; which was compleated at six. I then landed on the rock with the men; they proceeded to set up the shears and windlass, while I inspected the work; and found, according to Mr. Jessop's representation, every thing perfectly sound and firm, without the least perceivable alteration since we left it; except that the cement used the first year, now in appearance approached the hardness of the moor-stone; and that used the last year of the full hardness of Portland. By ten the hoisting tackle was fixed, and the spare hands, that were brought out to help with the mooring, returned to Plymouth; and we now proceeded to set the floor, not doubting but to compleat the whole of it this day.——The two remaining pieces of the outmost circle, which were left uncompleated last year, were soon set; and we proceeded to haul up the stones for the next circle (N° 4.) from the store-room; but instead of eight, I had the mortification to find that we had but *seven*, and unluckily the boat was gone home.——It was therefore the likeliest conjecture that the piece of stone wanting, had been driven out of the store-room door; and probably by the same sea that had floated the stone N° 2. mentioned § 262. from the top of the wall: and that this body of falling water, by making its way through the open ribs of the centre, had washed this stone out at the door, though it weighed between four and five cwt. I had no doubt but that it was missing when Mr. Jessop made his inspection in March; for finding those stones lying upon the store-room floor, piled up much in the same manner as we left them; he had never thought of counting them; not conceiving, but

* The work being now brought to such a period that it could go on with less interruption, I proposed that this year the companies should change only once a fortnight, which would occasion less loss of time, as well as give more equal opportunities, in having both spring and neap tides in the compass of each turn.

† This chain was forty fathoms, and weighed 36½ cwt.

that ſuch kind of weighty materials were very ſafely lodged in that place, the floor of which is nine yards above the top of the rock; and the border of the wall riſing up as a parapet of defence near eight feet higher.——The diſaſter of the loſs of N° 2. being foreknown, was eaſily repaired, by making another from the ſame mould; and which we brought out with us, and landed: the ſhorteſt way therefore to overcome this difficulty, appeared to be to ſend home one of the yawls, with orders, to ſend out a ſimilar piece belonging to the third floor; and we went on with ſetting what we had.

Friday July the 5th, we landed upon the rock at four A. M. and, having a very moderate breeze at N. W. I never ſaw the ſea more quiet about the Edyſtone. We proceeded ſo as to ſet two pieces of N° 2. but could go on no further with this part of the work till the arrival of the ſtone to ſupply the place of that which had been loſt.——We now began to fix up the new ſouth fender pile, which had been waſhed away in the courſe of the winter, though fixed with large iron bolts in the firmeſt manner we could. This was compleated at eleven; we then quitted the rock and retired on board the buſs, the *firſt* time, for *want of work*.——At noon we eſpied the Edyſtone boat about two leagues from us, but the breeze being now from the ſouth, as, it has been obſerved, generally happens in the middle of the day in fine weather, we ſent the remaining yawl well manned to bring out the wanting piece, which arrived this afternoon, and in the evening was ſet, with ſeveral others. On Saturday morning we landed at four, and ſoon ſet the two remaining pieces, which finiſhed the firſt floor. We then cleared away the centre, and ſent it on board the buſs.

267. HITHERTO we had got up our ſtones by firſt landing them into the entry-door from the *rock* ſhears, as we had uſed from the beginning; and after that hoiſted them up the well-hole, by a tackle upon the triangle, by hand; but on finiſhing the vaulted floor over the firſt room, many of the pieces of ſtone of the ſuperſtructure being too large to go through the man-holes in the centre of the floors, I contrived and got prepared an additional pair of ſhears, which being placed upon the top of the work, would of courſe be made to riſe with it. The idea of this kind of ſhears will be formed by inſpecting Plate N° 14. at the third ſtage; which we now ſet up, and applied accordingly. In this way the ſtones were hoiſted from the boats, as high as they could be, upon the rock ſhears; then a tackle depending from the top ſhears juſt mentioned, hooked hold of the pieces, and hoiſted them up to the top, on the outſide; and to facilitate this ſecond ſtage of hoiſting, as the work was gradually becoming higher and higher, and the hoiſting with tackles by *hand* not attended with expedition, (ſee note on § 232.) a temporary windlaſs for working it, was fixed in the ſtore-room, as is ſhewn in the ſame plate.——While thoſe things were fitting up, the Weſton arrived at noon on Saturday the 7th of July; and in little more than an hour, her cargo, conſiſting of twelve pieces of Courſe XXX. of near a ton each, was laid upon the firſt vaulted floor, without fear of, or finding, the leaſt degree of ſettlement, though only finiſhed that morning. For this ſervice we employed three men at the rock windlaſs, and two at the ſtore-room windlaſs. The Weſton had not got out of the Gut, before we experienced a change of weather, the wind beginning to freſhen at N. E.; and ſcarce was the firſt ſtone ſet, before our attending boats became ſo unquiet in lying near the rocks, that we found it adviſable to quit the work; however, having procured ſome ſubſtantial ſhelter, we now ventured to leave our mortar buckets, tools, and looſe materials, ſtowed away in the ſtore-room, which was indeed a great eaſement to us when, in conſequence of bad weather, it became neceſſary to quit the rock. As we had now the wind and tide both againſt us, we had a hard pull with our oars to get on board the buſs; which however we happily effected.

The weather being now attended with the uſual uncertainty, upon Sunday the 8th of July only five pieces of Courſe XXX. were ſet; but having ſtaid till Mr. JESSOP and his company were perfectly verſed in the mode of proceeding, I took my paſſage to Plymouth; having firſt eſtabliſhed, that they ſhould quit the work at night; for the building being now raiſed to a competent height, with ſufficient ſhelter to ſcreen the men at high water, in moderate weather; as the day-light now afforded as many hours as the men could poſſibly hold out to work; and as we had always found one hour in the day to be worth two in the night; it ſeemed no longer neceſſary to work by night, except when the unloading of the veſſels or other particular ſervice, ſhould require.

263. VARIOUS

268. VARIOUS weather prevented the out-company from making any great progress; however, finding, from accounts, that it would be likely to fall to the lot of RICHARDSON's company to *lead* in the chains of the second floor (he not having done this part of the work before) I determined to accompany them. We sailed on Tuesday the 17th, and after a bad passage arrived at the buss in the evening, and at low water landed with the company. I found the work at Course XXXIII. six pieces set, and four upon the work, unset, but which were scarcely got out of hand, when the swell came on so violent, that we found it difficult to get on board our yawls. The remainder of this course was still on board the Weston, which had taken it in on the 14th instant.——This evening, between ten and eleven, the Edystone boat arrived, having on board a part of the second floor; and brought me a message from Lord EDGECOMBE, that *Prince* EDWARD *Duke* of YORK was desirous of seeing the model of the lighthouse. However desirous I might be to gratify the curiosity of his *Royal Highness*; it yet seemed of still more consequence, that Mr. RICHARDSON and his company, should set right about the work of the second floor; Course XXXIII. being the first chain course thereof.

Wednesday the 18th of July, betwixt three and four, all hands landed, unloaded the Weston of her cargo, and set the remaining six pieces of Course XXXIII. and by noon the first chain was leaded in. This company having therefore now completed one of the chain courses; having set up the centre last year; and learnt the use of the new tackle by the stones just hoisted, and the whole method of proceeding, I took my passage to Plymouth on board the Weston, and arrived in the evening.

269. THURSDAY the 19th of July I carried the model, drafts, &c. to *Mount Edgecombe*, when the *Duke* of YORK was pleased to express great satisfaction. I had the honour of dining with, and attending his *Royal Highness* after dinner to Mill Bay, where the cove and cornice courses being together, with the balcony rails, and two courses of the lantern upon the platform; his *Royal Highness* was struck with the great strength and solidity of the work; and was much pleased with the machinery for facilitating the operations of the work-yard.——Being now at liberty, and wishing if possible to see RICHARDSON's company put together the second floor; that I might not be disappointed by a calm, in case there was not wind to carry out the Assistant, which was also ready, I hired a six-oared barge; for which, as it afterwards proved, I had occasion. We rowed out at half past two in the morning, and at six I landed upon the rock, finding RICHARDSON and company at work. They had completed the second chain course of the second floor, had got up the centre, and one of the boat's cargoes upon it, ready to begin the arch, which was now immediately proceeded with; and the day being quite serene, a sea breeze going round with the sun, and further cargoes of stone for the floor being delivered in due time, all went on without interruption.

270. SATURDAY the 21st of July, the morning quite fine, the company landed between three and four, and this forenoon the second floor was finished; so that notwithstanding several interruptions from weather, a whole room with its vaulted cover was built complete in seven days.——The above being effected, the company proceeded in course of work; and the entry and store-room doors with their iron work being brought out with the last boat, the carpenter proceeded to fit the same to place; and I set about leading the door hooks into the jambs, the holes for which had been made at the close of last season; but found they had unluckily forgot to send out a quantity of block tin, that I ordered, for the purpose of giving the lead a proper hardness, to prevent their shaking loose; to make, according to Mr. RUDYERD, a coarse kind of pewter. This was a disappointment, as it was one of the operations, the mode of which, I had in view to ascertain by coming out the last time; however, that I might not lose the opportunity, after some consideration the following expedient occurred to me; I melted down all the pewter plates and dishes that we could muster on board the buss, and mixing them with a proper quantity of lead, it answered my purpose; and the fixing of four hooks was accordingly accomplished. The composition I afterwards used for leading those in, was one pound of block tin to three pounds of lead.——The hooks were let into the stone *Lewis* or dovetail fashion, and were *keyed* in hot; and, like the cramps and chains,

run in with oil; and while hot, the external part of the iron was tarred over. And, having now ſeen this work in the ſituation I intended when I went off, I returned to Plymouth.

271. THE weather being quite fine, and the work going on with every degree of expedition that could be wiſhed, on Thurſday July the 26th, I propoſed to go out in the Aſſiſtant, as I expected to arrive there by the time the third floor was completed. Previous to my departure, the Maſter called upon me, to acquaint me that the ſeaman who belonged to his boat, and was to have laid in it all night, was miſſing this morning: and I dare ſay my reader, after what has been ſaid on this head, will wonder that the occaſion of his abſence could poſſibly have once more happened. Concluding he had been impreſſed, Mr. JESSOP went out with the Maſter, on board the men of war in the Sound, and found him on board one, from whom we ſhould leaſt have expected ſuch a detainer; and whoſe Lieutenant refuſed to deliver him without the Captain's order, who was then on ſhore. I thereupon found myſelf under the neceſſity of waiting perſonally on the Captain, who very politely diſmiſſed him at my requeſt; but this incident, from the turn of tides, prevented my arrival at the rock till ſix o'clock the next morning: when, being Friday the 27th, I found Mr. RICHARDSON had finiſhed Courſe XL. (ſee Plate N° 9.) being the ſecond chain courſe of the third floor; for which he was fixing the centre. Having ſeen this done, and the floor begun; having examined what had been done ſince I was laſt there, and finding all right; I returned in the ſame veſſel to Plymouth; and on Sunday the 29th that floor was completed: ſo that in a courſe of thirteen days two entire rooms with their proper covers were built; and, except ſix pieces of ſtone, all by one company.

Mr. RICHARDSON and company were proceeding with the work, when they were relieved by Mr. JESSOP's company on Monday the 30th; having then compleated two courſes of the fourth room: but this company was leſs ſucceſsful, for on Tueſday the weather came on ſo adverſe as to oblige the Aſſiſtant to quit the tranſport buoy, and to come home with her cargo in.——This day, the 31ſt of July, the copper ball, of two feet two inches diameter, with its neck and air pipes, was perfected at Plymouth.

272. THE weather turning out turbulent, and at beſt uncertain, it was Monday Auguſt the 6th before I thought it neceſſary to go out again: but at this time the cove Courſe XLV. being in hand, which comprehended two circular chains, I landed at ſix in the evening, and found four pieces of this courſe ſet; and this evening we ſet three more; it was not however till ten at night on Wedneſday, that this courſe was got out of hand, by the leading in of its two chains.——This day I was preſented, during a conſiderable part of it, with a *Phænomenon* new to *my* obſervation: we had light breezes at the weſt, and frequently drifts of thick fog, which, as the ſun ſhone out, preſented to us upon the top of the building, a rainbow making an *entire Circle*, except where cut off below us, by the ſhaft of the column.

Thurſday Auguſt the 9th in the morning we ſet up the *elliptical* centre, for ſetting the balcony floor; and the Weſton came into the Gut with her cargo; which, though conſiſting of only ſix pieces of ſtone for that floor; yet the wind coming ſuddenly freſh at eaſt, and the tide riſing, it occaſioned ſuch a ſwell in the Gut that ſhe preſently began to roll gunnel *to*, and while the third piece *was hoiſting*, parted her two *Faſts** to the eaſtern rocks, (ſee Plate N° 14;) ſo that being now left to the mercy of the eaſt ſwell driving her againſt the rocks, ſhe muſt have immediately been torn to pieces, had it not been for the *Fender Piles*: upon this accident I ordered both the windlaſſes to be *laſhed*, the ſtones remaining in ſuſpenſion, and all hands to her aſſiſtance; and happily got her out of the Gut, without other damage than to the upper works of her *Quarter*. When ſhe got to the tranſport buoy, there was ſuch a *cockling* ſea, that ſhe had not rode above half an hour, before the three remaining pieces began to ſhift their places, which obliged her to get under ſail and return to Plymouth.——Having ſeen the firſt ſtone compoſing the arch of the balcony floor got into its place, and having given Mr. JESSOP directions for proceeding, the wind by

* Short cables, or hawſers, for ſteadying or faſtening a veſſel, which are proportioned in ſize to that of the veſſel, and the ſtreſs expected.

this

this time was become ſo freſh as to oblige all hands to leave the rock; and I being wanted at Plymouth, to put forward the work of the *Copper* roof of the lantern, I went on board the Edyſtone boat, that waited for me under ſail.——This day the fog frequently came on ſo thick that the veſſels at the tranſport buoy could not be ſeen from the houſe.

273. MONDAY Auguſt the 13th RICHARDSON's company went out; and the next day, finding the work advancing towards a completion of the main column, upon which would come in courſe the fitting of the balcony rails, I attempted to go out the 15th, but was driven back by ſtreſs of weather: however, on Thurſday Auguſt the 16th, I got out to the buſs, landed with the company, and the Weſton was delivered of her cargo; and now all the heavy pieces belonging to the cornice being got upon the top of the building; and every thing but what would go through the hatchways or *Man-holes* in the centre; the moveable ſhears, that had gone up with us, from the top of the firſt room, were taken down and ſent home.——The interior area of the balcony floor I found completed, and we ſtruck the center from under it. We now proceeded to ſet its outermoſt circle of ſtones, which finiſhed the cap of the main column, ſee Plates N° 9; and N° 11. Fig. 9. being parts of the *Corona* or cornice: and we fitted the windlaſs in the ſtore-room, ſo as to hoiſt the ſtones of the lantern through the hatchways.

Friday Auguſt the 17th the laſt pieces of the *Corona* were ſet, and therewith the main column compleated.——I now examined the perpendicularity of the whole building, by letting fall a plumb-line from the centre of the man-hole in the balcony floor to the centre of the bottom of the well-hole, being 49½ feet; and found it to fall a ſmall matter to the eaſtward of the centre of the well-hole; as near as I could determine it, not more than ⅛th of an inch. I then meaſured the perpendicular heights of the ſeveral parts of the building, and found them as follows:

	Feet.	Inches.
The ſix foundation courſes to the top of the rock — —	8	4½
The eight courſes to the entry-door — — —	12	0½
The ten courſes of the well-hole to the ſtore-room floor —	15	2½
The height of the four rooms to the balcony floor — —	34	4½
Height of the main column, containing forty-ſix courſes —	70	0

274. WE now proceeded this day to ſet up and lead in the balcony rails, and completed them; but having no ſtone, we proceeded to make the holes preparatory for hanging the *Ports** for the windows; and having brought out a temporary cover for the man-hole of the balcony floor; I this day applied it to uſe; in conſequence of which, when Mr. RICHARDSON had got the ports hung ſo as to keep the ſea from coming in at the windows, he would be enabled to lodge with his company in the houſe.——The temporary cover of the man-hole was as follows: a ſhort tub of about a foot high was made *without* a bottom; and the ſmaller end of it being ſized as near as poſſible to the man-holes of the floors; it was driven into that of the balcony; and by the time it was driven about four inches; the compliancy of the wood to the ſtone rendered it quite tight; then the reſt of its height, forming a border, and ſtanding about eight inches above the floor, would prevent water from dripping into the rooms through the upper man-hole or hatchway; and having alſo provided another tub, about nine inches deep, having a ſtrong bottom in it, and ſo much more in diameter than the other that it would, when inverted, cover it; this being applied as a cover, would in the greateſt ſtreſs of weather defend the building from the entry of water at the top, and this was the ſame that I intended to have uſed, to make good the joint within the firſt vaulted floor, in

* *Theſe* in a dwelling-houſe would be called window-ſhutters; but as they were here made in the ſtrongeſt manner, with double plank, as the port-holes for ſhips are cloſed; being in like manner intended to reſiſt the violent action of the ſea, are ſtill (as they uſed to be) called *Ports* in this lighthouſe. Properly ſpeaking, I underſtand the openings are the *Ports*, and the ſhutters the *Port lids*.

caſe

caſe my propoſal of keeping a light the laſt winter, had been approved of, and executed*.——The Edyſtone boat arrived with the firſt courſe of ſtone for the lantern, and was unloaded this evening.

Saturday the 18th of Auguſt, we all landed in the morning at four, and proceeded to ſet the firſt courſe of the lantern; which being in a courſe of work, and having left directions with Mr. Richardson for the remaining part, including the ſtone ſtairs in the well-hole; I returned to Plymouth to expedite the work that was wanted to be done to complete the lantern, and arrived there at noon.

275. AMONGST the numberleſs vexations and diſappointments met with in the courſe of this work, not only from the elements, but from the negligence and inattention of others; it was not one of the leaſt, that the Carrier employed to bring the work of the lantern by *land* from London (for no other reaſon but to obviate the *uncertainty* and diſappointment that might attend the ſea), had, to ſerve his own convenience, left the greateſt part thereof at *Exeter* a week before; and I found it was not yet come the preſent week; which prevented our finiſhing the laſt courſe of ſtone from the platform, that was to receive the iron ſill of the lantern. The *Rabbet* was indeed rough cut in the ſtone, and was a plain piece of work; but, as I had never truſted to any thing *fitting* at the Edyſtone, but what had firſt had its parts brought together at Mill Bay, I did not think it prudent to diſpenſe with this rule, without *abſolute* neceſſity: for, the fitting or adapting the parts of matter together, comes under no calculation in point of time; as, from circumſtances, much time may be required for the purpoſe, when little is expected. This evening however the work of the lantern arrived; which deſirable event greatly alleviated the chagrin I had felt.

Tueſday the 21ſt of Auguſt the iron *Ground Sill* of the lantern, or *Cap Sill* of the wall, was brought to Mill Bay; and was tried and fitted to the LIId courſe, which, being the laſt, was made ready for going to ſea.——This day I thought it proper to write to the *Corporation* of Trinity House, to acquaint them with the ſtate of the building, and therein expreſſed my hopes that the lantern would be ſoon completed, if the weather continued moderate, ſo as to be capable of exhibiting a light in its proper place; and the houſe made completely habitable, and proof againſt wind and weather, without the aid of temporary contrivances.

276. THURSDAY the 23d of Auguſt. For ſome time paſt I had employed a copper-ſmith in preparing the copper for the roof, ſo far as he could do it, without having the iron work to which it was to be fitted. The platform therefore being now cleared from all the ſtone-work, the upper ſill of the lantern was put together upon it; as alſo the iron ribs that gave the figure and ſtiffneſs to the plates of the roof; and the copper-ſmiths began to fit the copper roof thereto; ſee Plate N° 12: it being only neceſſary here to ſay, that the plates being of 3½lb. to the ſquare foot, and of conſequence ſomewhat ſtubborn; to prevent all uncertainty in forming them at their hips to the proper figure, I choſe them to be *mitre-jointed* at the angles; and this joint being covered with a ſtrip of copper, or *ſaddle-piece*, of about three inches in breadth, it was eaſy to fit it to both plates, and render that eaſy that otherwiſe would have been difficult. This ſaddle-piece was therefore fixed upon the angles with a *double* row of copper nails; and the whole being rivetted together, the cupola, when finiſhed, would become one piece, and water-tight, like a boiler.

Friday Auguſt the 24th we had the welcome news by one of the boats, that this day Mr. Richardson compleated Courſe LII.: ſo that the ſtone-work was now ready for the reception of the metal part of the lantern; and alſo that he was proceeding with the ſtone ſtairs.

277. MONDAY the 27th Mr. Richardson and company arrived from the Edyſtone, and gave account that they had lived in the houſe ever ſince the 23d inſtant, and found it very warm and comfortable; much more ſo than the buſs's *hold* and cabin. That he ſet the laſt ſtone of the lantern, being that making the door-head, on Friday the 24th; and then a part of his hands were employed in fixing and completing

* This was intended as an additional ſecurity, beſides an entire cover or platform of wood, as mentioned § 255.

the

the fixture of the iron-work of the window *Ports*, while the other part were fetting the ftone ftairs: and laftly, that they had put on the cap-ftone of the ftair-head, and finifhed every thing belonging to the mafonry on Sunday evening the 26th of Auguft. However, when all was done, though all was very quiet within the houfe, they found the fea fo unquiet about the rocks, that the yawls could not come alongfide them that evening; and that it was with fome difficulty they quitted their habitation, and got on board the bufs this morning.

278. THE progrefs we had made this feafon could not fail to animate our further proceedings; for from the 5th of July to the 26th of Auguft, both inclufive, we had completed twenty-three ccurfes, including the greateft part of four vaulted floors, fix circular chains, and in the whole 470 principal pieces. ——Having brought the work to this defirable ftate, the next day I difmiffed all our mafons and tinners, except eight of our beft hands, who being ufed to the place, I kept to affift the joiners, fmiths, plumbers, copper-fmiths, glaziers, painters, &c. whom it was neceffary to take off before we could make an entire finifh; and who being new hands unaccuftomed to the place, I judged would act with more courage, by having feafoned men amongft them.

279. AFTER this time I was thoroughly employed in forwarding the works of the lantern; but we had very foon a change of weather, fo much for the worfe that though the feamen were ordered out the 29th, to try to fweep for and recover the moorings we had loft in the courfe of the two preceding years; an hard gale of wind and rain from S. W. coming on, they were obliged to return without attempting any thing.——During this time, however, an opportunity was taken by the feamen of landing in the houfe, and of wetting the infide of the rooms all over with water, which I directed to be done, in order to feed and harden the cement, and prevent its drying too haftily; as it was not like the outfide, fubject to be afterwards wet by the fea: but the weather never admitted of any opportunity of fweeping.

On Tuefday the 4th of September, when the work of the cupola was going brifkly on in the yard, the foreman of the copper-fmiths was taken fo ill that he was obliged to leave his work.——This day I received a letter from the Secretary to the TRINITY HOUSE, dated the 1ft inftant, acquainting me that the *Corporation* defired me to inform them of the day I was *certain* a light could be exhibited in the light-houfe, that they might advertife the fame; and that the night I fhewed the light I fhould acquaint Mr. SYMONDS, Mafter of the *Floating-Light*, not to exhibit it any longer. To this I anfwered, that though I had met with fome difappointments, yet I hoped the lantern and cupola would be ready to carry off that week; and that I fhould endeavour to complete the whole with the utmoft expedition; and when ready would acquaint the *Corporation*; and concert a proper fignal with the Mafter of the floating-light, in cafe accefs to him fhould be impracticable. That as the feafon was advancing, and the weather growing more precarious, it might not be in my power *abfolutely* to fix the day I could exhibit a light, till the day itfelf arrived: in which cafe, I fuppofed it to be their pleafure that it fhould be done, giving the proper notices that they had directed; but if I mifapprehended their directions, I defired not to be left in doubt.

The next day the fecond copper-fmith, with his affiftants, finifhed the clofing of the joints at the angles; and, that no time might be loft (wanting the proper workmen), on the 6th I worked myfelf all day at the cupola, affifting in rivetting on fixteen angle pieces of iron in the infide, in the nature of knee timbers of a fhip, for ftiffening the plates. When thefe were in part finifhed, the fecond copper-fmith was alfo violently feized with a *dry Cholic*, in the fame manner as the firft had been. The next day, he being incapable of proceeding with the work; and I very anxious to get what remained to be done at the cupola difpatched; as it prevented the iron ribs, &c. from being withdrawn from the cupola; I again went to work, along with the third copper-fmith; and on Saturday the 8th this part of the bufinefs being accomplifhed, the whole iron frame of the lantern was in the afternoon put on board the Wefton ready to go to fea, whenever the wind and weather would permit; it having been invariably bad ever fince the firft inftant.——As there was now nothing to prevent our proceeding to fix the frame of the lantern in its place but bad weather; nor any thing to prevent the cupola from following it as foon as fixed, except the joining of the ball to the neck of the cupola; and finding that the copper-fmiths who had hitherto ferved me were

not

not likely very foon to be effective; I requefted another brazier of Plymouth, to lend me a journeyman to complete this part of the work. But fuch is the amazing narrownefs of mind of fome perfons, that he pofitively refufed us, though he owned the man could be of no ufe to him the next day, being Sunday: however, on application to *Commiffioner* Rogers, he immediately granted leave for the brazier of the yard to affift us in that, or any thing elfe we might want. Accordingly, on Sunday evening the cupola was got ready for fea, its ball being fitted; but the weather ftill continued fo very bad, that the *Duke* man of war of eighty guns, having parted her moorings, very providentially drove directly into Mill Bay, and grounded on the foft mud; from whence fhe was, on tide of flood, got off without damage.

280. IT was not till the 12th inftant that we were able to look out to fea further than to fupply the feamen on board the bufs with provifions: in this interim I received Mr. Shuttlewood the *Secretary*'s letter, in anfwer to mine of the 4th inftant, informing me, that to remove any doubt which might arife, he was directed by the *Corporation* to acquaint me, that I was to fix the day of lighting, fo as to enable them to give a week's notice by advertifement; and, that I might be certain of the day, proper perfons were to remain in the houfe upon the rock, after the lighthoufe was finifhed, to light it on the day appointed.

281. EVERY thing immediately wanted to the completion of the houfe being got ready and put on board two of the boats, together with all neceffary hands; the morning of Wednefday, September the 12th, at one o'clock, we weighed anchor, in a thick fog, without a breath of wind; a breeze, however, fprung up, and we arrived at the bufs at five; but the wind being now frefh at eaft, neither of the boats could go into the Gut; I therefore took the opportunity of landing in a yawl to infpect the houfe; and had the fatisfaction to find, that all the ftone work had been finifhed by Mr. Richardson and his company in the manner I had ordered it: but by nine o'clock the wind was grown fo frefh, and raifed fuch a troublefome fea, that the boats were obliged to return without being unloaded; and, as nothing could be done without their cargoes, I took the opportunity of returning, to expedite what was wanting to be done on fhore, leaving the workmen on board the bufs.

September 13th. My copper-fmiths being ftill unable to work; this morning Mr. Knighton, the brazier from the *King's Yard*, began to work upon the copper funnels for venting the fmoke from the kitchen fires. The next day at noon the weather became fo favourable as to admit the boats to go out, and I arrived in the evening, but ftill could not land on account of the ground fwell: however, all the working hands at low water had taken an opportunity of getting into the houfe, with their beds, victuals, &c. as they had been directed to do.

282. SATURDAY September the 15th, between three and four in the morning, the Wefton was got into the Gut, and delivered of her cargo, confifting of the pillars, fafhes, and frame-work of the lantern; and though the turn of the tide made it impracticable to get the Edyftone boat into the Gut, yet, as her cargo confifted chiefly of the joiners materials, thefe being light, were landed by help of the yawls: and now the workmen being eftablifhed in the houfe, along with a great variety of materials, every one went to the occupation allotted; to recount the particulars of which, would be equally uninterefting and tedious.——I gave my principal attention to the eftablifhing the frame of the lantern upon a bed of lead, and the fcrewing of it carefully together; feeing that every joint was filled, and fcrew covered with white lead and oil, ground up thick for paint; and every crevice fo full, that the bringing the fcrews *home* made the white lead matter to ooze from every juncture; thereby to exclude all wet and moifture, and fo as to prevent the iron-work from rufting. To this purpofe I took to my aid Roger Cornthwait, one of the fubmoft alert of the mafons; this being in reality, after the parts were fitted together by a fmith, more the fubject of mafonry than that of fmith's work.——The attention of Mr. Jessop was chiefly confined to the other artificers: and the rooms being fo much encumbered with materials and ftores, that there was fcarcely room for the workmen; he and myfelf, as the weather was now promifing, went to our former lodging on board the bufs.

283. SUNDAY

283. SUNDAY September the 16th was remarkably fine; ſo that by the evening the whole frame of the lantern was ſcrewed together, and its ground-ſill was reſted upon a bed of lead; which was done in the following manner. The whole frame being ſcrewed together, was raiſed from its bearing upon the ſtone about [illegible]ths of an inch, by a competent number of iron wedges; and adjuſted by them to an exact perpendicular. Both the ſtone and the iron were taken care to be oiled before they were applied to each other; and one of the eight ſides, having its wedges withdrawn, was run with hot lead; and making a place for it to overflow, as much could be uſed as would competently heat both the iron and ſtone, to bring them to a cloſe bearing with the lead; then on the lead's cooling, as the frame became ſupported on one ſide by the lead, the wedges of a ſecond ſide were withdrawn, and treated in the ſame manner, and ſo ſucceſſively till the whole reſted upon a ſolid baſement of lead. It was not ſuppoſed that the ſucceeding maſs could be ſufficiently heated to re-melt the ends of the parts already leaded, as in the caſe of the chains; but being heated ſo as to bring them to a cloſe contact, this I judged ſufficient, as the lead ſo applied had no other intent but to bear *weight*, and give the frame of the lantern one ſolid uniform bearing.

284. MONDAY the 17th. This morning was alſo exceedingly fine; and the Weſton being in ſight, which was appointed to bring out the cupola, we began to ſet up our ſhears and tackle for hoiſting it. This perhaps may be accounted one of the moſt difficult and hazardous operations of the whole undertaking; not ſo much on account of its weight, being only about 11 cwt. as on account of the great height to which it was to be hoiſted, clear of the building; and ſo as, if poſſible, to avoid ſuch blows as might bruiſe it. It was alſo required to be hoiſted a conſiderable height above the balcony floor; which, though the largeſt baſe we had for the ſhears to ſtand upon, was yet but fourteen feet within the rails, and therefore narrow, in proportion to *their* height. The manner in which this was managed will in a great meaſure appear by the repreſentation thereof in Plate N° 14. (ſee the uppermoſt ſtage); but is more minutely explained in the technical detail of that plate.——As the legs of the ſhears that had been uſed upon the rock would have been in the way of the cupola, they were now removed, as being done with there, and were uſed as a part of this machinery.——About noon the whole of our tackle was in readineſs; and in the afternoon the Weſton was brought into the Gut; and in leſs than *half an hour* her troubleſome cargo was placed upon the top of the lantern without the leaſt damage.——During the whole of this operation, it pleaſed God that not a breath of wind diſcompoſed the ſurface of the water; and there was the leaſt ſwell about the rocks I had obſerved during the ſeaſon.——This work did indeed require good weather, and we had it; or otherwiſe we muſt have poſtponed it, till it had at leaſt *ſeemed* promiſing; but yet we were *prepared* for ſomething otherwiſe than *perfect* tranquillity: for, beſides that our ſhears and tackle were ſo well laſhed down and ſtayed, that it was not a ſmall blaſt of wind that would have carried them away, I had it in contemplation (if it had been needed) to have appointed a couple of men to go up upon the cupola, with ſtaves in their hands, who could, in moderate weather, have defended it from the wall.——This evening the cupola was ſo far got fixed, with its ſcrews, that the tackle was caſt off from it: but this was ſcarcely got done before the wind began to blow freſh at E.

Tueſday September the 18th, in the morning, the wind was at S. E. with intervals of thick fog; however, betwixt thoſe, I had the ſatisfaction, with my teleſcope, to perceive the Edyſtone boat, on board of which I expected the *Ball* to be; and which being *double gilt**, I had ordered the carriage of it to be carefully attended to. The wind and tide were both unfavourable to the veſſel's getting ſoon near us; therefore, being deſirous to get the ball ſcrewed on, before the ſhears and tackle were taken down, one of the yawls was diſpatched to bring it away. This being done, and the ball fixed, the ſhears and tackle were taken down, which took up nearly as much time as was employed in ſetting them up; that is, near twelve hours each, in the whole, to do the work of an hour.——I muſt obſerve, that by choice, I ſcrewed on the ball with my own hands, that in caſe any of the ſcrews had not held quite tight and firm, the circumſtance might not have been *ſlipped over*, without my knowledge; being well aware, that even *this part* would at times come to a conſiderable ſtreſs of wind and ſea; and which could not be replaced without ſome diffi-

* The leaf gold was made on purpoſe, being four times the ordinary thickneſs; beſides which, after the firſt coating of gold was on, a ſecond was laid upon it, with a view to make it as laſting as poſſible; and over all a coat of *[illegible]*.

U u   culty,

culty, in case any thing should fail*.——I now looked upon it that we might think ourselves secure of finishing the lighthouse this year.

By this time the joiners had set up and completed the three cabin bedsteads, (for their plan, and position betwixt the windows, see Plate N° 11. Fig. 8.) The house being now less encumbered, the morning of Wednesday the 19th, the wind fresh at E. and the weather threatening to cut off the communication between the house and the buss; Mr. Jessop and I removed our beds and stores into the house, and took possession of two of the cabin beds; which we had no sooner done, than it blew so hard, that the yawl was obliged to leave us, and retreat to the buss.

285. On Friday the 21st all the copper sash frames were got completely fixed in, and ready for receiving the glass. In this work we were somewhat retarded; for the carrier that brought down the work of the lantern (besides disappointing us in time) having carelessly laid very heavy things upon the boxes that contained the sash frames; by the continual working of the carriage, two of them had been broken; and though I got them carefully repaired at Plymouth, yet I judged it expedient to order two new ones from London in readiness, which might at any time be changed for the others, if they happened to fail; but (on account of the late bad weather) these new ones coming, so as to be sent out to us before it was necessary to put them in, I set Mr. Jessop to drill, screw, and fit the new ones, which occasioned the loss of time just mentioned. All the sash frames, in like manner as the iron work, were screwed in with white lead and oil; as I judged that the best means, not only of preserving the work, but of keeping out the wet. ——This day the Weston brought out two glaziers and two copper-smiths; they spoke with us, but it blew so hard a gale that they were obliged to return.——On Saturday the Weston came out again, and brought only one copper-smith, the other having been taken ill of the same distemper, which was said to be *epidemic*; but the wind was still so fresh at E. that there was no landing; they therefore put him and the two glaziers on board the buss.

286. On Sunday morning the 23d, the yawl came to the house and landed the two glaziers and the copper-smith, with their utensils and materials; the former began to glaze the lantern, and the latter to fit and put up the funnels. This day, with my assistant the mason, I began to fix twenty-four iron cramps; that is, three to each rib of the roof, and which were obliged to be fixed after the roof was together; and being fixed inside, and surrounding the ribs, served to key home the plates of the cupola to the ribs. For this purpose small wood wedges were used, as being more supple, elastic, and compliant than wedges of metal, and therefore more suitable to this particular purpose. This day also the Edystone boat brought out and landed a plumber with his utensils and materials.——The most considerable work for the plumber, was the covering the whole balcony floor with thick plates of lead; and which extended from the top of the plinth, or first course of the basement of the lantern, quite down to the drip of the *Corona*. They were fitted on separately in sixteen pieces, and soldered together, in place, with strong ribbed joints; and, to prevent the sea from laying hold of them at the drip, and beating them up, they were turned under about 1½ inch; and being near half an inch thick, I judged them sufficiently stubborn to prevent being unripped: I took care myself to put the finishing hand, by *batting* them closely to the stone underneath, by the *gentle blows* of a *small* hammer. In this work the copper-smith assisted the plumber.——Though the joints of the balcony were all very carefully filled and pointed up with our cement, which of consequence would render it *water-tight* in the common acceptation of the word, yet this being a *level* part, the water of the sea beating up in time of storms, would come down with such violence, and in such quantity, upon it; that, to prevent the possibility of the least exudation of moisture down into the rooms, arising either from the calcareous nature of the cement, or any want of closeness in any part of the upright joints, I judged it

* It may not be amiss to intimate to those that may in future have occasion to perform the same operation, that the scaffold on which this was done, consisted of four boards only, well nailed together, at such distances as to permit it to be lifted over the ball when done with. It rested on the cupola, encompassing its neck, and Roger Cornthwaite placed himself on the opposite side, upon it, to balance me, while I moved round to fix the screws.

proper

proper to have this part covered with lead in the manner mentioned, and of such a thickness that, when once done, the wear of the feet, &c. should not produce the necessity of a renewal in many years.

Thursday the 27th, the lead work upon the balcony and corona being now entirely finished, and the cupola completely keyed home to the ribs; the straps and bolts were applied at each angle of the lantern, for screwing it down to the floor of the balcony: but the copper-smith, who had again begun to work upon the funnel, was taken ill, so that he could not proceed; and one of the masons was taken ill also.

287. FRIDAY September the 28th. Since Sunday last the works of the lead and glass were going on very well, the weather in general having been moderate and dry. This day the Joiners finished their work, which consisted of the following articles.——Three cabin beds to hold one man each, with three drawers and two lockers in each to hold his separate property, which were fixed in the upper room or chamber. (See plan thereof, Plate N° *11.* Fig. 8.) In the kitchen, besides the fire-place and sink, were two settles with lockers, a dresser with drawers, two cupboards, and one platter case. (Fig. 7. of the same plate shews how these were disposed.) In the lantern, a seat was fixed to encompass it all round, the door-way excepted, serving equally to sit upon, or stand to snuff the candles; and to enable a person to look through the lowest tier of glass panes at distant objects, without having occasion to go on the outside of the lantern into the balcony.——Besides the above, the joiners had fixed the ten window frames with their sashes; that is, two in the upper store-room, disposed N. and S. and four in each of the rooms above: all which were bedded in putty, and falling into rabbets cut for them in the original formation of the stone, they could be at any time removed, and replaced at pleasure, as they were fastened in only with two wooden pins above, and two below, driven into holes bored in the stone. And it is here to be noted, that though, for fixing up and steadying the several articles in their places, something of fastenings to the walls were frequently necessary; yet, wherever any thing was to be affixed to them, it was never done by driving any thing into the joints, but always by drilling holes with a jumper into the solid of the stone, deep enough to answer the end required; and then, if *iron* plugs or bolts, they were either driven, upon a very gentle taper till they became fast, or were fixed in with lead; or, as was generally the case with the inside work, holes were bored in the solid, and oaken plugs being driven therein, and sawn off even with the surface of the stone, iron holdfasts could be very properly and effectually driven into those wooden plugs, by which means the disturbing of any part of the cement was avoided.

288. IT is to be observed, that in the *present* edifice I fixed the *Beds* in the uppermost room; and the *Fire-place*, which constituted the kitchen, in the room below it; whereas, in the late house, the upper room was the kitchen, and the beds (which, as I have understood, were upon common bedsteads) were placed in one of the rooms below. The former disposition was doubtless adopted, because the funnel for the smoke would be the shortest; but, as I was informed that in moist weather, the beds and bedding were generally in a very damp disagreeable state; I proposed to remedy this evil, by lengthening the funnel into the room, below the top room, by which means the copper funnel passing through the upper room, its surface being warmed by the smoke and heated air within, would communicate a genial warmth to the upper room through which it passed; and, as air when warmed has a natural tendency to ascend, whenever the copper cover was taken off, that closed the man-hole or passage from the kitchen to the bed-chamber, (and which, indeed, except at nights, would generally be the case) the warm air of the kitchen would ascend through the bed-chamber, into the lantern, and be vented there by the air-pipes made to discharge the hot air and smoke from the candles. This disposition has perfectly answered the end, as nothing can be more completely dry than the two habitable rooms. Nor are the store-rooms below, subject to any moisture, to the injury of the stores, being in reality much drier than those of the former building were said to have been. Indeed this is not to be wondered at, if it be considered, that the encompassing walls are wholly of moor-stone, which is a substance that does not admit of any humidity into its pores, as wood will do: and there is nothing of *Parget* or plaster in the whole building; for every stone fulfils its place inside and out; the piece of stone that makes the outside, being worked fair within, makes the inner surface of the room; and the

the ſame ſtones that are trod upon, as the floor in the room above, reach through and form the cieling of the room below.

289. THIS afternoon the Edyſtone boat came out, and brought out two cheſts of candles for the lights, and other ſtores. She alſo brought out ſixteen croſs bars for the windows, with a couple of ſmiths to fix them, and which were prepared as far as they could be on ſhore: but as by miſtake they had only made half the number I wanted, the order being for ſixteen *pair*, I found it neceſſary to ſend them home to forge and prepare the reſt, while I proceeded, with ſuch help as I had, to fit thoſe we had got.——This boat was to have brought out a painter, who promiſed to come; but hearing of ſo many being taken ill at the Edyſtone, he refuſed to come off. I therefore ſet one of the maſons to work in painting the outſide of the roof of the cupola. The copper-ſmith and the maſon who had been taken ill yeſterday, continuing unfit for work; they, with the three joiners, and the two ſmiths, returned back to Plymouth this evening, in the Edyſtone boat.

After the boat was gone, and it became ſo dark, that we could not ſee any longer to purſue our occupations, I ordered a charcoal fire to be made in the upper ſtore-room, in one of the iron pots we uſed for melting lead; the intent of which was, that as the croſs bars muſt exactly fit their reſpective places in point of length, anſwerable to the diſtances of the ſcrews wherewith the copper ſaſh frames were ſcrewed to the iron pillars of the lantern, there could only be prepared on ſhore, holes made at one end; leaving the other to be marked to its place. In conſequence, all theſe holes muſt be bored here; and to facilitate this operation, by *annealing* the *blank* ends of all thoſe bars, they were made red hot all together in the charcoal fire. Moſt of the workmen were ſet round the fire, and by way of making ourſelves comfortable, by ſcreening ourſelves and the fire from the wind, the windows were ſhut; and, as well as I remember, the copper cover or hatch put over the man-hole of the floor of the room where the fire was: the hatch above being left open as a funnel for the heated vapour to aſcend. I remember to have looked into the fire attentively, to ſee that the iron was made hot enough, and not over-heated: I alſo remember I felt my head a very little giddy: but the very next thing of which I had any ſenſation or idea, was finding myſelf upon the floor of the room below, half drowned with water. It ſeems, that without being further ſenſible of any thing to give me warning, the *Effluvia* of the charcoal (being from my ſituation more expoſed thereto than the reſt ſo ſuddenly overcame all ſenſation, that I dropped down upon the floor; and, had not the people hauled me down into the room below, where they did not ſpare for cold water to throw in my face and upon me, I certainly ſhould have expired upon the ſpot.

290. THE next day, *Michaelmas*-day, was diſtinguiſhed by the whole glazing of the lantern being completed; and conſequently now the houſe was in a condition to exhibit a light.——I proceeded with my *Maſon* to bore the holes, and fit the bars; in doing which I found we made ſuch good diſpatch, that I doubted not but we ſhould have them all fixed before we received any more from the ſmith; and this day, not having been diſtinguiſhed by any other event than what is above-mentioned, it may be a proper place to mention what my intention was reſpecting theſe croſs bars.——They were not indeed a part of the original deſign. I had conceived that the main upright ſtandards of caſt-iron (ſee Plates N° 12, 14, and 16.) having their feet or claws ſtrongly ſcrewed down upon their *Ground-ſills* and to their *Cap-ſills*, which were of wrought iron, four inches broad, and almoſt an inch thick; theſe, together with the great number of ſcrews, faſtening the copper ſaſh frames thereto, would form ſo ſtrong a frame, that no power leſs than what would overſet the whole lantern, could make any material derangement of its figure: yet, when I afterwards conſidered, that all the bars, both great and ſmall, were either perpendicular or horizontal, and conſequently nothing to oppoſe the *racking* of the frame; the violent actions of the ſea, though not ſufficient to break any of the parts, yet might be ſubject to produce ſuch kind of twiſting, agitations, and vibrations, as that by preventing the panes of glaſs from being at reſt in the putty, might prevent their fixing therein, with that ſolidity which I wiſhed. For, though underneath the putty in every pane, there were ſix braſs pins, driven through holes drilled acroſs the bars, by way of retaining in the panes excluſive of the putty; yet

yet to keep them as ſteady as poſſible, from the cauſes of vibration juſt mentioned, I determined to place a pair of *Croſs Bars* behind each ſaſh frame, ſcrewed thereto in a firm manner. In conſequence, each face of the octagon having two ſaſhes in height, the whole number of ſaſhes was ſixteen; and there were thirty-two bars: which, to make little obſtruction to the light, were not only placed ſo as to be the leaſt poſſible in the way, where the candles were commonly to be put, but were at a *medium* leſs than an inch in diameter; being ¾ of an inch near the ends, and 1¼ inch in the middle. Theſe bars have in reality completely anſwered the end intended.——The next day, September the 30th, the glaziers had ſcarcely finiſhed the puttying of all the windows of the rooms below, when the principal one was taken ill; however, he got that part of the work out of hand.

291. MONDAY October the 1ſt I completed the fixing of the firſt eight pairs of croſs bars begun on Saturday; and, leſt weather, or any accident, ſhould prevent the reſt from being fixed, ſo ſoon as intended, I diſpoſed theſe eight pairs ſo as moſt effectually to contribute to the general purpoſe: for this reaſon I fixed them upon the N.E. S.E. S.W. and N.W. faces of the lantern, leaving the intermediate faces without any; by which means their ſtrength became equally diſtributed *.——This day alſo the copper funnel was finiſhed, by the help of the *plumber*; and on being tried by lighting a fire, was found fully to anſwer. The tackle was alſo fixed for raiſing and lowering the *Chandeliers*; and thoſe being hung, (ſee Plate N° 12.) there was now nothing to hinder our making trial by lighting the candles, while it was *day-light*, to ſee that every thing, regarding the light, operated in a proper manner. Accordingly this afternoon we put up twenty-four candles into their proper places, and continued them burning for three hours; during which time we had a very effectual trial; for it had blown a hard gale of wind at S. E. all day, which ſtill continued; and keeping a fire at the ſame time in the kitchen, they both operated together without the leaſt interference; not any degree of ſmoke appearing in the lantern, or any of the rooms: and by opening the vent-holes which I had cauſed to be made at the bottom of the lantern, for occaſional uſe, it could be kept as cool as we pleaſed; whereas, in the late lighthouſe, this uſed to be complained of, as being ſo hot, eſpecially in ſummer, as to give much trouble by the *running* of the candles.

Tueſday October the 2d, the wind freſh at E. the Weſton came out with two perſons to be light-keepers; but, as they could not land, they were put on board the buſs.——Letters brought by the Weſton were delivered in the houſe by means of a *Keg*. This I got made, with an intention to convey proviſions and ſmall ſtores into the houſe, at ſuch times as a boat might come near the rocks but not be able to land. It was made very ſtrong, with one of the heads to take out, and fit like a plug; ſo as to be water-tight when driven in with a piece of canvas. This being carried by the wind and ſea to the leeward of the houſe, could be taken up by a boat in that ſituation: and we found it to anſwer whenever we had occaſion to uſe it. The Weſton alſo brought out eleven more of the croſs bars; which not being able to land, were left on board the buſs; and, as I was deſirous of getting them as ſoon as poſſible, we at low water got a rope from the houſe, by the keg, to the yawl; and to this faſtening the bars, they were ſunk with the keg, and therewith drawn into the houſe.

292. WEDNESDAY October the 3d, we began to fix the *Conductor* for lightning, (§ 158.) As the copper funnel reached through the ball, and from thence came down to the kitchen floor, above forty feet, (ſee Plate N° 9.) I conſidered this as containing ſo much metal, that if ſtruck with lightning, it would thus far be a ſufficient conveyance; then joining the kitchen grate to the leaden ſink by a metal conveyance, the ſink pipe of lead would convey it to the outſide. From the ſink pipe downwards, which being on the N. E. ſide, was conſequently the leaſt ſubject to the ſtroke of the ſea; we continued the *electrical* communication by means of a ſtrap of lead about 1½ inch broad and ¼ths thick, fixed on the outſide by being nailed to oaken plugs, drove into *two* jumper holes in the ſolid of each courſe; the prominent angles of the ſtrap being *chamfered* off, it was bedded and brought to a ſmooth ſurface with putty. At the foot of the leaden ſtrap, an eye-bolt of iron was driven into the rock; and to this was fixed an iron chain, long

* Was this part of the work to do again, or the like to be wanted, the croſs bars would moſt commodiouſly be caſt as a part of the copper ſaſhes; and are ſo repreſented in Plates 9 and 12. But not intended to interfere with the glaſs panes.

enough

enough to reach at all times into the water; its lower end being left loose to play therein, and give way to the stroke of the waves: by this means an electrical communication was made from the top of the ball to the sea.——This day we learnt from the buss, that one of our intended light-keepers, by the rolling of the buss, had fallen, and put out his shoulder; and that the other being intimidated, refused to come into the house.

293. THURSDAY October the 4th, the wind at N. W. and moderate; the Edystone boat came out with stores and water, which were landed, as also some more of the cross bars.——The season being now advanced towards that which we had always found to grow very *precarious*; and every thing being now completed about the house that we could judge *essentially* necessary to the exhibition and maintenance of a light; I immediately agreed with three of the workmen to abide in the house, and keep the light till proper persons could be engaged with and sent off: I therefore now thought it time to take the opportunity of dispatching an express by the Edystone boat to Plymouth, to be forwarded to the *Corporation* of TRINITY HOUSE, giving notice for Tuesday the 16th of that month, as the day of lighting the house; which allowed twelve days for the passage of the express, and advertisements for a week previous, as ordered by the Corporation: and at the same time I dispatched the yawl, with a letter of notice to the same purport to *Captain* SYMONDS, Master of the *Floating-Light*.——The sick glazier, and the man with the dislocated shoulder on board the buss, returned with the boat to Plymouth.

Friday the 5th of October, all the cross bars were got fixed that we received yesterday. There being a great sea about the rocks, with wind at S. W. I could, by resting steadily against the wall of the lantern, perceive a sensible motion from the action of the sea. This I did not wonder at, having felt a steeple sensibly move by the ringing of bells; but I was quite surprized to find, that such heavy seas as now rolled over the *adjacent* rocks, *without touching* the building, produced a motion nearly as sensible. This, however, fully convinced me of what I had for some time been led to think, that the Edystone rocks have a very sensible degree of *Elasticity*.

Saturday October the 6th, the wind was at S. W. but become very moderate. The ground swell, however, that came home, frequently this day broke up as high as the windows of the kitchen, but I could not perceive *that* to produce the least sensible motion in the building.——This day the plumber completed every thing in *his* way about the balcony.——At low water the yawl brought the light-keeper who had remained on board the buss; and who having in some degree conquered his fears, made an apology for not coming before, which I thought it prudent to admit of.

Sunday October the 7th. After so severe a visitation of sickness amongst the workmen *, all those remaining in the house, that stood their service, were employed in clearing the rooms ready to take in the winter's stores: except those who were employed in giving the outside parts the *second Coat* of paint, since being fixed in place.——This day the electrical communication for the lightning was completed.

294. MONDAY October the 8th in the morning, the Weston arrived at the transport buoy; being loaded with further stores for the winter; and had the remainder of the cross bars on board: these were immediately landed with the yawl; but the ground swell was too great to admit the boat to venture into the Gut; and the Edystone boat appearing in sight, which was also laden with stores, she was ordered to deliver them on board the buss. This being done, and it appearing doubtful when the Weston might be able to deliver her cargo in the Gut, she was ordered to follow the same example. As soon therefore as the tide was fallen away sufficiently, to render it practicable for the yawls to come into the Gut, a number of hands were employed to bring the stores from the buss, and land them in the house; and in the course of this tide the whole business was performed, four casks of water only excepted.——This evening the second coat of paint was finished, and the cross bars all completely fixed. A time-piece I had provided, was set up and put in motion †; and as nothing material now remained to be done, we determined, as the

* There were now but few remaining hearty; of this number, however, were Mr. Jessop and myself.

† A meridian for the setting of the clock, would naturally arise from observing when the sun-beams of the south windows, directly tended to the opposite ones, as this would point out the time of noon. This Time piece, by a simple contrivance, being made to strike a single blow every half hour, was intended to warn the keepers to snuff the candles.

wind

wind and weather were then favourable for unmooring the buſs, to leave the houſe in poſſeſſion of the perſons appointed to keep the light, and remove on board the buſs the firſt opportunity: and, leſt time ſhould be ſhort on our removal, and another opportunity might not occur before the day of lighting; this evening, with the aſſiſtance of Mr. JESSOP, I gave full orders and inſtructions to HENRY EDWARDS and JOHN MICHELL both tinners; and who were the only perſons that had continued ſteadily to act as *labourers* from the beginning. Thoſe, therefore, being perſons upon whom I could depend; and who had ſeen and aſſiſted in the lighting of the houſe in the day time the 1ſt inſtant, I could have no doubt but that they would fully inſtruct the perſon entered as *Light-keeper*; and that my directions would be punctually obſerved, and the houſe lighted according to its deſtination the 16th inſtant, in caſe I could not myſelf be preſent, as I propoſed to be, if wind and weather permitted.

295. TUESDAY the 9th of October, in the morning, before one o'clock, the yawl came into the Gut with the remaining caſks of water, and began to remove the men, with their beds, tools, and neceſſaries; which being performed, Mr. JESSOP and myſelf, with all hands, were got on board the buſs at four.——The wind was then S. E. and very moderate, the ſky ſerene, and every thing appearing promiſing, we began to unmoor. We had ſcarcely got the eaſtern anchor from the ground, when clouds began to gather from the S. W. and the wind ſhifting into that quarter, threatened an immediate ſtorm: however, as my maxim always was, *to proceed till there was ſomething to ſtop us*, we went on; and fortunately, though it looked very diſmal and threatening all the time, it did not blow outright; and the more diſmal it looked, the more anxious we were to get out of the way of it.——In heaving up our moorings we were much ſurprized to find the eaſtern chain *parted* from the weſtern; but by applying to the buoy of the weſtern anchor it was got on board; and in heaving in the bridle, we found one of the links more than half worn through, by fretting againſt the rocks; it being as bright as if ſhorn by a file; ſo that in all probability the next hard gale of wind muſt have broke the buſs adrift.——At four in the afternoon having got all our moorings on board, we hoiſted ſail; and it now coming on a freſh gale of wind at S. W. it drove us right into the Sound; and the tide being alſo in our favour, we never had ſo quick a paſſage in the *Neptune Buſs*; for in leſs than *three* hours, we were come to an anchor in *Plymouth Harbour*, with a flowing tide, to the great joy and ſatisfaction of all concerned.——And thus, after innumerable difficulties and dangers, was a happy period put to this undertaking, without the loſs of *Life* or *Limb*, to any one concerned in it; or accident, by which the work could be ſaid to be *materially* retarded.

C H A P. IV.

Comprehending an Account of OCCURRENCES, *ſubſequent to the bringing Home the* NEPTUNE BUSS *at the End of the Seaſon* 1759, *to the preſent Time.*

296. IT perhaps will not be thought the leaſt commendation to the ſtructure of the Edyſtone Lighthouſe, that this will not be one of the *longeſt* chapters in the whole work. In reality, very few occurrences have happened regarding it in the whole of this interval; and I truſt it will be thought the very beſt part of the account, that in the courſe of *thirty* years, that have elapſed ſince the commencement of this chapter, it ſtill remains in the ſame good condition, in which it then was: however, it may be proper, herein to take notice of ſeveral matters, that did not naturally fall into the courſe of the preceding narrative.

The very evening after we got in with the buſs, it began to be very bad weather from the S. W. and which continued till Monday the 15th; ſo that had we not got clear of the houſe, and unmoored when we did, in all likelihood we muſt have ſtaid there till then.

As

As Monday 15th proved more moderate, preparations were made, and every thing got ready to go out the next morning, in order to be prefent at the lighting of the houfe; but that morning it again began to blow at S. W. to a degree which rendered the attempt needlefs; and the night appointed for the lighting was ftormy; which weather continued till Thurfday the 18th, when preparations were again made to go out, and all ftores were got on board.

297. FRIDAY October 19th. This morning appearing promifing, though little wind, I went on board with Mr. JESSOP, ROGER CORNTHWAITE the mafon, (whofe particular activity in this building, I have had reafon to notice and commend) JOHN WATT, painter and glazier, and JOHN HATHERLEY. This laft I had agreed with to go out as light-keeper, upon the old eftablifhment, inftead of JOHN MICHELL, tinner, who only entered till one could be got. We went out in the Wefton, being accompanied by the Edyftone boat, as being the fmalleft and the lighteft; and therefore the moft eafily managed in the Gut. ——We had all our feamen, and alfo one of the yawls attending. About noon, having had but little wind, we got to the tranfport buoy; which we had not unmoored, intending to leave it to ride as long as it could, as it might be of fervice in the attendance upon the houfe during the fucceeding winter.——As it was then about half flood; that is, about the turn of the tide toward the eaft, we did not think it prudent to attempt to lay either of the boats alongfide the rocks, but landed in the yawl, and had the fatisfaction to find *all well*.——HENRY EDWARDS gave account that they lighted the houfe, as they were directed, early on Tuefday evening the 16th, and had continued the fame the two following evenings; and that they found the lights to burn very fteadily, notwithftanding it blowed very hard, efpecially on the night of lighting.——That they had the greateft feas on Friday, Saturday, and Sunday, preceding the lighting; and that then the waves broke up fo high, that had they not been thrown off by the *cove courfe*, they would have endangered the breaking the glafs of the lantern: but that, notwithftanding the broken fea went in great quantities over the ball, yet no water came into the lantern by the funnel, the air-pipes, or otherwife; except that a very fmall leakage came in, by an upright joint in the ftone-work of the lantern, which they fhewed us, and which we eafily remedied.——They informed us, that the feas had broke up, during almoft the whole time of our abfence, fo high upon the houfe, that they were not only obliged to keep the *ports* of the windows fhut to windward, but alfo to keep the joints well ftuffed with *oakum*; for otherwife, the great preffure of the water made its way through the joints thereof, even of the *uppermoft* chamber. That however, upon the whole, they had been both warm and dry. They further informed us, that when the feas broke up the higheft, they had experienced a fenfible motion, fomething like what we had all obferved from the hole in the rock, in hard gales of wind at E.; but that being but juft fenfible thereof, it occafioned to them neither fear nor furprize.

This afternoon we landed a further fupply of coals, water, and fmall ftores, by means of the yawl, which completed the intended winter's provifion for fix months*.——On this occafion I fhall take the opportunity to obferve, as intimated § 58. the wages of the light-keepers had, for many years paft, been eftablifhed at £. 25 per annum, finding their own provifions of *eating* and *drinking*.——I found it a matter of complaint through the country, on my firft going down to Plymouth, that the light-keepers had at various times been reduced to the neceffity of *eating the Candles*; and therefore, it feemed very much to be wifhed, on lighting the new houfe, that fome fcheme might be hit upon, whereby the neceffity of fuch fhocking viands might be avoided; and the remedy, with the greateft part of the obfervers, feemed mighty eafy; "Let them have greater wages, whereby they may be enabled to buy a better ftock of provifions:" or, "Let the proprietors furnifh them with victuals."——On confidering this matter over and over, it did not

* Account of Stores laid into the Edyftone Lighthoufe, in October, 1759, by the Proprietors, as a *Winter's Stock*.

Coals, [illegible]	64 bufhels.	Large candles	10 chefts.
Water, [illegible]	Nº 16	Small ditto	1 ditto.
[illegible]	Nº 2	Bifcuit	3 cwt.
Salt beef	2 cwt.	Boiling peafe	2 bufhels.
—— pork	1 ditto.	Oatmeal	2 ditto.

N. B. The above is according to Winchefter meafure, but the cuftom of dry meafure at Plymouth, is denominated according to [illegible] *Winchefter*.

not appear that either of theſe expedients would anſwer the end. *£.* 25 *per annum* ſeemed to many a very bare ſubſiſtence; but yet, being near upon 10*s.* a week, it was conſiderably more than the country price of labourer's wages, as I found it. A labourer on ſhore has houſe rent to pay, houſhold goods to provide, and maintain, as alſo fire and candle. In *this* ſituation, he is at no expence, but merely meat and drink, and a few cloaths; of which he is not in need of many changes: it is plain, therefore, that it was not want of ſufficient wages that cauſed the complaint, but want of ſufficient foreſight. I have given many inſtances, in my narrative of the progreſs of the building, that the high wages we were *obliged* to give, to induce *ſtout* labourers to face the perils of the ſervice, did not engage them to ſecure themſelves with a ſufficient ſtock of proviſions. Even for thoſe ſhort intervals they were likely occaſionally to ſtay, their ſea ſtock was ſo ſlender that they were repeatedly obliged to come home, *after ſharing their laſt pound of bread.*——Nor did it appear that things would go better if the *Proprietors* were to provide ſuſtenance for the light-keepers: for, on enquiry of the moſt elderly people, I underſtood, that formerly, as ſeems intimated by Winstanley, the houſe was provided by the proprietors*. By degrees the light-keepers got into the practice of embezzling the ſtores, and bartering them for ſtrong liquors, then alledging that they grew bad, and that they were obliged to throw them into the ſea; ſo that the eating of the candles was an early complaint; and which at that time ſeemed likely to be obviated by allowing them wages to victual themſelves, as had ever ſince continued.——The moſt likely expedient therefore that occurred to me, was, for the proprietors to put into the houſe a ſtock of *Sea Proviſions* ſufficient to laſt three men for ſix months; which ſtock of proviſions being the property of the proprietors, the light-keepers were to provide for themſelves as *they liked*; the boat being to attend them as before: this ſtock of proviſions being only lodged there, by way of ſecuring them from ſtarving.——Of this they might take what they had occaſion for, being accountable only for what was wanting, at the ſeaſon when the ſtock ſhould be overhauled. In this way there could be no *want*, or foundation of complaint of *badneſs* of the proviſion; nor yet any *embezzlement* of the ſtore: and provided it was laid in of the beſt kind, and the men only charged with what was conſumed, at the *wholeſale* price, it would come to them ſo much cheaper than any victuals they could provide, that it would be greatly their intereſt to uſe it; as it would enable them to live conſiderably cheaper in reſpect to ſuſtenance, than they could poſſibly do on ſhore. In effect, none would remain unconſumed, or be any loſs to the proprietors, unleſs ſome of it ſhould turn out *really* bad; which would be a trifle to them, as it would ſeldom happen.——This being propoſed to the proprietors was readily agreed to; and in this view the ſtock of proviſions, already ſpecified in the note to this ſection, was laid into the houſe; and was found fully to anſwer: and, the light-keepers being at liberty to get a joint of *freſh Mutton*, or piece of *Beef*, or a caſk of *Ale*, whenever opportunity admitted, and they *choſe*, all diſſatisfaction about the proviſions was totally prevented.——In this way matters went on for ſeveral years, till at length, by the aſſiduity of John Bowden, they found themſelves ſo frequently enabled to get *freſh Proviſions*, and the light-keepers *ſeldom charging*, that they chiefly depended thereon; laying in themſelves a ſmall ſea ſtock of ſalt proviſions, to be uſed on emergencies; inſomuch that the agent became no longer troubled in providing for them.

298. IN this viſit of the light-houſe we began to give the outſide faces of the upright pillars of the lantern a coat of paint, of a *lead colour*, the ſame as the *Cupola*, and *Balcony* rails, had originally been done.——Theſe uprights being before painted white, the ſame as the ſaſh frames; I had obſerved, on firſt ſeeing them at a diſtance, on our paſſage home on the 9th inſtant, they produced an unpleaſing effect: for theſe pillars inſtead of appearing *more* conſpicuous, by reaſon of their *white* colour, in reality appeared *not at all*: for, being of the colour of the ſky, not forming a ſufficient contraſt with the light ſeen through the glaſs, the *Cupola* appeared *unſupported*; like an *Umbrella* at a diſtance.——This circumſtance I find particularly noted in my Journal; to the intent, that any one hereafter, who ſhould in like manner think to improve the colouring of the lantern, might not fall into the ſame error that I had done.——We had however ſcarcely finiſhed one of the faces before a ſtorm of hail came on at N. W. which prevented our proceeding; and alſo cut off all communication with the veſſels. Upon this we began to give the inſide

* "But by good providence, then two boats came with *proviſions*, and the *family* that was to take care of the light; and ſo ended this "year's work." § 20.

inside of the cupola another coat of paint, as this could not well be repeated next season, on account of the coat of soot, that long before that time it would acquire; and perhaps prevent an adhesion with the former coat. This evening our two *hands* worked therein for three hours after the candles were lighted, yet so perfect was the ventilation, that though their work was principally in the roof above the candles; they did not experience the least inconvenience from smoke.——This afternoon the floating-light vessel sailed from her moorings, and coming near the rock, gave us *three Cheers*, which we very heartily returned. ——This evening Mr. Jessop and myself exercised all the light-keepers in their turns to trim and snuff the candles, and render them perfect therein: for, however easy and trifling such a business may seem, there are circumstances, which neglected, the effect of the light would be greatly impaired *.——This night I took up my lodging in one of the cabin beds, and found as I had done before, that when all was shut in, and otherwise quiet, the noise of the sea breaking upon the rocks made it seem as if there was a violent storm: and being now more still than before I had used to be, from having fewer workmen; I had persuaded myself before morning, that it really was so. I was therefore surprized, on getting up, to find that the sea was more quiet than it had been the preceding evening.

Saturday October 20th. This morning being fine and dry, we finished the outside painting; and also fixed an iron hand-rail to render the passage more safe and easy from the steps cut in the rock to the foot of the ladder, see Plate N° 8: and *lastly*, our mason ended those rough steps.——As every thing was now done, that a further time would have induced me to do; the laying on a coat of *Amber Varnish* over the whole painted work, excepted; which the season would not admit of, on account of the coats of paint not being sufficiently hardened; and as the general care and superintendance of the building was to be committed to Mr. Jessop, I had no difficulty in leaving this matter to him to be done the next spring. Having therefore read over and explained the *Instructions* I had received from the proprietors, for the light-keepers, fairly ingrossed; and hung the same up in a frame for their guidance; and also given every instruction I could think of, and every exhortation that I could devise, to a diligent discharge of their duty, I took my leave of the building and of the light-keepers; who were Henry Edwards, Henry Carter, and John Hatherley.

299. AT noon we went on board the boats and sailed; but the wind being northerly, and not so fresh as we could have wished it, we were full twelve hours turning to windward upon our passage; so that it was Sunday morning, October 21, before we arrived at Plymouth.——During this passage the air was remarkable clear: and we were about seven or eight miles distant from the house at the first lighting this evening. The light at first appeared very strong and bright to the naked eye, much like a star of the first magnitude. Its lustre diminished as we increased our distance, till it came down to a star of about the third magnitude; after this it ceased to diminish, and on the contrary seemed to *increase*; this I could not but wonder at: however, at length it became a matter quite out of doubt, as to the fact, it being obvious to the whole company. We saw it in this manner till we were passed the anchoring place of the men of war in the Sound, that is, near the island of *St. Nicholas*, where having ceased looking at it for a small space of time, on renewing our look out, it had now totally disappeared.——Though this was a *Phenomenon* I did not expect, yet I had casually made an observation, some time before this was apparent, that led me to a ready explication of it. I observed, that while the light was diminishing with the distance, and yet had a *sensible* elevation above the horizon, a kind of luminous appearance was seen upon the surface of the sea, directly under the star-like appearance of the light; and though the surface of the water was very far from that of a plain *Mirror*, yet, as the top of every wave would appear to be tipped with light, in that very oblique direction, they would all become nearly united in the observer's eye. Now when the *elevation* of the object becomes too small to be discerned, as separated from the luminous reflection, this will become united with the direct light, so that they will appear *at one*; and in consequence increase, till their union becomes perfect; but in going a little further on, till the main light is intercepted by the sea; that is, till it is in reality sunk below the apparent horizon, then both the direct and reflected light will be intercepted, and vanish together.

* This would be the case, if they should neglect to put the *Chandeliers* to their due height; by the interposition of the horizontal bars.

300. DURING

300. DURING my stay at Plymouth, which was not above a fortnight longer, (that is, till the accounts of different tradesmen were settled) I generally visited the *Hoa* every clear evening, being curious to observe what appearance the light made from thence. It was a fact universally agreed in, that the light in the old Lighthouse had *never* been discerned from thence: whatever appearance therefore it now made, was at least so much gained by the different fabric of the lantern; the candles themselves, their disposition, and number being the same as before*. I found it required the air to be clear to see it at all, and then it appeared like a star of the fourth magnitude; but when the air was very clear, it appeared as a star of the third magnitude, and doubtless could have been seen several miles further: and, as it has been shewn, that under favourable circumstances of the *Luminous reflection*, the light may be seen at sea much stronger, it is probable also at a greater distance, than it can from a *great* elevation at land.

301. IN the times of stormy weather, that happened during this interval at Plymouth, I took several opportunities of viewing the Lighthouse with my telescope † from the *Hoa*, and also from the *Garrison*, both of which places are sufficiently elevated to see the base of the building and the whole of the rock at low water in clear weather: and though I had had many occasions of viewing the unfinished building, when buried in the waves, in a storm at S. W.; yet never having before had a view of it under this circumstance, in its finished state, *I* was astonished to find that the account given by Mr. WINSTANLEY did not appear to be at all exaggerated. (See § 19.)——At intervals of a minute, and sometimes two or three; I suppose when a combination happens to produce one overgrown wave ‡, it would strike the rock and the building conjointly, and fly up in a white column, enwrapping it like a *sheet*, rising at least to double the height of the house, and totally intercepting it from the sight; and this appearance being momentary, both as to its rising and falling, one was enabled to judge of the comparative height very nearly, by the comparative spaces alternately occupied by the house, and by the column of water, in the *field* of the telescope. ——Of this column, I made an eye-sketch at the time: and must further observe, that while I was in the Lighthouse, during the last interval of finishing, in which time we had more than one hard gale that obliged us to shut the windward ports of the uppermost rooms; I particularly noticed the manner in which the waves begun to *gather*, as soon as they came so near the house as to be sensible of the sloping rocks underneath them, (see § 6.) Those waves by degrees towering higher as they came nearer, formed a deep hollow sea at the foot of the building; and then falling into it, struck it with all imaginable fury. Combining this appearance with what I saw on shore, I have endeavoured to give the reader some sort of idea thereof by the figure in the *Frontispiece*.——All representative drawings, however, though from an accomplished pencil, must be inadequate to this subject. The exhibition being *momentary*, and the building for that moment *entirely hid*; the relation betwixt the column and the building, the principal thing desired, could not have been expressed if so represented; and thinning away the column on one side, as here done, so as to let the building appear, takes off from the magnitude of the column; and in a *drawing*, its appearance being *permanent*, it so nearly coincides with that of a *Jet d'eau*, that it will necessarily suggest this idea, better than what it is intended to represent: I must therefore refer such of my readers, as may happen to have the opportunity, to satisfy themselves, by taking a view of it from the *Garrison* or *Hoa* with a good *Telescope*, as soon after a storm at S. W. as the air comes tolerably clear, but not later than the day following §.

* *Viz.* 24 candles at once, whereof 5 made 2lb.; and they were snuffed every half hour. See Note to § 60.——I take this opportunity of mentioning, that the *Lamp Oil* specified in note * to § 297, was an article never provided before. As it will keep good much longer than candles, it was intended to remedy the possibility of the want thereof. There were therefore twenty-four *Lamps* made to go into the *Chandeliers*, in place of the *Candlesticks*: but as the burning of the lamps was found to produce a greater *Soot* upon the inside of the glasses, than candles, though no apparent smoke attended either, the lamps were never used but in cases of a necessity.

† This glass was originally fitted up for me in 1756, by Mr. JOHN DOLLOND, in his best manner at that time, with a common double convex object glass; but when I came to town the latter end of the year 1757, he fitted it with an *Achromatic* object glass.

‡ This is what I suppose the vulgar attribute to the TENTH WAVE.

§ This momentary *Spout* of the Edystone may perhaps be best compared with the momentary *jet of boiling water*, said to be 19 feet diameter in the orifice, and at times to rise 92 feet high, thrown from the Fountain *Geyser* in *Iceland*; described in VON TROIL's Letters, English Edition, page 259—261. To this account, however, I own I could have given but little credit, had it not been confirmed to me by my honoured friends Sir JOSEPH BANKS, the late Dr. SOLANDER, and Dr. LIND, who were eye-witnesses of it.

Occurrences

Occurrences after leaving Plymouth.

302. THE year 1759 concluded with a series of very stormy weather; and it was not till the month of January succeeding, that there was any prospect of the boat's going off. I have a letter from Mr. JESSOP, dated Plymouth 13th January, 1760; in which he mentions, that upon the 8th instant the Edystone boat went off, wind at E. and moderate, but a great swell. They got thither at four o'clock in the afternoon, but could not land. However, going to the west side of the house, they conveyed some *small* stores into it by means of the *keg* (see § 291); and by it received a letter from HENRY EDWARDS, directed to Mr. JESSOP. The purport of it was to acquaint him, that they had had such very bad weather, that the sea frequently ran over the house, so that for twelve days together they could not open the door of the lantern, or any other.——He says " the house did shake as if a man had been up in a great tree. The *old* " *men* were almost frighted out of their lives, wishing they had never seen the place, and cursing those that " first persuaded them to go there. The fear seized them in the back, but rubbing them with oil of tur- " pentine gave them relief." He further mentioned, that upon the 5th December at night they had a very great storm; the wind being at E. so that the ladder which was lashed below the entry-door broke loose, and was washed away. Also upon the 13th there was so violent a storm of wind, that he thought the house would overset: and at midnight the sea broke one pane of glass on the S. E. side of the lantern*. That they had had a very melancholy time of it; having had besides, a great deal of thunder and lightning.

Mr. JESSOP further informed me, that upon the 10th the boat went out again; but the wind at east blowed too fresh for her to be gotten into the Gut; that with some difficulty they landed some fresh provisions by means of the small boat; the candles, water, and beer, they could not land; but as there were several chests of candles, of the original store, remaining, and a sufficient quantity of water, there could be no real want for some time.——Mr. JESSOP, however, did not give entire credit to what EDWARDS had related in regard to the house having so great a motion; as SMART and BOWDEN told him, that they could not see that the mortar in the joints had *started*.

303. A LETTER from Mr. JESSOP of the 13th February following, relates that upon the 8th the Edystone boat went off to the house, and landed four chests of candles, and an half hogshead of beer. That J. BOWDEN told him he went all over the house, to see if it had received any damage by the storms, but found nothing amiss; the pane of glass mentioned by EDWARDS excepted. In short, he found all in order, the house clean, and the people well. The south pile was gone, but the north one remained firm. (See Plate N° 14.)

304. SOON after this a *violent* storm happened at S. W. I was informed that *Admiral* BOSCAWEN had mentioned to the *Admiralty*, that it was the greatest storm that had been known, by the oldest person on board his ship. I therefore expected a still more formidable account from Mr. JESSOP of its effects upon the Lighthouse. But no account being received in course of the post, I wrote to him the 21st of that month, desiring that, as soon as possible, enquiry might be made into the state of the house; as likewise whether it has more motion, with the wind at E. or at S. W.; and whether they were sensible of the sea's striking the cornice.——To this I received an answer, March 2d, that SMART and BOWDEN had been off the 29th of February, to land stores; that they stayed at the house two hours, and viewed it all over carefully, inside and out; but could not discover any of the mortar started, nor the joints anyways cracked: and that all the damage sustained by the *last* storm was, that the *electrical* strap, which went from the sink-pipe down to the rock, was washed away (see § 292.) The glass of the lantern was all found; the pane excepted that was before mentioned. HENRY EDWARDS said the sea went all over the house, which caused a motion much the same as when the wind was at E. and he could perceive no

* A number of boards cut to the size, had been provided; which might be put in from the *inside* in case of such accident, till a proper repair with glass could be made: as had been usual in former times.

difference

difference when it ſtruck the cornice, or otherwiſe. The light-keepers, it ſeems, had now pretty well got rid of their fears; as they were all well, and made no complaint.

305. EVERY thing now appearing to go on ſucceſsfully and in courſe, I heard nothing more concerning the Lighthouſe till the 8th June, 1761, of which date I received a letter in *Yorkſhire* from Mr. WESTON. In this interval my faithful aſſiſtant Mr. JESSOP had departed this life, leaving an unblemiſhed character behind him; and Mr. RICHARDSON had been appointed *Surveyor* of the Lighthouſe in his ſtead. Mr. WESTON deſired to be adviſed, concerning the renewal of the painting, and alſo reſpecting the reſtoration of the *Electrical* ſtrap; both of which remained undone. ——In anſwer, I recommended that the painting ſhould be done by a proper painter; and not by the light-keepers, as he had ſuggeſted: and that the original colours ſhould be preſerved.——That with regard to the *Conductor* for the *Lightning*; as in our hurry in finiſhing, we had not had time to form a *groove* in the wall, wherein to bury the leaden ſtrap, as originally intended; we contented ourſelves with *two* faſtenings at every courſe, as mentioned § 292; the want of which groove, had doubtleſs been the occaſion of its being waſhed away from the wall. However, to render it now ſtill more effectual, I recommended a ſmall round bar of copper, or braſs, of about half an inch diameter, to be formed; and to bury it in a groove made by the point of a pick, fixing it with ſmall copper ſtaples at every courſe, to the plugs that had been uſed for fixing the lead. This bar to be bedded in putty, and covered with the ſame, ſo as to make all fair and fluſh.

306. THE ſtorms which the building had now ſuſtained, without material damage, convinced us, and every one, of the ſtability of the *Stone-Lighthouſe*; except thoſe (who were not a few) that had taken the notion, that nothing but WOOD could reſiſt the ſea upon the Edyſtone Rocks; who ſaid, that though they allowed it was built *very ſtrong*, yet if ſuch a ſtorm as had deſtroyed WINSTANLEY'S *Lighthouſe*, was again to happen, they doubted not but it *muſt* ſhare the ſame fate.

The year 1762 was uſhered in with ſtormy weather, and indeed produced a TEMPEST of the firſt magnitude, the rage of which was ſo great, that one of thoſe who had been uſed to *predict* its downfal, was heard to ſay; *if the Edyſtone Lighthouſe is now ſtanding, it will ſtand till the* DAY OF JUDGMENT: and in reality, from this time, its exiſtence has been ſo entirely laid out of men's minds; that, whatever ſtorms have happened ſince, no enquiry has ever been made concerning it *.

Mr. RICHARDSON, though a very ſound hardy maſon, was not a man converſant in literary deſcriptions. The pen was therefore, on this occaſion, taken up by my very valuable and ingenious friend Dr. JOHN MUDGE; who gave me two letters upon the ſubject of this ſtorm; and which, coming warm from the heart, ſo much exceed any thing I can compoſe, that I cannot do ſo well as to inſert them.

" DEAR SIR, *Plymouth*, Friday 15th January, 1762.

" Accept my moſt ſincere congratulations on the ſafety of the *Edyſtone*; as well from the danger that has threatened it, as that I think the dreadful ſtorm it has withſtood, will for ever remove any anxiety about its being injured in future, by the united force of the wind and ſea.——It blew very hard the beginning of laſt Monday night, but increaſed with incredible fury towards Tueſday morning; when about ſix, partly from the long ſoutherly winds, but principally by its concurring with the ſpring-tides, it afforded the moſt horrible ſcene of devaſtation. This tide roſe full two feet higher, than when the *Victory* was loſt, and when the *Fiſh-houſe*† was carried away; or than was ever known in the memory of the oldeſt man living. The ſeas came in bodily over the *Barbican* wall, but one wave with ſuch irreſiſtible violence, that it ſwept away the parapet, below its foundation; and in its return carried off five people then upon it, all of whom

* Witneſs the ſtorm in which the *Halſewell Indiaman* was loſt!——And though the public papers were full of the immenſe damages done by it at *Plymouth*, and in the *Sounds* (in particular a ſhip in the harbour that broke looſe, and beat down a [illegible], will be very well remembered) yet not a ſingle word was ſaid about the *Edyſtone Lighthouſe*.

† The *fiſh-houſe* was a building ranging acroſs the mouth of *Sutton Pool*, which may be called the *interior harbour* of Plymouth. Betwixt the weſt end of the *fiſh-houſe*, and the moſt projecting eaſtern end of the Jetty, or ſhort pier, called the *Barbican*, an opening was left of about 65 feet wide; by which the ſhips entered.

were drowned. The new *Lammy Pier* was swept clean away *. Prodigious losses have been sustained by the shopkeepers on the quays; as in some of their shops near the *Barbican*, the water was as high as their *counters*; and the quays themselves are in so ruinous a condition, and so much of them carried away, that had the gale continued till the next tide, it is highly probable some of them would have been wholly swept away, and the houses with them.

"In the midst of this confusion there was no less than six large merchant ships wrecked in the very harbour, some of which were beat to pieces, but all lost; and this in the short space of 300 yards, betwixt *Teatshill* and *Frankfort*.——There were nine men of war in the Sound; several of which were constantly firing signals of distress. Some cut away one, others two, another three; and one lost all her masts and her bowsprit. Three of them only escaped with all their masts standing; one of which, to avoid immediate destruction on the south side of *Mount Batten*, was by the great dexterity of the pilot brought in within the *Fisher's Nose*, and ran ashore under the *Lammy*: but this was when the ebb had made considerably; so that she was safely got off the next tide. But it exhibited a very uncommon appearance; as I believe it was the first time that ever a man of war was seen in that place.——In the *Hamoaze* the men of war were all this while firing signals of distress; and some of them ran foul of each other. The sea came over the dock gates, into the dock where the *Magnanime* was; but as there did not come in enough to float her, it did no considerable damage. The new dock was likewise filled.——I will only mention one circumstance more, to give you some idea of the extreme agitation of the sea: the *Froth* of it flew clean over the walls of the *Garrison*; and in such quantities, that in one situation a centinel was obliged to quit his post.

"In the midst of all this horror and confusion, my friend may be assured, that I was not insensible to his honour and credit; yet, in spite of the high opinion and confidence I had of his judgment and abilities, I could not but feel the utmost anxiety for the *fate* of the Edystone: and I believe poor RICHARDSON was not a little uneasy.——Several times in the day, I *swept* with my telescope from the Garrison, as near as I could imagine the line of the horizon; but it was so extremely black, fretful, and hazy, that nothing could be seen; and I was obliged to go to bed that night, with a mortifying uncertainty. But the next morning early I had great joy to see, that the *Gilded Ball* had triumphed over the fury of the storm; and such a one as before I had not a conception of.——I saw the whole so distinctly from the bottom to the top, that I could be very sure the lantern has suffered nothing.——It is now my most steady belief, as well as every body's here, that its inhabitants are rather more secure in a storm, under the united force of wind and water, than we are in our houses from the former only."

307. I RECEIVED the above letter in *Yorkshire*, where we had had very stormy weather; the account of my friend was therefore equally agreeable and astonishing: yet, notwithstanding his letter announced the general safety of the building; and that nothing very bad could have happened, even to the lantern, I could not conceive, that his expression *the lantern had suffered nothing*, could be strictly and literally true; I therefore wrote in return, desiring he would send me a circumstantial account of the damages, after the house had been *visited*. The following is an extract of his second letter, dated *Plymouth* the 24th January, 1762.

"The boat went off, with an intention to land, on Friday sennight; but there was so great a sea, and the wind being too much to the south, they desisted till the next day; when the wind being a point to north of the west, and better weather, they got near the house, landed their things, and had a long conversation with the people.

"[illegible] tell me, that the ladder was carried away †; and some small matter of putty, which was cracked by the l[illegible]st summer's heat, was washed off from the lantern. This was all that the violence of the

* A[illegible] of small vessels laying against the *Victualling Office*, which is built upon the ground called the *La*[illegible] *Fisher's Nose*; a prominent point of rock so named.

† T[illegible] from the top of the rock to the entry-door, was at first a common ladder, like that of a *Lamp*[illegible] at the same time it was firmly lashed to Iron *Eye-bolts*, drove into the [illegible] before-mentioned instances, appearing not sufficient to resist the storms, I have since ordered it to be [illegible] so that when it is not in use, it may be drawn into the entry, and laid in the passage.

sea

ſea had effected; that there was not ſo much as a ſingle pane of glaſs broke. That the lantern was ſecured by (that perfection of ornament) the *Cornice*; which, when the ſea roſe to the top of the houſe, blanched it off like a *ſheet*. They inſiſted on it, that the ſea went *bodily* over the top, for, that it came in through the vents of the ball, and filled the ſockets of the candleſticks*. They were aſked whether they had been under any uneaſineſs; they ſaid, not in the leaſt, as the houſe had not been affected by it in any other way than they had before experienced.——The ſtorm in the evening of Monday begun at the ſouth-eaſt, and then they felt very ſenſibly a tremor from every ſtroke of the ſea; ſo that while it continued there to act upon the natural cavern in the rock †, it gave them ſome uneaſineſs; which though they now believed unneceſſary, yet they could not help wiſhing it was filled up.——Now, though I look upon this as a proof, that no ſtorm will ever affect the houſe, as it is a plain ſmooth ſurface; and though a leſs ſea has a greater influence on the rock at low water, than a mighty one has upon the houſe itſelf; yet I muſt ſay, that I concur with them in wiſhing it was done; and that for two reaſons: One is, I ſhould be glad to ſee every, the leaſt appearance, of defect, removed; and the other, that I ſhould hope it would give me a chance of ſeeing my dear friend once more, here. In earneſt, I wiſh you'd complete the rock too, as well as the houſe; for ſo many vibratory ſtrokes, can do it no ſervice.

" You ſeem to have been greatly affected by the little I have ſaid of the horror of this Storm; but believe me, it cannot give you even a tolerable idea of it. It has, upon a moderate computation, done above £. 80,000 worth of damage in the Harbour and Sound: and I cannot help repeating again, that I am very ſure you may for ever rid yourſelf of an uneaſy thought of the houſe, as to its danger from *wind* and ſea."

" P. S. I broke open this letter to mention a whimſical circumſtance, that comes in my head: One of the articles (beſides ſugar, ſome flour, &c. which they landed at the houſe) was a *Gallipot of putty*, to repair, as I ſaid, the *only derangement* the houſe had ſuffered."

308. IN the year 1766, having a call to *St. Ives* in *Cornwall*, I gladly ſeized the opportunity of viſiting my friends at Plymouth, and the Lighthouſe: on this occaſion, I was commiſſioned by the *Gentlemen Proprietors* of the *Edyſtone*, to inſpect that building, and report my obſervations; which were as follows.

Extract of the REPORT *of* JOHN SMEATON, Engineer; *concerning the State and Condition of the* Edyſtone Lighthouſe, *from a View thereof, taken the 10th Auguſt*, 1766.

HAVING carefully inſpected this Edifice, I had the ſatisfaction to find, that no one part had in the leaſt degree given way to the rage and violence of the ſea; but that the maſs of building was found and firm as at firſt: nevertheleſs there appeared ſome matters, that I thought worthy of regard: which are in order as follows.

The cement every where below high-water mark; and from three to ſix feet above it, was perfectly entire, as left by the *Trowel*, and ſeems changed to the colour and conſiſtence of *Iron-Stone*.——From thence to ten or twelve feet above high-water mark, the cement appears here and there to be ſomewhat impoveriſhed in the joints, or fretted; and I obſerved that this was more ſo on the *Eaſt* ſide than on the *Weſt*: above the parts laſt deſcribed, the cement appears perfectly fluſh in the joints, quite to the top, as left by the trowel, being no ways altered in colour or conſiſtence.

From the above appearances it ſeems to me, that thoſe parts of the building that are generally wetted every tide, are in the higheſt degree of preſervation; thoſe that are wetted ſeldom, are nearly the ſame; but thoſe that are frequently wetted, but not always, have ſuffered moſt by the alternate action of the ſun, wind, and of the ſea ſalts: was this to go on ſeveral years longer, nothing is likely to happen that would materially affect the ſtrength of the building; yet in a ſtructure of ſo much conſequence, and which can ſo eaſily be reſtored to its primitive ſtate, it would ſeem negligence to let it remain unrepaired.

The *electrical* conductor is compleat down to the rock, as to uſe; but of the chain that hangs from the top of the rock into the water, about half of the lower part is gone; by its wearing away with ruſt, and

* This might poſſibly happen by the falling of a detached maſs of water into the *Vents* made for the clearance of the ſmoke.

† See Plates N° 6, 8, and 14.

beating

beating againſt the rocks. I have ordered a new one to be made of ſtronger iron. From the rock, for about twelve or fourteen feet upwards, the communication is by *Braſs* bars let into the houſe ſide, in a little groove or gutter, in which they lie buried in putty *; and which ſeem to ſtand very well; the reſt of the outſide communication is by the original ſtrap of lead, that I fixed there †; but as about half a yard of the lower part of the lead is getting looſe, I ordered Mr. RICHARDSON to let in another length of braſs bar, like the former; and ſo on, as the lead fails.

The balcony rails have as yet ſuffered very little, conſidering their expoſure: but as flakes of ruſt ſeem gathering under the paint, I ordered it to be knocked off with proper tools before a freſh coat of paint is laid on.

The whole of the lantern is in remarkable preſervation, ſcarcely a ſpeck of ruſt appearing on the outſide, and only a few ſpecks within; which are chiefly upon the ribs, and knee pieces under the cupola; theſe ſpecks I ordered to be firſt ſcraped off, and then freſh paint laid on.

I was much ſurprized to ſee the gilding of the ball, which, notwithſtanding its expoſure, and the ſmoke of the whole houſe going through it, appears as bright as it did the firſt day it was ſcrewed on. The lantern has always continued remarkably water-tight, not the leaſt wet ever beating through any part of it; except in high ſtorms; and what gets in between the glaſs and the copper frames, by the drying and cracking of the putty; but this ſo ſeldom and ſo little, as ſeems not worth regard.

The loops and crooks of the doors and window ports have ſuffered moſt of all by the ruſt; and particularly thoſe parts of the iron that are on the *inſide*; but as all *theſe* things are renewable at pleaſure, they are not to be eſteemed of any conſequence; eſpecially as they ſeem likely to laſt many years.

The *Cavern* in the rock on the eaſt ſide, ſeems exactly in the ſame ſtate I left it. In hard gales of wind at eaſt, it is ſaid to cauſe a wonderful noiſe; and a ſenſible tremor in the building: but though it makes more noiſe, the light-keepers ſay it does not affect the building, with ſo ſenſible a *vibration*, as the heavy ſeas from the S. W.; and yet even thoſe are not much more than to be readily perceivable in the greateſt ſtorms ‡. Whether this cavity in the rock may ever prove of any detriment to the building is not to be determined with certainty: all that can be ſaid, is, that hitherto it does not ſeem to have been of any hurt thereto. I could undertake to fill it up and make it ſolid, at the expence of about £. 250, beſides my own attendance, if it was thought worth the charge.

Beſides the pleaſure of finding all the main *Stamina* perfectly ſound and firm, and every thing elſe likely to endure for many years to come; I had the ſatiſfaction of finding every thing in the inſide ſo perfectly neat and clean, that it ſeemed as if it had not been a twelvemonth in uſe.

J. SMEATON.

Austhorpe, 30th Auguſt, 1766.

308. FROM this time nothing further occurred till the year 1777, when having a ſecond call into *Cornwall*, I again took the opportunity of viſiting *Plymouth*: and though I had no commiſſion to inſpect, &c. yet my own curioſity prompted me to viſit the Lighthouſe: and I had the great ſatisfaction to find that Mr. RICHARDSON had ſo well attended to my laſt inſtructions; and its condition was ſo nearly the ſame as in the year 1766, that very nearly the ſame report would have ſerved; every thing was neat and clean, and in good condition; no other change or repair having happened, except that of repeated paintings of the metalline parts, which appeared ſtill in high preſervation. This viſit to the Lighthouſe was in the month of September.

310. IN the year 1787, having a call to *Plymouth Dock*, I again took this opportunity of gratifying my curiosity by inspecting the Lighthouse; and also spent some days in getting the necessary *Trigonometrical* operations for determining the real distance of the *Edystone* from the *Ramhead*, from *Plymouth Sound*, and from *Plymouth Harbour*: and though I did not find them materially different from what I had put them down in the former part of this work, § 4. (which was then printed) as deduced from bearings, compared with the maps of the adjacent coasts, from whence Plate N° 2 was compiled: yet, observing some contrariety in the results, I was desirous of settling this matter from more authentic materials, than my opportunities would give me leave to collect while the Lighthouse was building and finishing. The particular result of these operations I shall give with the *technical* description of Plate N° 18.

311. MY visit to the house was the 3d August, 1787; and I then had the satisfaction to find both stone and iron so very nearly in the same state, as I had found and reported it twenty-one years ago, in the year 1766, that I was agreeably surprized: the only thing in which I could perceive a change, was, that the cement in the upper works was in most places sensibly corroded. I could not, however, estimate the quantity in general, at more than one sixth of an inch, that the present mortar surface wanted of *flush* with the face of the *Granite*. Had the whole building been of *Portland* stone, and supposed, in such a situation, to have lost of its *whole substance* an equal quantity: had the mortar wasted equally, the whole would have been a fair surface.——Of all the lower parts, including the whole work of the year 1757, being the first year's building, and which is generally wet every tide, there did not appear on this last visit to be the diminution of a grain of sand, but they appeared exactly as the same parts are reported to be in 1766: that is, the mortar having the appearance of *Iron Stone*; the *Limpet* shells, and sea weeds, fixing indiscriminately upon the mortar and the stone. But above that, as the eastward joints are more sensibly affected, and somewhat irregularly; to about the height of the entry-door, and after that are pretty uniformly in the degree I have already related; I am much inclined to suppose, that in raging storms the sand is raised from the bottom, and mixed with the water, and being driven violently against the building, may be capable of grinding, and making an impression upon what is compounded with calcareous matter, (however hard it may be, and in reality is) that it cannot make upon the *Moorstone*: which nothing seems to affect but a considerable degree of fire.——This is, however, not the case on the S. W. side; though that sustains the first stroke of the sea: for the *sea-weed* fixing itself the highest on that side, becomes a defence to the joints in this part.

Since my visit in 1777, the very *careful* and *diligent* Mr. RICHARDSON departed this life.——Mr. RICHARDSON, during life, remained sensible what patience and assiduity were necessary, during the course of the work of the first and second year, not only to repair the *pointing* when injured by a rough tide; but to *look to it* again and again till it had *stood* a *rough* tide: On the present visit I was disgusted with seeing the joints, in several places of the second year's work, made up with glazier's putty, which was an expedient of the light-keepers, when the masons mortar did not happen to stay on, after their departure. This, though it would often stay in the joint when the mortar would not; yet, being of *unctuous* matter, it hinders the union of the proper *cement* with the stone, and becomes a means of preventing those joints from being made compleat and flush in the way they were at first. It also disgraces the work with party-coloured mortar.

312. AS the *Iron Work* still endures with very little apparent injury, having had a coat of paint every two years; and this standing remarkably well, in spite of its exposure to the sea-salts, many persons have been curious to know the manner in which this part of the work was originally performed.——I then conceived the exposure of the *rails* in particular to be such, as to require every advantage that could be put in practice: and after considering the matter, I determined upon the following method; which, as it appears to have succeeded, I dare say my reader will like to know.——I had observed, that when iron once gets rust, so far as to form a *Scale*, whatever coat of paint or varnish is put over this, the rust will go on progressively under the paint, unless it is eradicated by being knocked off, and scraped.——The most effectual way therefore seemed, to endeavour to apply the *protective* coat, before any rust could be formed.

After the rails were made in eight compartments, and screwed together, I ordered that they should not come out of the smith's shop, till they were to undergo the following operation.——A fire was made,

made, though not very ſtrong, yet extenſive enough to heat the whole of a compartment together, tolerably equal, till the iron came to about, or rather above, a *blue* heat; this part was then removed and another applied; and while it was heating, a couple of men with bruſhes, *ſtruck* over the ſurface of the former with raw *Linſeed* oil. This at firſt would ſmoke, and nimbly run into every joint, crevice, and flaw in the iron; and the operation was continued, till every part had at leaſt been gone twice over; and the oil would begin to lie fluid on its ſurface. It was then ſet by to dry; and the reſt followed in the ſame manner. The next day, if properly done, the ſurface of the whole would appear to be covered with a thin coat of varniſh. The doing this to *purpoſe* is what the main matter conſiſts in*. As ſoon as it was well dried a couple of coats of common white lead and oil paint were given: after theſe were dry, the Rails came down by ſea to Plymouth, and from thence were carried out, and ſet up upon the Lighthouſe; and there, as I have related, they were finiſhed with a *couple* of coats more, in place.——Doubtleſs by theſe carriages, the coats laid on at *London*, were a good deal ſcratched, and in point of *appearance* ſpoilt, but in point of utility were little the worſe: becauſe, it was only the *prominent* parts that could be ſcratched and rubbed; and therefore the bruſh could not fail to make theſe good, in *preference*; and, as they would get two coats in *place*, they muſt be conſidered as ſufficiently covered; whereas, all the intricate, retreating parts, would have the whole *five* coats remaining entire upon them.

313. ON this viſit I found the luſtre of the ball was conſiderably diminiſhed. But as the *Gilding* was perhaps the only part of the whole work that was *merely Ornamental*; and as much coſt did not attend it, in its firſt application; as it has laſted thirty years in good ſplendor, and is not yet wholly effaced; it may be alledged, that it has ſufficiently anſwered every purpoſe there was in view at the time: and whenever it ſhall appear to be *neceſſary* to renew it, I doubt not but *ways* and *means* will be found.

In examining the ſkirt of the leaden cap, turned under the *drip* of the *Corona*, that I had carefully batted to the ſtone (ſee § 286): on the ſouth-weſt ſide I found it to hang down more than an inch. On enquiring whether the great ſtorms had any ſenſible effect upon it, I was told by the light-keepers, that in the ſtorm of January 1786, (remarkable for the loſs of the *Halſewell Indiaman*) the lead was conſiderably raiſed up, by the action of the ſea, on the ſouth and S.W. ſides; but that they had beat it down again, as well as they could. ——Of this I apprized my reſpected friend HENRY TOLCHER, Eſq. the *Agent*; and that it would be neceſſary to ſend off an intelligent workman, to *bat* the lead carefully to the ſtone under the drip, as at firſt; and that where it was become too broad, it might be cut narrower.——I conceived that the feet, and other bodies that are continually making impreſſions, and ſtriking ſmall blows upon the balcony floor, had in time ſtretched out the lead: and its own weight would alſo contribute to encreaſe the effect.

314. BEFORE I conclude this narrative I wiſh to meet an enquiry, that has very often been made with a degree of ſurprize: How is it poſſible to find men that will ſeclude themſelves from the *world*, and the *comforts* of life, for ſo ſmall a conſideration, as a ſalary of £.25 a year; when I found myſelf under the neceſſity of giving ſuch high wages to the *workmen* employed in erecting it? intimating, that it might rather be conſidered as the *alternative* for condemned *Felons*, than an appointment for which people would make *intereſt*.——The caſe is, the Lighthouſe is ſupplied with light-keepers from a different ſort of men to thoſe, the queſtion ſuppoſes †. A man while he is in his youth and ſtrength generally enters into the engagements of a family, and an induſtrious man ſo ſituated, no conſideration would hire to part with his *liberty*. But when he comes to be above the age of *Sixty*, and has ſtill his bread to earn by his own labour; an *eaſy birth*, in which he can get as much as he could do formerly, becomes a very eligible thing; eſpecially to thoſe who are not otherwiſe encumbered. To elderly *Seamen*, it may be conſidered as an *Aſylum* ſomething like equivalent to *Greenwich Hoſpital*.——Formerly there were ſeldom leſs than half a dozen appli-

* A perſon repeating this proceſs, if he finds the oil not to be dry like varniſh the next day, may conclude; either, that he has continued the *ſtriking* with oil too long, till the iron was too cold; or, that he had not heated it ſufficiently.

† I was applied to in the courſe of the *laſt* ſeaſon, by a *philoſopher* kind of man, to be one of the *light-keepers*; obſerving, that being a man of ſtudy [illegible] he could very well bear the confinement, that muſt attend it: I aſked him if he knew the ſalary: he replied, no, [illegible] very handſome. When I told him it was £.25 a year, he replied, he had quite miſtaken the buſineſs; he [illegible] *liberty* for ſo low a price; he could not have ſuppoſed it leſs than three times as much.

cants

cants upon the agent's liſt, ready to ſupply a vacancy; and as no one was under a neceſſity of ſtaying longer, than till, after giving notice of his intention to quit the ſervice, a freſh man was ſent out to fill his place, thoſe vacancies happened frequently. At preſent they happen ſo rarely, that very few think it worth while to apply. John Ireland, who is the *ſenior* of the preſent ſet, entered with me in the year 1756 as a *ſeaman*. When the building was finiſhed, John, being ſtout, hearty, and *willing to work*, ſhipped himſelf on board a trading veſſel, and continued for ſome time to uſe the ſea. However, a few years more of hardſhip, and *advance* in life, occaſioned him to change his mind; and, I believe, on Edwards quitting, he entered. I found him there in the year 1766; in the year 1777; and on my laſt viſit in 1787.—— The *ſecond* man I alſo found there in my viſit of 1777; and the preſent *third* man, who was at this time taking his *month* on ſhore, (ſee § 57) I was told had been a light-keeper *four* years; and had ſucceeded one who had been there *fourteen* years; and who neither being very old nor very infirm, probably would have been in the Lighthouſe at this time, had his death not been *premature*, which occaſioned the vacancy*. ——Theſe facts, more ſtrongly than any arguments, prove that this Lighthouſe as an *Habitation* (ſingularly ſituated, expoſed, and circumſtanced as it is; and where water was never known to freeze) is not only remarkably *healthy*; but really *comfortable* to a degree, that renders it *eligible* to a certain claſs of men; who do not conſider their abode there as any infringement upon their *liberty*, becauſe they well know it is in their own power to put a period to it, whenever they chuſe.

* As the death of this man exhibits a remarkable *trait* of *human nature*, on this account I inſert it. In the fourteen years that he had been here, he was grown ſo attached to the place, that for the two ſummers preceding he had given up his *turn* on ſhore to his companions, and declared his intentions of doing the ſame the third; but was *ever perſuaded* to go on ſhore, and take his *month's turn*. He had always in this ſervice proved himſelf a decent, *ſober*, well-behaved man: but he had no ſooner got on ſhore, than he went to an *Alehouſe*, and got intoxicated. This he continued the whole of his ſtay; which being noticed, he was carried in this intoxicated ſtate, on board the Edyſtone boat, and delivered in the Lighthouſe, where he was expected to grow ſober; but after lingering two or three days, he could by no means be recovered. The reflections ariſing, I leave to my reader.

---

315. THE following words, letters, and figures, were ſunk into the Moorſtone with the point of a pick.

Upon the firſt ſtone of the foundation - - - - - 1757.

Over the Entry-door - - - - - - 1758.

Round the upper Store-room, upon the courſe under the ceiling,

EXCEPT THE LORD BUILD THE HOUSE
THEY LABOUR IN VAIN THAT BUILD IT.
Psalm CXXVII.

Over the ſouth window, on the outſide of the dwelling room, or kitchen - 1759.

Upon the outward faces of the octagon baſement of the lantern,

⚜ • NE • *door* • SE • S • SW • W • NW.

Upon the laſt ſtone ſet, being that over the door of the lantern on the eaſt ſide,

24th Augt 1759.
Laus Deo.

GENERAL

GENERAL ABSTRACT *of the Progress of the Work of the* EDYSTONE LIGHTHOUSE.

DATE.		Time upon the Rock. Hours.	Days and Hours.		Number of Pieces of Stone.
1756. August 5.	Began to cut the Rock for receiving the foundation.				
November 22.	The principal parts thereof being completed; the *Neptune Buss* quitted the moorings; after which she was driven out to sea by a storm, to the westward of the *Land's End*. Returned to *Plymouth* the 26th.				
	In this year the time out upon the work was 110 days = 15 weeks 5 days: and upon the Rock — — — — —	348½	14	12½	
1757. June 12.	Landed the first stone.				
August 11.	Completed the first six foundation courses. — — —	342½	14	6½	123
October 1.	Finished three courses of the solid shaft, consisting of 53 principal pieces each; and one stone let into the Rock, to make good a *chasm* therein over the *Cavern*. — — — — —	288½	12	—½	160
	In this year the time out upon the work was 113 days = 16 weeks 1 day: and upon the Rock — — — —	631	26	6½	283
1758. July 2.	Landed the first principal piece of course X. being the first stone this season.				
August 8.	Completed the *Entire Solid* up to the Entry-door, inclusive of course XIV.	237	9	21	265
September 24.	Finished the solid to the Store Room floor, inclusive of course XXIV. —	416½	17	8½	383
October 7.	The last stone of this year's work was fixed; having completed the walls of the *Store Room*, consisting of 78 principal pieces; and set 14 pieces of the first *vaulted Floor*. — — — —	127½	5	7½	92
	After which, on the 8th, the *Neptune Buss* parted her cable in a storm, and was driven into *Torbay*; from whence she got into *Dartmouth Harbour*: and afterwards returned to *Plymouth*.				
	In this year the time out upon the work was 99 days = 14 weeks 1 day: and upon the Rock — — — —	781	32	13	740
1759. July 5.	Landed and began the work of this season.				
August 16.	Completed the *Balcony Floor*, and therewith the *Main Column* — —	502	20	22	398
—— 26.	The *Basement* of the Lantern, the stone Stairs in the *Well-hole*, and all the stone work completed. — — — —	119½	4	23½	72
October 9.	The *Lantern*, and the *whole* of the *Building*, with its equipments, completed: the workmen left the house, with three light-keepers and proper stores therein; with orders to light the house upon the 16th. Unmoored the *Neptune Buss*, and carried her into *Plymouth Harbour*. — —	292	12	4	
16.	This evening, according to the appointment of the *Corporation* of TRINITY HOUSE, the light upon the Edystone was *rekindled*.				
	In this year the time out upon the work was 99 days = 14 weeks 1 day: and upon the Rock — — — —	913½	38	1½	470
	Totals of the four years; out upon the work 421 days = 60 weeks 1 day: upon the Rock — — — —	2,674	111	10	1,493

Besides the larger Pieces of stone above specified, the *mass* of *Masonry* inclosed the following smaller parts; which the *regularity* of the construction enables to particularize.

- 75 Large cubic *Joggles* and *center-plug* stones.
- 162 Cubic *Joggles* of 6 inches, used in the *Well-hole* courses.
- 399 Flat *Joggles* in the courses of the rooms and lantern.
- 399 Joint stones in D° ——— ———.
- 1,300 Oaken *Trenails* of 1¼ inch diameter used in the solid.
- 4,570 *Pairs* of oak wedges for steadying the stones of the solid.
- 8 Large circular chains, two used at each vaulted floor.
- 221 Strong iron cramps, used in the walls of the rooms and lantern.
- 5 D° — — in the foundation, in consequence of accidents.

N. B. The whole time intercepted betwixt the *first stroke* upon the Rock, and leaving the Lighthouse compleat, was 3 years, 9 weeks, 3 days.

And the whole time from the Fire taking place, in December 1755, to the rekindling of the light, October 1759, was 3 years, 10 months, 16 days.

The whole time of working upon the Rock (being 111 days, 10 hours) amounts scarcely to SIXTEEN WEEKS.

APPENDIX.

A P P E N D I X.

Containing an Account of the Establishment of the present Lights *upon the* SPURN POINT, *by Direction of the Honourable Corporation of* TRINITY HOUSE, *Deptford Strond,* LONDON.

316. IN the year 1676 a patent was granted by *King* CHARLES II. to JUSTINIAN ANGELL, of *London, Merchant*, enabling him to *continue, renew*, and *maintain* certain lights that he had erected upon the *Spurn Point*. Which lights were erected at the request of the masters of ships using the *northern Trade*; who, in their petition to his *Majesty*, represented that a very *broad long Sand*, about six or seven months before, had been discovered to have been thrown up near the mouth of the river *Humber*, upon which they had had great losses; and by means whereof they failed in great danger in the night; and that having considered, that lights erected upon the *Spurn Point* would in future prevent such danger, this had induced them to apply to Mr. ANGELL, as being the proprietor of the *only* piece of ground, that was adapted to the purpose; and who, at their request, had erected two lights thereon; which the petitioners found to be not only of great benefit, but an *absolute safety* to all navigators on that coast.

In process of time, the *Broad Long Sand*, complained of in the petition, became itself a dry land at high water; and which continued to increase considerably: for, antecedent to the year 1766, the lights thus established by Mr. ANGELL were, by the gradual extension of the real point of the *Spurn*, become *now* at so very great a distance therefrom, that the masters of ships loudly complained, that the said lights were so far from being of that benefit they originally had been, that they were become detrimental to them; by inducing them to suppose themselves more near to the *point* than they in reality were. In fact, that they were *deceived* thereby, and in consequence many very great losses had lately happened *.——Wherefore an application was made to parliament in the year 1766, promoted by the *Corporations* of the TRINITY HOUSES at *Deptford Strond*, and *Hull*, for removing the said lights; and an act passed in consequence, *Anno sexto* GEORGII III. *Regis, Cap.* 31. "*An act for taking down and removing certain Lighthouses now standing near the* Spurn Point, *at the mouth of the* Humber, *and for erecting other fit and convenient Lighthouses instead thereof*;" whose preamble sets forth, that JOHN ANGELL, of *Stockwell*, in the county of *Surry*, Esq. was owner of three fourth parts of the said Lighthouses, duties, and profits; and that LEONARD THOMPSON, of *Sheriff Hutton* in the County of *York*, Esq. was proprietor of the other fourth share thereof. That Mr. ANGELL having been applied to by the said *Corporations*, and also by the said Mr.

* The spot of ground called the *Spurn Point*, seems to have undergone great changes; for in CAMDEN's time, about a century before the petition for erection of lights, there seems to have been no more than a pretty sharp *Head* of *Land*, that did not extend far from *Kilnsey*, and was then called *Spurn* HEAD. His words are "*Inde in ipsa promontorii Lingula quæ maxime in Oceanum contrahitur &* SPURN HEAD *dicitur* "KELNSEY *visitur viculus*." CAMDEN's *Britan.* 8vo. Edit. 1590. p. 580. It seems therefore gradually to have been drawn out to a greater length, and to a sharper point of land; taking the name of *Spurn* POINT, upon which the *lighthouse* was erected, and to which the *broad long sand* afterwards attached itself, and became dry land in the shape of a *Spoon*, which form it still retains.——There is also an obscure tradition current, that upon a flat of ground just within the *Point* that now but just *dries* at low spring-tides, there stood a considerable town called RAVENSPURN: and some pretend they have seen traces of its foundations.

THOMPSON,

Thompson, to change the situation of the said Lighthouses, so as to answer the ends and purposes for which they were originally designed; and this application having been ineffectual, it is thereby enacted; That the said Leonard Thompson should be intitled, as soon after the first day of June 1766 as conveniently could be, to erect two new and sufficient Lighthouses, with suitable offices and conveniences, at or near the said *Spurn Point*; according to such plan and estimate, as the *Master*, *Wardens*, and *Assistants* of the said *Corporation* of Trinity House, *Deptford Strond*, should by writing under their common seal specify, appoint, and approve of: and in the mean time, and until the said new Lighthouses should be completed, to erect two *Temporary Lights*, as near as may be to the respective places where the new Lighthouses shall be appointed to be built: and, as occasion might require, to enlarge, contract, alter, or remove the same, with the consent, and by the direction, of the said Corporation so signified. The said Lighthouses to be subject to the visitation of the *Trinity Houses* of *Deptford Strond* and of *Hull*.

317. MATTERS being in this state, the *Corporation* of Trinity House, *Deptford Strond*, did me the honour to request my attendance to meet a Committee of their body, appointed to proceed to the *Spurn Point* to take a survey, and give directions in respect to the situation and erection of two new Lighthouses; and of temporary lights, pursuant to the act of parliament lately passed for that purpose. Accordingly I met John Barker, Esq. and Thomas Bennet, Esq. the Committee appointed, at *Hull*, the 22d June 1766; and the next day attended them, and a deputation of the *Trinity House* of *Hull*, to the Spurn Point by water: when the gentlemen of the said Committee, after examining the ground, and hearing every matter of information that was offered to them, fixed the places for the two *Lighthouses*; and also for the temporary lights, as near the extremity of the point of the Spurn, as they could with the appearance of safety be built; and which situation was at the distance of more than a mile from the old Lighthouse: all which they proposed to lay before their Board for their concurrence.

They particularly enquired from me, considering the ground where the proposed Lighthouses were to stand, being a sand thrown up by the sea, in the course of less than a century, whether I could undertake to erect Lighthouses of *Brick* thereupon: and particularly, if one of them was to be ordered of 90 feet high to the center of the light?——To this I answered; That though the ground whereon they proposed to erect the lights was *new Ground*, in comparison of that whereon the present Lighthouse stood; yet, as it appeared to be of the same quality, whereon that had already stood 90 years, without apparent crack or settlement; I did not doubt of making a foundation, at least as much more firm than that of the old one, as the new building should be more lofty; and that it would stand, as long as the ground remained, that it stood upon: and in regard to *this*, it was the unanimous opinion of the whole company, that as the *Spurn Point* was a piece of ground that was *rapidly increasing*, there would be no danger of the ground being washed away. Therefore the judgment would be, to place the new lights as *near* the present point as possible, that there might be the greater course of years before the land, that doubtless *would be added*, should cause the necessity of a *second removal*.

In respect to the temporary lights; having then examined the *low light* machine, called a *Swape* *: though that was scarcely capable of hoisting the light above 25 feet above ordinary high water, yet, I doubted not but to produce a machine upon the same principle, so much more complete, that it should hoist the light 50 or even 60 feet high if required: and which I recommended to their consideration.

* The lights then subsisting, though in the original *patents* and the present act they are called *Lighthouses*, yet it does not appear that the [illegible] was ever exhibited otherwise than upon a *Swape* (a north country term for a *Lever*, when fixed upon a centre, and acted upon by [illegible], and which works in a way, very similar to that by which water is drawn by a bucket out of such wells as are not deep, in the [illegible] about *London*, and many other places: and which machine, as the coast wore away, being moveable, was now placed upon the beach near [illegible] water mark.

The *Great Lighthouse* was a strong octagon building of brick; and its light, also hoisted on a *Swape*, was a naked coal fire, which, [illegible] from the wind, was subject to burn with very different and unequal lustre: and it is related by the master of this Lighthouse, [illegible] of 1703 (when that of the *Edystone* was beat down) he "verily believed his tower (20 yards high) would have [illegible] down, and the tempest made the fire in it burn so vehemently, that it melted down the iron bars on which it was laid, [illegible] they were forced, when the fire was by this means almost extinguished, to put in new bars, and kindle the fire afresh." [illegible]

318. IN the autumn following I received from CHARLES WILDBORE, Esq. *Secretary* of the *Trinity board*, the *Corporations* directions concerning the *Spurn Lights*, as follow:

The Situation, Heights, Dimensions, &c. of the new Lighthouses *and* Temporary Lights *to be erected at the* SPURN POINT; *as agreed on at a* General Court *of the* Corporation *of* TRINITY HOUSE, *held 12th July*, 1766; viz.

The lights to be in a N. W. and S. E. direction; and to be 300 yards asunder.

The great Lighthouse to be placed on the Spurn Point, at a distance from high-water mark (at common spring-tides) of 90 yards, in a N. E. and S. W. line; and 150 yards in a N. W. line, within the *Spurn*.

The small Lighthouse to be 116 yards distant from high-water mark in a S. E. line, without the Spurn.

N. B. The breadth of the land from sea to sea, in a N. W. and S. E. line, is 566 yards; and the soil is the same as in other places, where the sand grows up from the sea; viz. gravel mixed with sand, and a moderate quantity of shingle.

The Lighthouses to be built with *Brick*: the large one to be 90 feet high, from the mean surface of the ground to the center of the light.——The small one to be 50 feet high; that is, 40 feet lower than the other: both with *inclosed Lanterns* for *Fire Lights*.

The two *Temporary Lights* to be placed in the same direction as before mentioned; 250 yards asunder; and to be 23 yards to the S. W. of the ground marked out for the Lighthouses.

The Great Temporary Light to be 50 feet high } both with *Swapes* for coal fires.
The small one - - - - 35 feet high }

It will be necessary to have a platform from one light to the other, for the men to walk on in the nights; about three feet wide, with a rail on each side *.

319. THE beginning of the ensuing year I produced to the Board a set of *Designs* for the erection of the two Lighthouses; and of two temporary *Light Machines*, conformable to the foregoing directions; and estimates for the same: which being considered by the Board, were approved, and passed the *common seal* of the Corporation, the 21st February 1767. Those being afterwards delivered to LEONARD THOMPSON, Esq. he proceeded to the execution thereof; and in the course of that season, built two *Temporary* Light *Machines*, according to the designs †; as also dwelling-houses, and conveniences for the residence of the light-keepers: which being lighted, according to due notice given, were found to answer the end so completely, in point of situation, height, and construction, that the trade seemed entirely satisfied therewith.

The temporary lights being thus established, and Mr. THOMPSON finding difficulties in getting a contract for the erection of the *Lighthouses*, two years elapsed without further progress; after which, in virtue of a *Proviso* in the said act, the *Corporation* of TRINITY HOUSE, *Deptford Strond*, became entitled to execute the further purposes thereof; and to this being also requested by Mr. THOMPSON, advertisements for contractors were put forth; and at a meeting of the Corporation, of the 7th April 1770, Mr. WILLIAM TAYLOR, of *York*, appearing to be the lowest proposer, was declared the *Contractor*; and afterwards articles of agreement were entered into in consequence.

320. THE 6th of May 1771, I had the honour to be appointed, by writing under the *Common Seal* of this *Corporation*, to be their *Surveyor*; for them, and in their behalf to *superintend, inspect, order*, and *direct* the execution of the works contracted to be done by the said WILLIAM TAYLOR, in such manner as I should see most conducive to answer the end proposed. In consequence of this appointment I visited the *Spurn Point* the following month, when Mr. TAYLOR had got together materials; but not having begun, it appeared to me, that since the year 1766, the sea had so far encroached upon the eastern coast of the *Spurn Point*, that the very place fixed for the *Low Lighthouse*, at 116 yards within high-water mark, according to the line of direction, was now in the very high-water mark itself. (See Plate 20, Fig. 2.) I

* The above resolutions, as well as what precedes, will be fully explained by the literary references to Plates N° 19, and 20.

† Plate N° 23, Fig. 2d, shews the elevation of the great temporary *Light Machine*. In its original state, its base was sunk into the ground, to keep it steady; but it is here shewn set upon walls, as it now serves for the *Low Light*.

therefore

therefore suggested to the Board, that it would be proper to shift the place of the Low Lighthouse, as they had marked it out, so as to be 80 yards more *inland*; or to N. W.: which alteration being approved, Mr. TAYLOR began the foundation accordingly.——And furthermore, as it was possible the sea might in process of time make an attack upon *this building*, I directed Mr. TAYLOR to drive as many piles under the outward circle of its base, as should bring them *close together*, and to drive them as deep as they could be got into this sand; which on trial was found to be about 9 feet *.

The 23d July the piling of this foundation was finished, and the brick work begun; but the Contractor had scarcely got the work up to the level of the ground, before he was interrupted by an attack from the *agents* of Mr. ANGELL; which shewed the necessity of an *amendment* in the *act*: the obtaining of which stopped the works for above a twelvemonth. The latter end, however, of the year 1772, the foundation of the High Light was begun: and, by the approbation of the Board, it was placed 60 yards more towards the N. W. than originally intended, to make up in part for the 80 yards we had given up upon the S. E. side. I did not think it prudent to take the whole 80 yards; because, though the N. W. coast had apparently *gained*, it did not appear certain, how much or how long it might continue so to do. The distance of the houses, therefore, as now settled, was 280 yards.

The beginning of February 1773, the foundation for the *High Light* was completed: and in December following, the Low Lighthouse was covered *in*; and the High Light got 40 feet high.

321. TILL my visit in June 1771, I never had gone to the Spurn Point by land; in consequence I had had no opportunity of remarking that the sea was incroaching upon the *whole Coast*, quite from *Bridlington* to the high grounds at *Kilnsey*. I then saw the coast was in a state of wear, but it was not till my visits in the year 1774, that there had been a sufficient interval, to ascertain the rate, at which the sea was annually washing away the high *clay* cliffs of *Kilnsey*: which, as near as I could then estimate it, was at the rate of 10 yards a year.——As the Low Light was then *erected*, the information naturally drawn from this observation came *too late*; for though I perceived that, as had been suggested in the year 1766, the *Point* of the *Spurn* was *increasing*, yet it was chiefly in *length*. I now found that the high-water mark was not in reality more than 40 yards from the center of the Low Light; I therefore concluded it could not be many years before an attack *must* be made upon the Low Lighthouse; but, as I had for some time considered the Spurn Point as an *appendage* to the high cliffs of *Kilnsey*; and formed from the waste of the lands to the North; therefore, at whatever rate the sea encroached upon these cliffs, by taking off parallel *Screeds*, this whole *appendage of the Spurn* must remove at an equal rate *westward*, upon the *average*. It, however, might alter some years more, others less, according to the casual influence of storms.

322. ACCORDINGLY, a great storm happening in January 1776, took away so much of the S. E. coast in general, that it not only took away entirely the *site* of the old Lighthouse; but first laid bare the circular *Court wall* of the *Low Light*; and then taking away the sand below its foundation, beat down one half of its circumference in a single tide; and ceased not till it had laid bare the *close piling* under the circumference of the main building, driven for its protection. (§ 320.)

On visiting Spurn Point on this occasion, I ordered down a quantity of *Hazlecliff* stone † to be deposited, so as to form a *sloping Bank* or *Bulwark* at the foot of the building, to break off the fury of the sea, till the season should come on when something more effectual might be done; and left the further progress and application of the same means to Mr. TAYLOR, who had constantly resided upon the place.

323. IN reflecting upon the observations I had made, and have already stated; I plainly perceived, that to defend this building against the future attacks of the sea, nothing less could avail than what would

* The design of the Lower Lighthouse, was perfectly similar to that of the Great Light, in respect to the *Lantern* and *Pipe Room*, but the Body of the Light itself being less, the diameter of the lantern, and all below, to its base, were proportionably less: so that being 40 feet lower than the other was intended, it consisted of fewer rooms in height; viz. a *Coal Vault*, in the base story, a *Dwelling Room*, *Pipe Room*, and Lantern.

† A kind of hard chalk-stone, got near the *Humber* side, above *Hull*, and much used in this country for all kinds of rough works, and defences against the waters.

defend

defend it as an *Iſland* at low water: this, though not impoſſible, would be ſo expenſive, as greatly to exceed that of rebuilding it, as often as it ſhould be beat down. I therefore adviſed the Board not to enter into any *formidable Expenditure*, but to give the injured parts a repair or re-eſtabliſhment, at the moſt moderate charge, that was likely to give the building a chance of its anſwering the end for which it was built, for a number of years: and, in this view, to rebuild the wall of a greater thickneſs; and *found* it as deep into the ſand, as it could *well* be got at a *moderate* expence; and then to fill the cavity between the wall and the houſe with *Hazlecliff* ſtone. Laſtly, to form a ſloping *Bulwark* of the ſame ſtone, againſt the outſide of the new wall: after this, with ſuch palliative aids, as prudence ſhould from time to time direct, to let it take its chance, to laſt as long as it could: and, at any rate, to ſet up the preſent *temporary high light machine*, in the line of *direction*; as ſoon as it ſhould be done with where it ſtood, by the lighting of the houſes. In this caſe, it might be applied as a *low light*, on an hour's notice; that is, as ſoon as any accident to the preſent *Low Light Building* ſhould make it neceſſary. This advice and opinion being approved by the Board, the ſame was put in execution, in the courſe of the following ſeaſon.

324. THIS accident did not, however, materially delay the progreſs of the work towards the lighting of the houſes; for at that time the Great Lighthouſe was covered in, the windows of the Lantern glazed, the *Hearth* ſet, and the balcony rails in their places: ſo that whilſt the interior works were proceeding, Mr. Taylor was employing other hands to rebuild and defend the wall as propoſed.

325. IT being the anxious deſire of the Corporations, and of the trade in general, that the houſes ſhould be lighted before the enſuing winter, I thought it my duty not only to forward this, but to give the Board the information, that from local ſituation I was able.——That in various parts of the *Weſt Riding* of *Yorkſhire*, there was dug a coal, of the ſpecies of the *Lancaſhire Kennel*, called here *Stone coal*, or *Cracklers*; which burns with a brighter and whiter blaze, than the ſtrong coal of *Newcaſtle* and *Sunderland* *, and therefore, it ſeemed to me, would be better adapted to the purpoſe of producing a light, and could be had at as low, if not a lower, price. The Board were pleaſed to order me to procure ſuch cargoes of *Stone coal*, as might be ſufficient for a full trial thereof, and which accordingly were procured.

326. UPON the 5th September 1776, the fires were kindled with *Stone Coal*, which exhibited an amazing light, to the entire ſatisfaction of all beholders.

As ſoon as the houſes were lighted, I immediately ordered the temporary High Light Machine, which I found ſound and firm, to be ſet upon the walls, that had been built in the direction of the lights; its centre to be 30 yards nearer the Great Lighthouſe than the centre of the Low Light; ſo that its diſtance from the centre of the Great Light, would ſtill be 250 yards.——Theſe walls, though ordered to be built in length, ſo as to be only capable of taking the baſe of the machine; yet whenever it ſhould want moving the walls could be lengthened, and the machine being then got upon rollers, would readily be moved to its deſtined place.

327. DURING the following winter it was found that ſometimes on firſt lighting of the fires in an evening, the funnels of the Lanterns would not vent the ſmoke ſo faſt as it was produced by the fires, but it accumulated in the Lantern. The chimneys were then of the ſame material as the roof, viz. *Elland Edge Flag-Stone*. Being willing to leave every thing complete, and finding that they would be conſiderably enlarged by making them of copper plate; the experiment was firſt tried upon the Low Light, which fully anſwering the end, the High Light was ſerved in the ſame manner; and it is ſo ſhown in the ſection of this building, Plate N° 21.

On viſiting Spurn Point, the 7th April 1777, I certified to the Board, that the *Lighthouſes* at *Spurn Point*, together with the whole of the works contracted to be done by Mr. Taylor, were fully completed and finiſhed.——Upon this viſit I had the gratification to find, not only that the lights had given

* As the Spurn lights had hitherto been made by fires expoſed to the fury of the wind, they doubtleſs required a coal of the ſtrongeſt quality; but as theſe lights were now to be ſcreened by Glazed Lanterns, a coal that would more freely yield its light ſeemed better adapted.

the utmoſt ſatisfaction; but that the Court-wall of the Low Light, was likely to endure for *ſome time:* for though it had had ſuch ſhocks, that the light-keepers had ſelt the tremor in the lantern, yet it remained ſound and firm.

328. CONSIDERING the inconvenience that this place ſuffers for want of freſh water; and that it is likely more and more to become inhabited, on account of the numbers that come on ſhore from the ſhips, lying in the Humber as an harbour; on this viſit I directed Mr. TAYLOR to ſink a *well*, to try to obtain either freſh water, or that which was ſo far free from ſalts, as to anſwer all ſubordinate purpoſes; and to be had *in plenty:* for here, the tops and roofs of the buildings are ſo impregnated with ſalts from the ſpray of the ſea, that the rain-water collected from the drippings thereof, is ſeldom without a very ſenſible impregnation. The experiment was not likely to be an expenſive one, and was ordered in virtue of an obſervation that had occurred in the courſe of the work.

Mr. TAYLOR being at liberty to uſe ſea water for wetting his mortar, ſunk a well near to each Light-houſe, when he began them; merely to obtain ſalt water *more eaſily*, than by fetching it from the ſea at low water; but was much ſurpriſed to find, that the water ſo obtained was but merely *brackiſh*, and that in all ſtates of the tide. On examining this circumſtance myſelf, I found further, that the height of the water in the well remained nearly the ſame, that is, at about the *half-tide* mark. That at the high water of a ſpring-tide, when the water flowed within the diſtance of 20 or 30 yards of the top of the well, the water in the well neither roſe ſenſibly higher, nor was it, to common obſervation, more brackiſh; though there was nothing to hold off the ſea, but a great maſs of porous ſand: and on the other hand, when the ſea retreated 150 or 200 yards, the water of the well during the time of low water became ſcarce ſenſibly more empty, nor did it grow ſenſibly more freſh.——Reflecting on the cauſe of this unexpected fact; it appeared to me, that whatever rains or ſnows fall upon the ſurface of the Spurn, conſiſting of about 98 acres, it all ſinks into the ground, and therefore muſt make its way to ſea by percolation through the pores of the ſand; and in its paſſage it will by degrees waſh off the ſalts adhering to the ſurface of the particles of ſand at their firſt depoſition: in conſequence, this happening repeatedly, the internal part of the *Peninſula*, which being ſuppoſed to have been the longeſt formed, muſt have had the greateſt length of time to have its ſalts waſhed off by the freſh water of the rains, would of courſe afford the freſheſt water when ſunk *into*, deep enough to pierce the *water bed*; and which probably would lie upon an higher level there, than near the border, on account of the neceſſary declivity for the paſſage of the water by percolation to ſeaward.——In conſequence of theſe ſpeculations, I ordered a *well* to be ſunk near the middle of the peninſula; and had the ſatisfaction to hear, that it anſwered expectation, being but *barely brackiſh*; for that cattle would drink it, and it ſerved every purpoſe of a family, except for human drinking, and waſhing of linen: nor could it be expected to be perfectly freſh, as the very rain muſt frequently have a conſiderable admixture with the ſpray of the ſea.——It appears then, that though a great maſs of ſand does not hinder a ſlow progreſſive motion by *percolation*, yet it reſiſts all great impulſes, to ſuch a degree, that, in the ſpace of a tide, the ſalt water has not time to make much progreſs in return. *Attraction* of *Cohesion*, therefore, between the particles of ſand and water, ſeems to perform the office of a *Stop-gate*, which ſuffers the eſcape of the water to ſea at a *medium height*; and, by preventing its ſpeedy return, ſuffers the downfall waters (like thoſe of a tract of country under artificial drainage by ſluices) to have a progreſſive motion from the internal parts towards their outfall *.

329. BEING upon a journey to *Hull*, the 5th October 1786, I went from thence to viſit the *Spurn*, and had the ſatisfaction to find every thing in order, and completely anſwering their purpoſe †.——

On

* Had Sir THO' HYDE PAGE been acquainted with what had here been done; it ſeems as if it would have led to an explanation of what he experienced at *Landguard Fort* in the year 1782: where he found that *good water* was produced by digging into a ſand at eight feet deep, and continued in great plenty to 12 feet deep; but by forcing the well down to 18 feet deep, the water that iſſued from the bottom became *entirely ſalt*. See his account *Philoſ. Tranſact.* vol. lxxiv. p. 16.

† I muſt however except the *well*, the water of which, it was my intention to have examined; and I had taken with me ſuch materials as my chemical friends adviſed, to have aſcertained the quantity of admixture of ſea ſalt in this water. But I was defeated in my inten-

tion

On this occasion I took a *Survey* of the *Spurn Point*, and Plate N° 20, Fig. 1st, is the plan deduced from thence; from whence it appears, that the foundation of the old Lighthouse, which was wholly within the unbroken land in the year 1771, was now 50 yards without the present border towards low-water mark: not the least vestige of it being to be seen. It was, therefore, by the united testimony of the *residents*, who referred to marks, that I was enabled to ascertain its place. In the year 1771, the land where it then stood had a considerable breadth, but now it lies opposite to the narrow *Isthmus*, which, after extending about a quarter of a mile to the N. Eastward of this site, becomes a naked *beach* or ridge; over which the sea breaks into the *Humber*, at high-water, in rough weather, with easterly winds, at spring-tides; and after running about half a mile in that form, attaches itself to a prominence of the main land, from *Kilnsey*; which was probably the *Spurn* Head of Camden.——This beach or ridge I found to have nearly the same appearance in 1786, that it had in 1771; only, it seemed to have grown longer, by encroaching southwards, upon the flat area of the Spurn Point *.

330. ON this visit, the original temporary light great machine was now in actual use; the Low *Lighthouse* having been for some time demolished, and, at this time, not the least trace left of its foundation †.

331. IN departing from the Spurn this last visit, I was struck with an appearance that I can scarcely satisfactorily account for. I did not leave the Spurn till some time after the Lights were kindled. The Low Light, though in itself a fire of much less bulk than that of the High Light, yet, at this distance, being *now* a naked light, without the interposition of glass, appeared more vivid and brilliant than the High Light. When I got about three miles off, near *Kilnsey*, they seemed nearly equal; but when I got to *Patrington*, nine miles off in a straight line, the lustre of the High Light was greatly superior: in this I could not well be deceived; because, in observing them for a considerable time when the fires were in different states, the brightness of the High Light when faintest considerably exceeded that of the Low Light when brightest: now the query is; If the glass diminished the lustre of the light in a sensible degree (as it must be expected) when *near*, why should it not do it *proportionably* at every other distance?

332. I HAD the great satisfaction to find at *Hull*, that the *Spurn Lights* were in such credit among the *Seamen*, that they were by them esteemed (on account of their clear and brilliant light) to be the best Lights in *Europe*.——It is said that vessels going round the *Point*, in a *dark night*, have the shades of their masts and ropes cast upon their decks: that vessels sailing northward gain sight of the *Spurn* before they lose sight of the *floating Light* of the *Dodgeon*, which lies off the great *Lincolnshire Wash*; and that frequently, the Great Light of the *Spurn* has been seen, in clear weather, from the high grounds near *Beverley*, which is a distance of 30 miles.

333. I SHALL close this account by an explanation of the principle whereon the *Air-draught* of this Lighthouse is performed: which, as I apprehend it is somewhat new, and succeeds well, the curious artist may not think undeserving of his notice.

tion and mortified, by finding that it was filled by bricks and rubbish, so that at eight feet deep, there was no water.—I was told, that as it was appurtenant to no one's tenement, and at a distance from them all; idle mischievous people, who frequently come on shore to saunter about, had amused themselves by throwing things into the water, to judge of its depth, till they had reduced it to that state: and as it was no one's business to clear it, each was willing to shift for himself; though all agreed it had been very useful.

* This Beach or Ridge has in its appearance some similarity with that of *Portland*; and, if I mistake not, it is formed, underneath the sand, of *blue clay*, such as the cliffs of *Kilnsey*.

† I found on enquiry, that after a repetition of storms, the Court-wall had given way, and an ineffectual attempt had been made to repair it. The main body of the building was soon after attacked; but it stood without the least crack or appearance of settlement, till successive gales had proceeded so far as to take away several of the piles in the *Circumference* of the base; insomuch, that, (according to their expression) an *Heifer* might have been drove under it, among the piles: but after remaining some time in that condition, in one single rough tide, it came down all at once, and the materials were in a great measure dissipated and buried in the sand. The *Machine* had then been some time in use.

The

The air being rendered ſpecifically lighter by the heat of a fire; if from thence it is introduced into a tube or *funnel* while in its heated ſtate, the abſolute gravity of this column is juſt ſo much lighter than a column of the external air of equal height, as is due to their difference of ſpecific gravity: and this difference of abſolute weight of the two columns, is a poſitive power by which the lighter one endeavours to aſcend up the tube, according to the laws of *Hydroſtatics*.——Now, if the air that is required to replenish the tube at the bottom, to fill up in *lieu* of what has aſcended, cannot enter it without paſſing through, or ſo near, a body of fire that it becomes heated thereby, this alſo becomes ſucceſſively rarefied; and thus a conſtant power, or *Draught* of air is generated.——This I look upon to be the common principle upon which the draught of chimneys and Furnaces depends: the tube of rarefied air being placed *above* the fire.

In this Lighthouſe the principle of *Air-draught*, or tube of rarefied air, is *below* the fire: for as the fire muſt of neceſſity be expoſed to full view, all round; being in a capacious Lantern the draught is cut off, or interrupted, above the fire; ſo that the funnel of the Lantern muſt be wide enough to vent all the ſmoke that is ſent up, as we have ſeen, § 327. In this conſtruction the *receptacle* for the cinders, being a large tube, over the top of which the fire-grate lies, no air can paſs through the fire-grate into the fire, but what comes from the receptacle; the air of which being heated by the cinders, that fall through the grate, has a tendency to aſcend, upon the ſame principle of rarefaction.——This receptacle is ſupplied by horizontal air-pipes, from the external air: and, that its operation may not be impeded by, but rather receive advantage from the wind; in every direction; the pipes, which are eight in number, are regularly diſpoſed with reſpect to the *compaſs*; and each has a ſlider to ſhut up ſuch as would be otherwiſe a diſadvantage. A further explanation of theſe matters will be found in the technical deſcription of Plate N° 21.

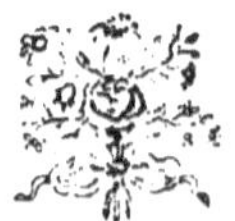

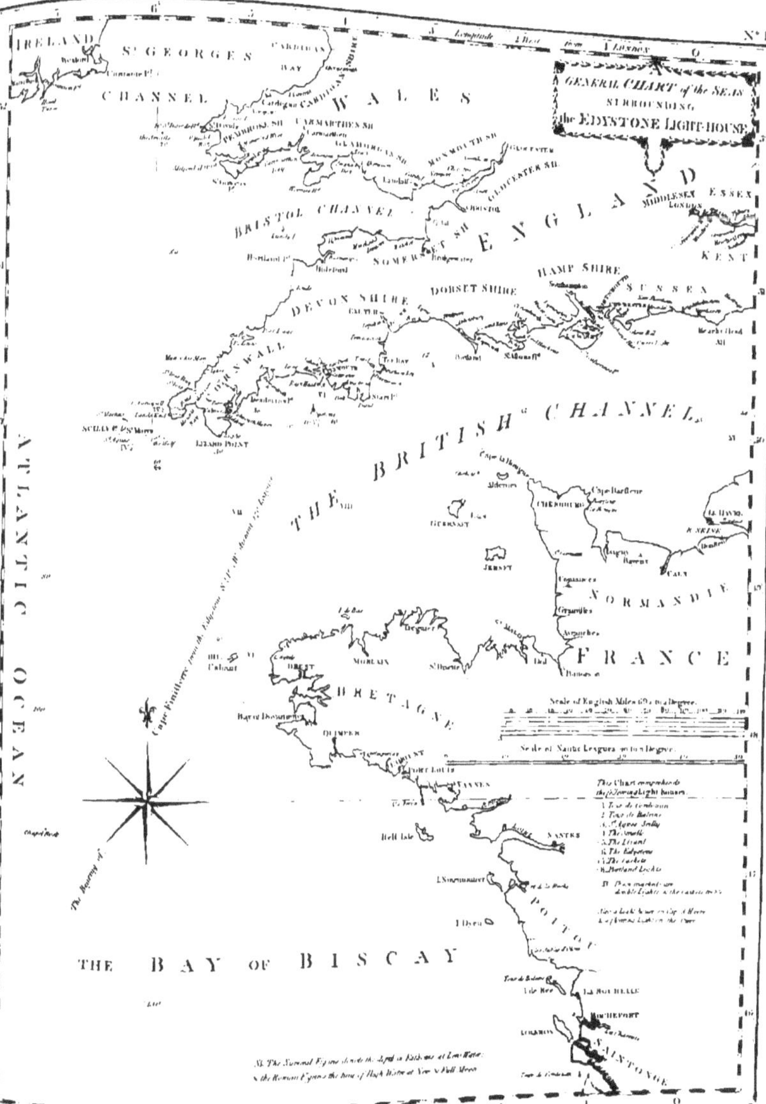

N° 1
A GENERAL CHART of the SEAS SURROUNDING the EDYSTONE LIGHT-HOUSE
IRELAND
S^t. GEORGES CHANNEL
CARDIGAN BAY
WALES
CARMARTHEN SH
GLAMORGAN SH
MONMOUTH SH
GLOCESTER SH.
BRISTOL CHANNEL
ENGLAND
MIDDLESEX
LONDON
ESSEX
KENT
SOMERSET SH
DEVON SHIRE
DORSET SHIRE
HAMP SHIRE
SUSSEX
CORNWALL
SCILLY
LIZARD POINT
THE BRITISH CHANNEL
ATLANTIC OCEAN
GUERNSEY
JERSEY
CHERBOURG
Cape Barfleur
CAEN
NORMANDIE
FRANCE
BREST
BRETAGNE
QUIMPER
PORT LOUIS
VANNES
Bell Isle
NANTES
POITOU
LA ROCHELLE
ROCHEFORT
SAINTONGE
Scale of English Miles 69½ to a Degree.
This Chart comprehends the following Light houses.
THE BAY OF BISCAY

MAP of the COASTS & COUNTRY opposite the EDYSTONE ROCKS. No 2

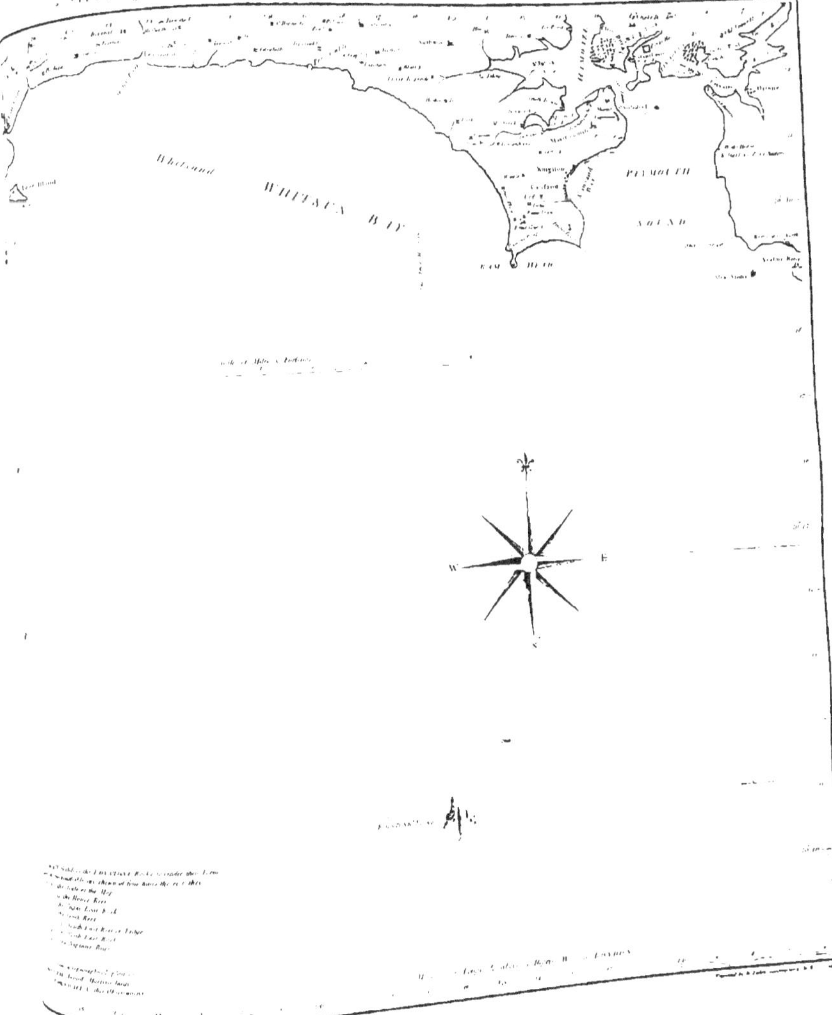

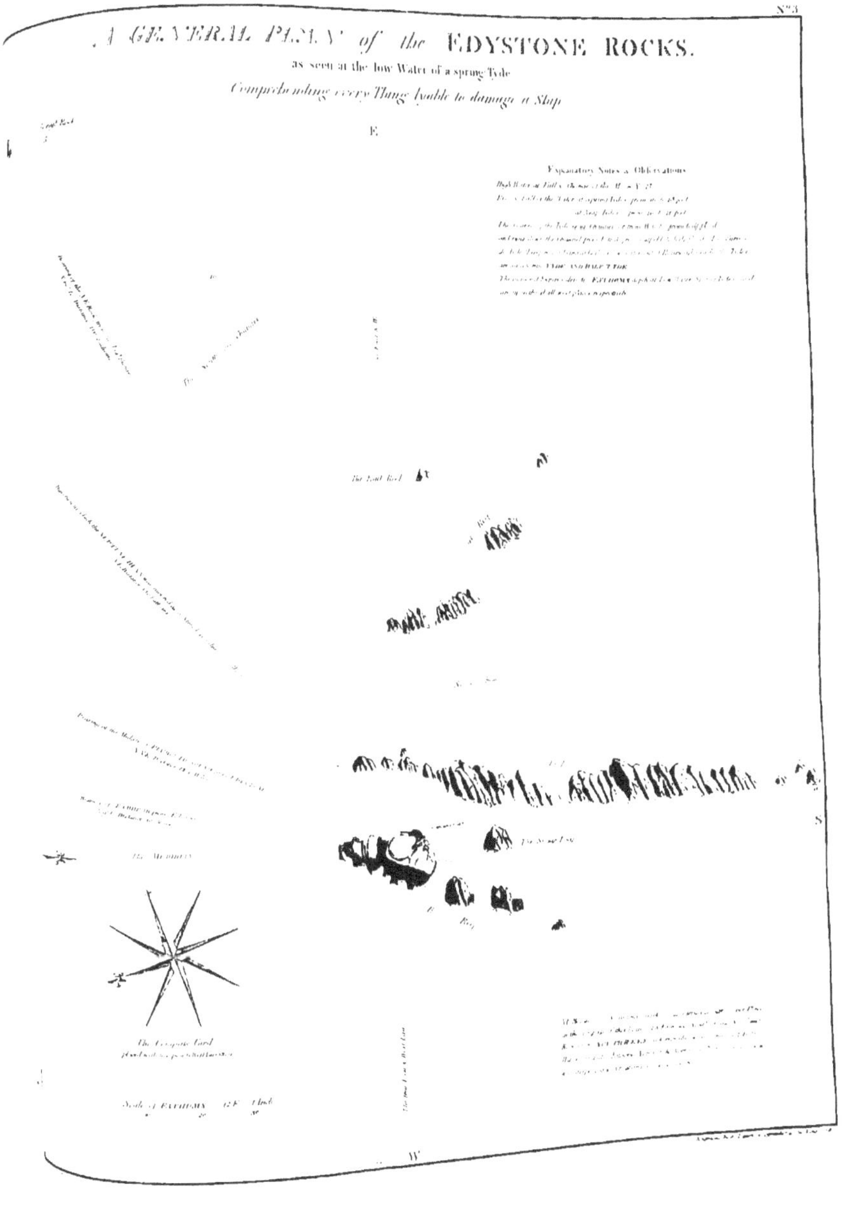

No 3

A GENERAL PLAN of the EDYSTONE ROCKS.

as seen at the low Water of a spring Tyde

Comprehending every Thing lyable to damage a Ship

E

Explanatory Notes & Observations

The East Rock

S

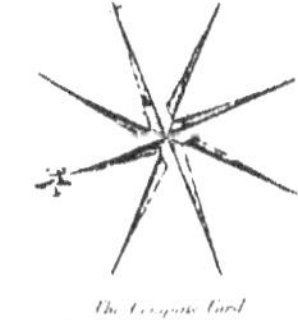

The Compass Card

Scale of FATHOMS

W

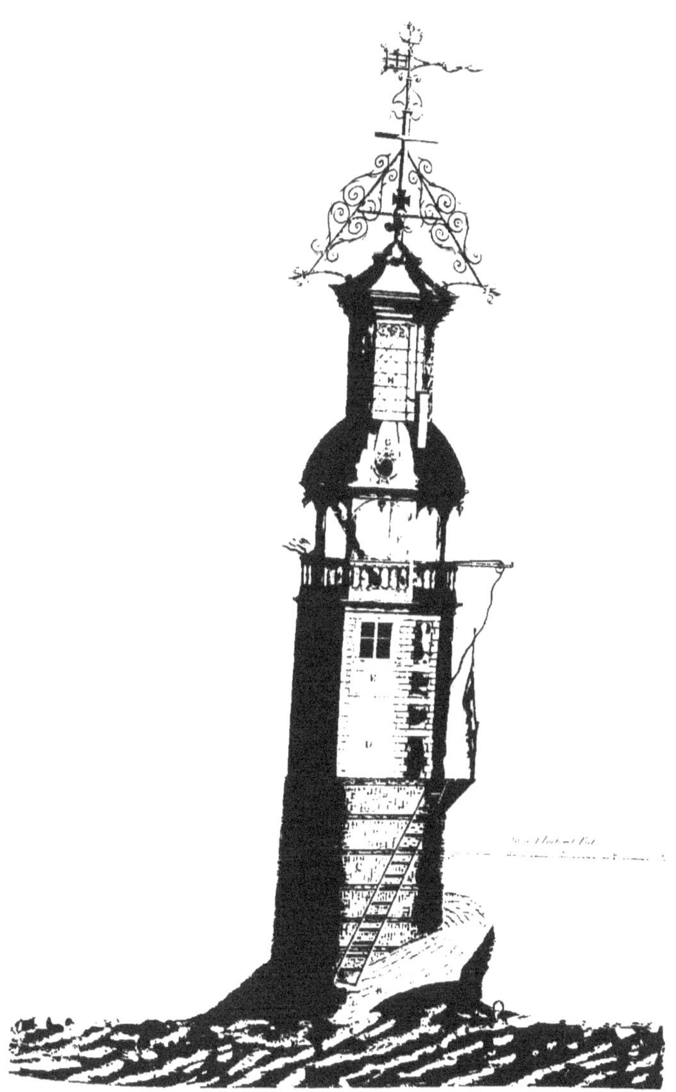

South ELEVATION of the ORIGINAL LIGHTHOUSE,
Built upon the EDYSTONE ROCK, according to the first Design of M.R WINSTANLEY.

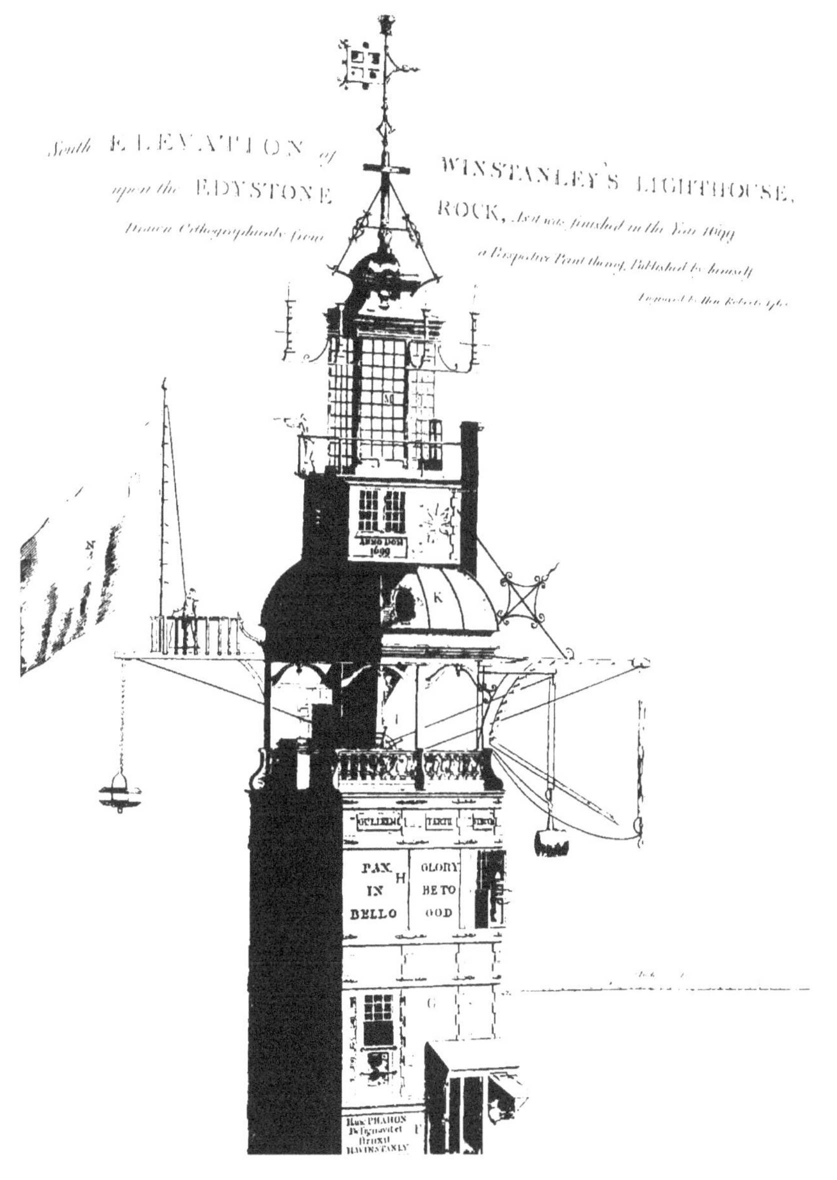
South ELEVATION of WINSTANLEY'S LIGHTHOUSE,
upon the EDYSTONE ROCK, As it was finished in the Year 1699
Drawn Orthographically from a Perspective Print thereof, Published by himself
ANNO DOM
1699
PAX
IN
BELLO
GLORY
BE TO
GOD

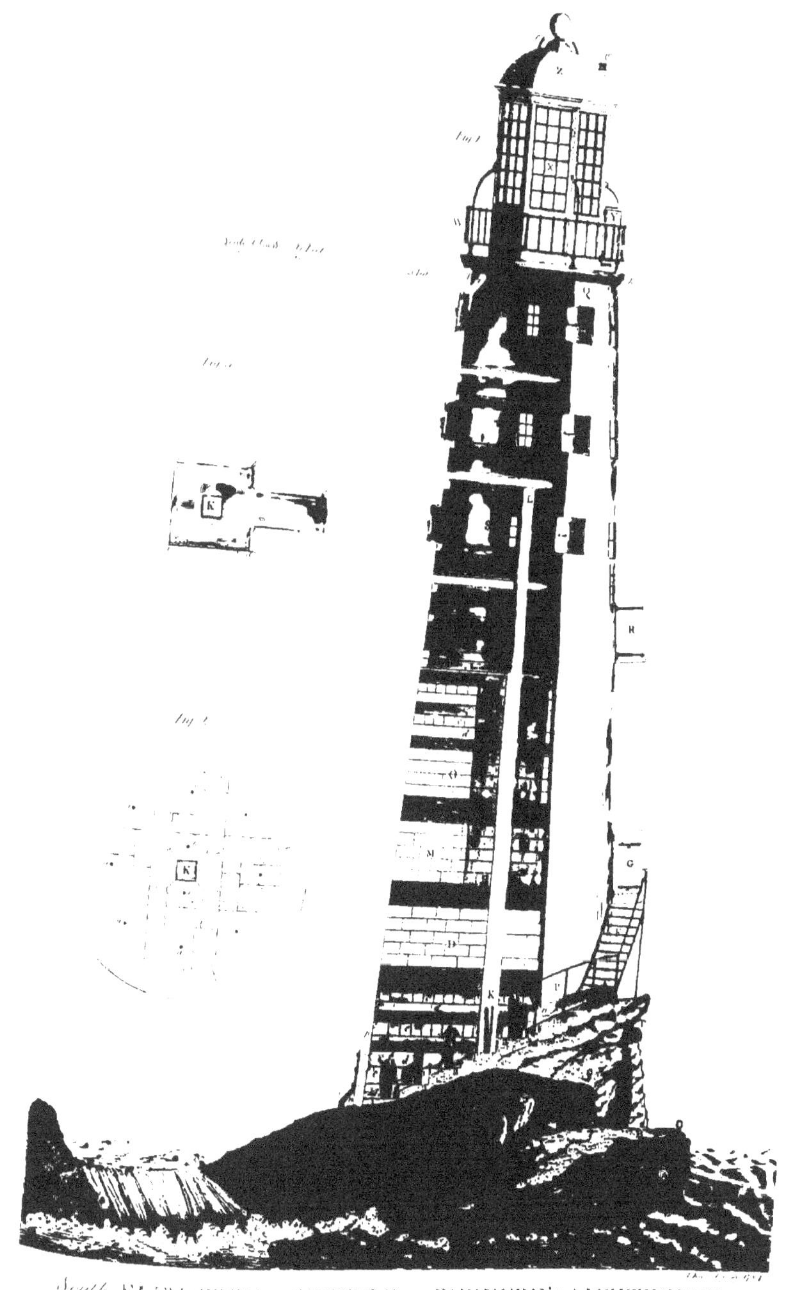

South ELEVATION & SECTION *of* RUDYERD'S LIGHTHOUSE,

Completed in 1709, represented as it stood previous to its demolition by Fire in the Year 1755

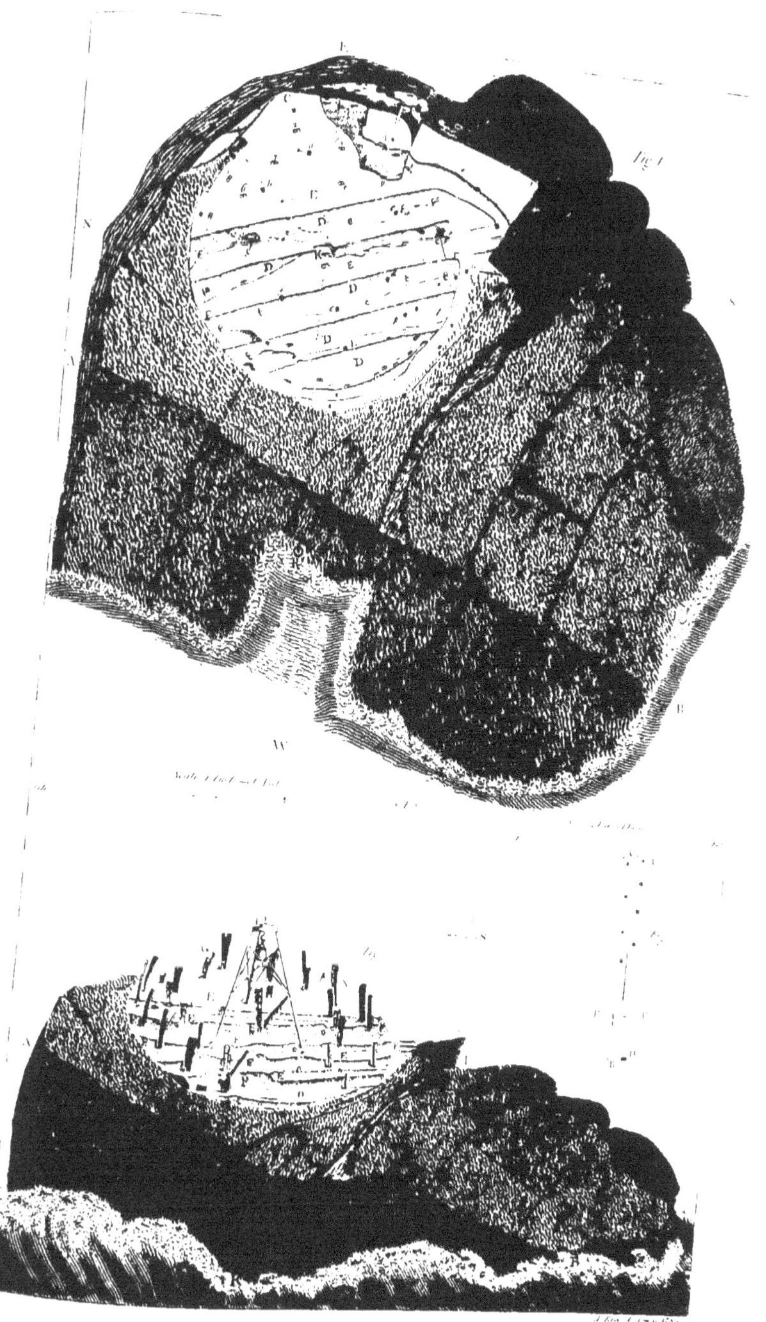

PLAN and perspective ELEVATION of the EDYSTONE ROCK,

Seen from the West, taken from the Model thereof mentioned

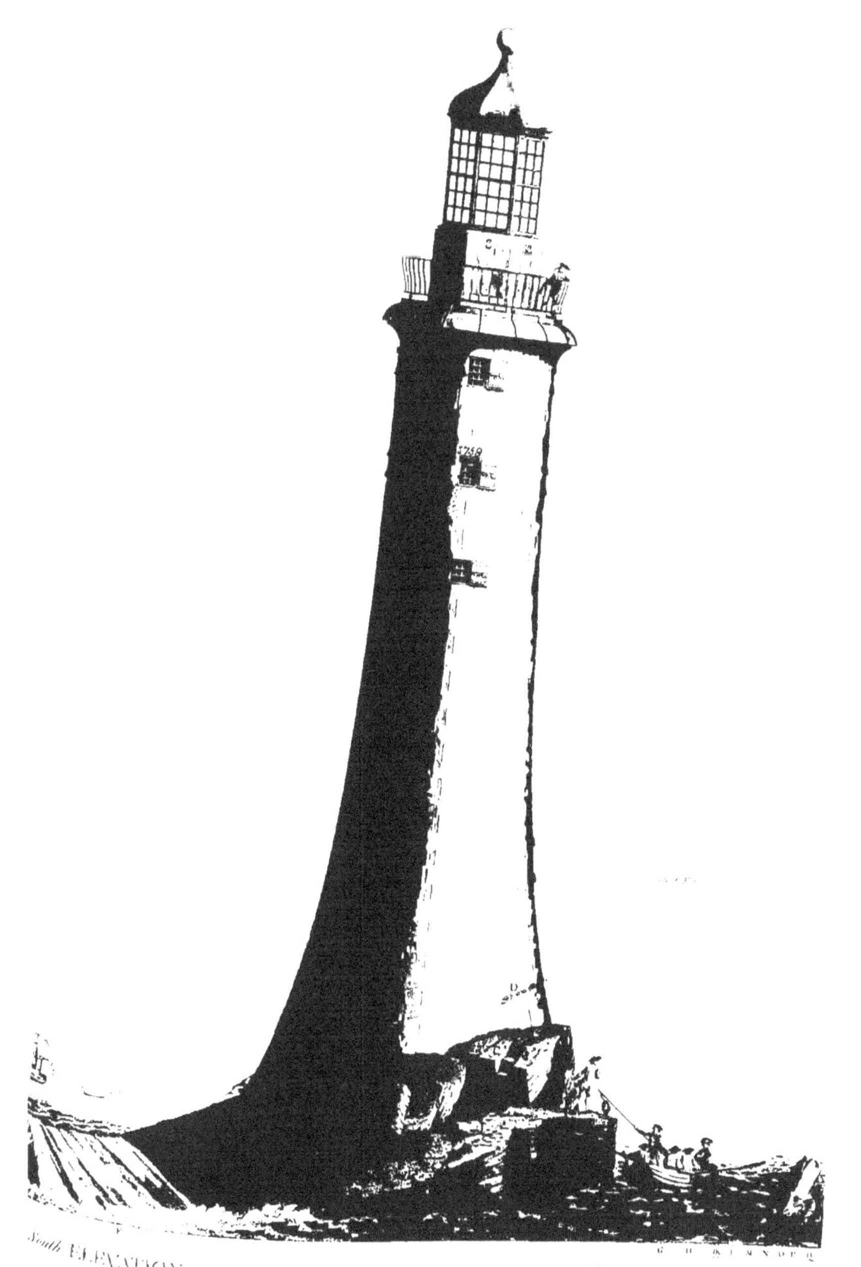

South ELEVATION of the STONE LIGHTHOUSE completed upon the EDYSTONE in 1759

Shewing the Prospect of the nearest Land, as it appears from the Rocks in a clear calm Day

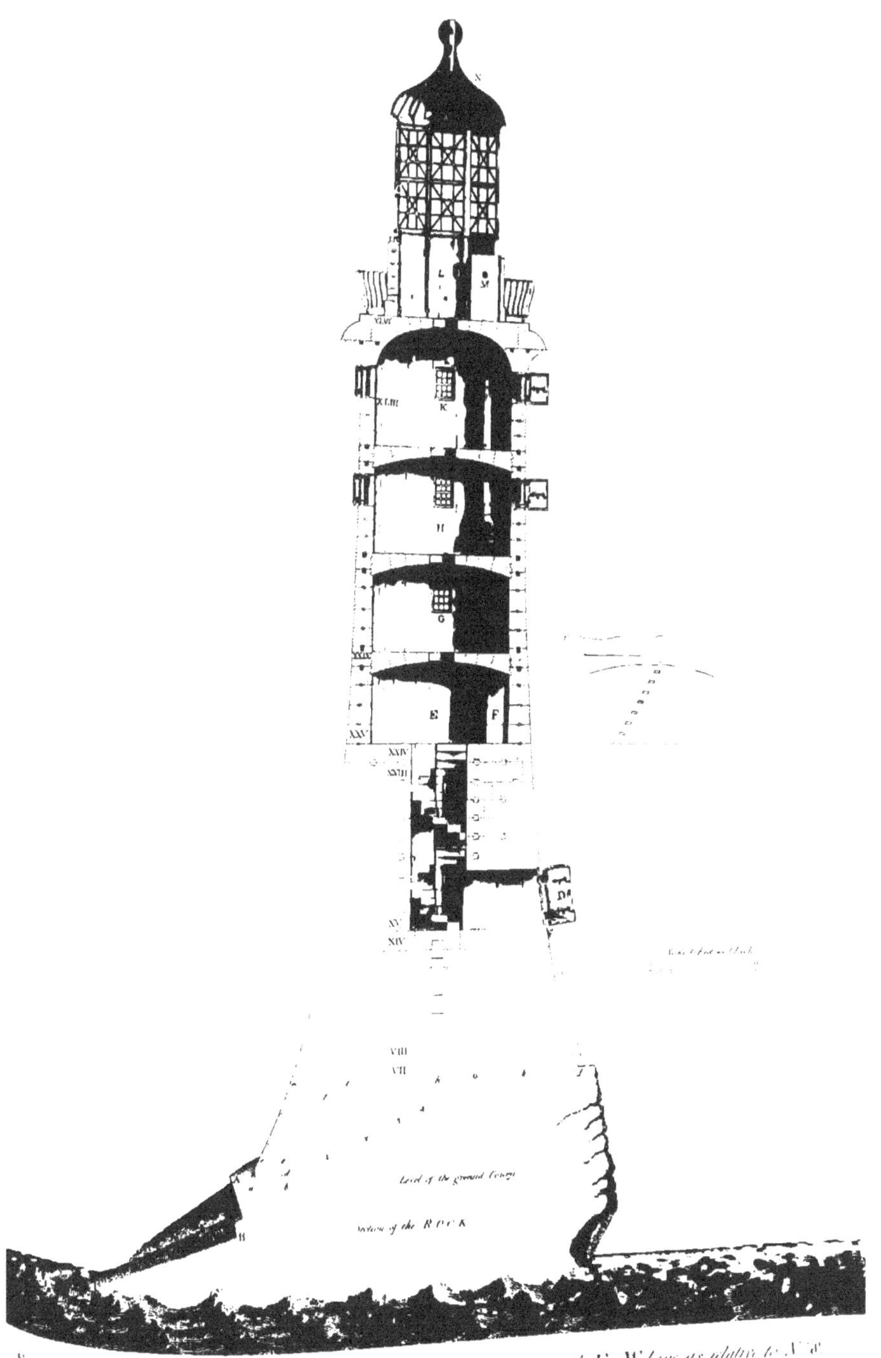

SECTION of the EDYSTONE LIGHTHOUSE upon the E & W Line as relative to N° 8.
on Supposition of its being LOW WATER of a SPRING TIDE.

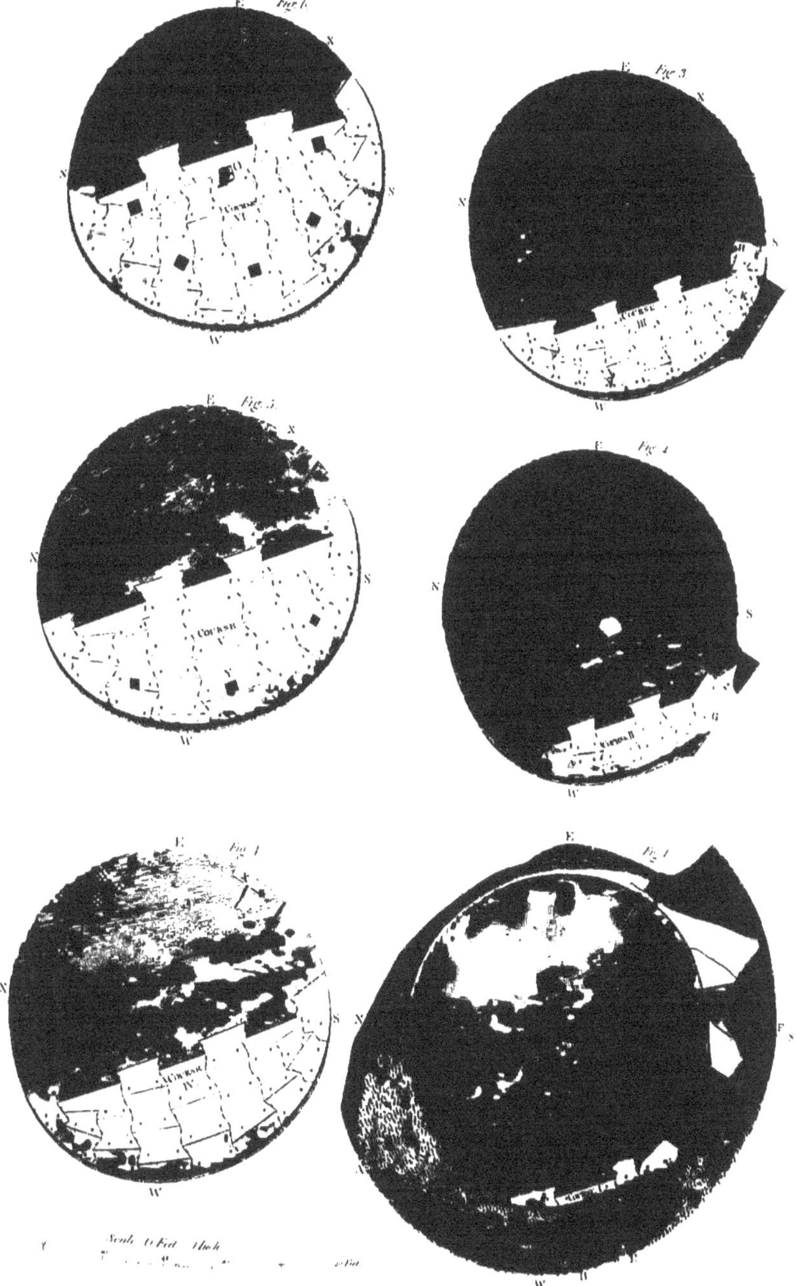

Fig. 6
Course VI
Fig. 3
Course III
Fig. 5
Course V
Fig. 4
Course II
Fig. 1
Course IV
Fig. 1
Scale 10 Feet 1 Inch

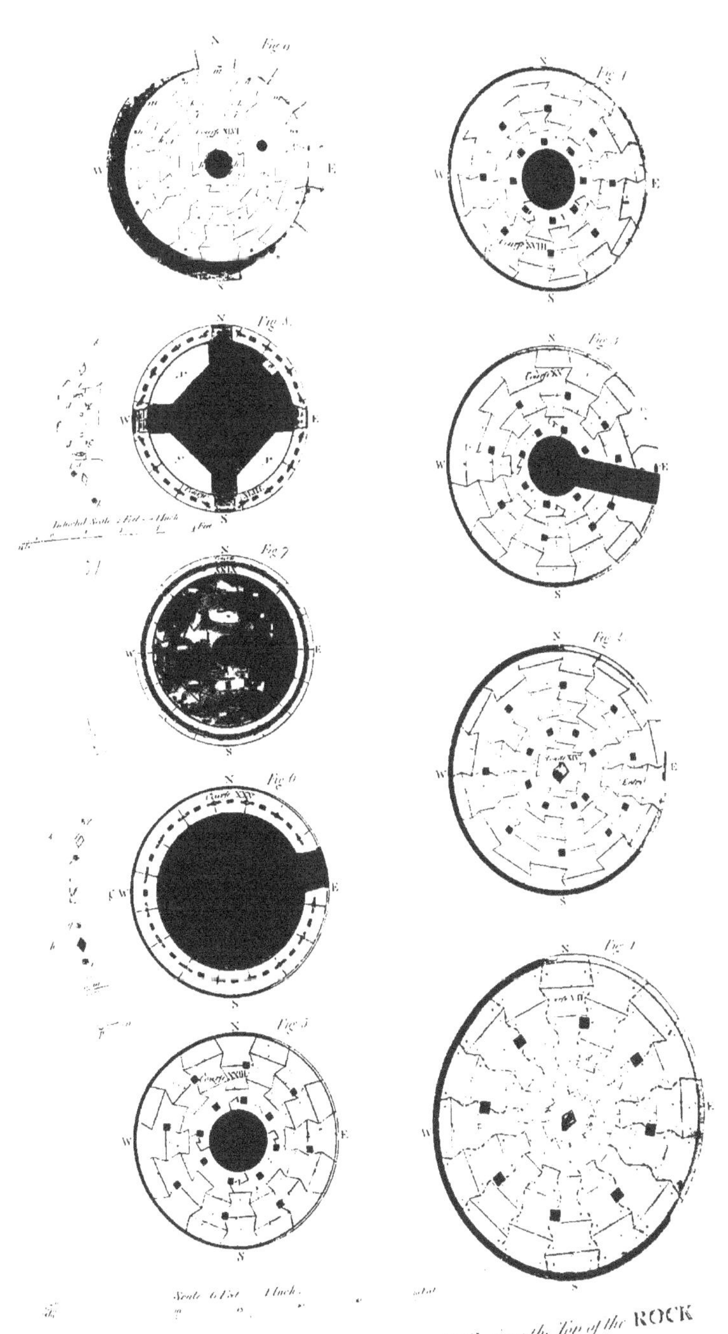

PLANS of all the Different COURSES from the Top of the ROCK to the Top of the BALCONY FLOOR inclusive.

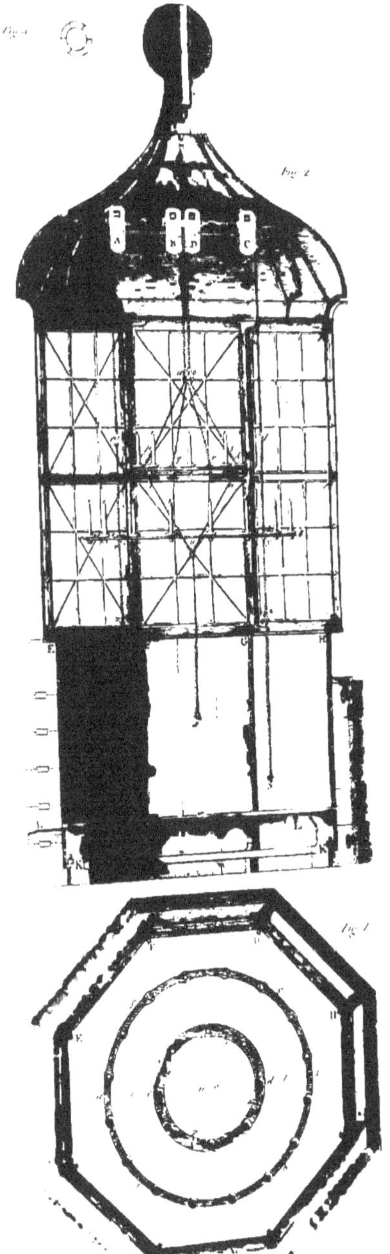

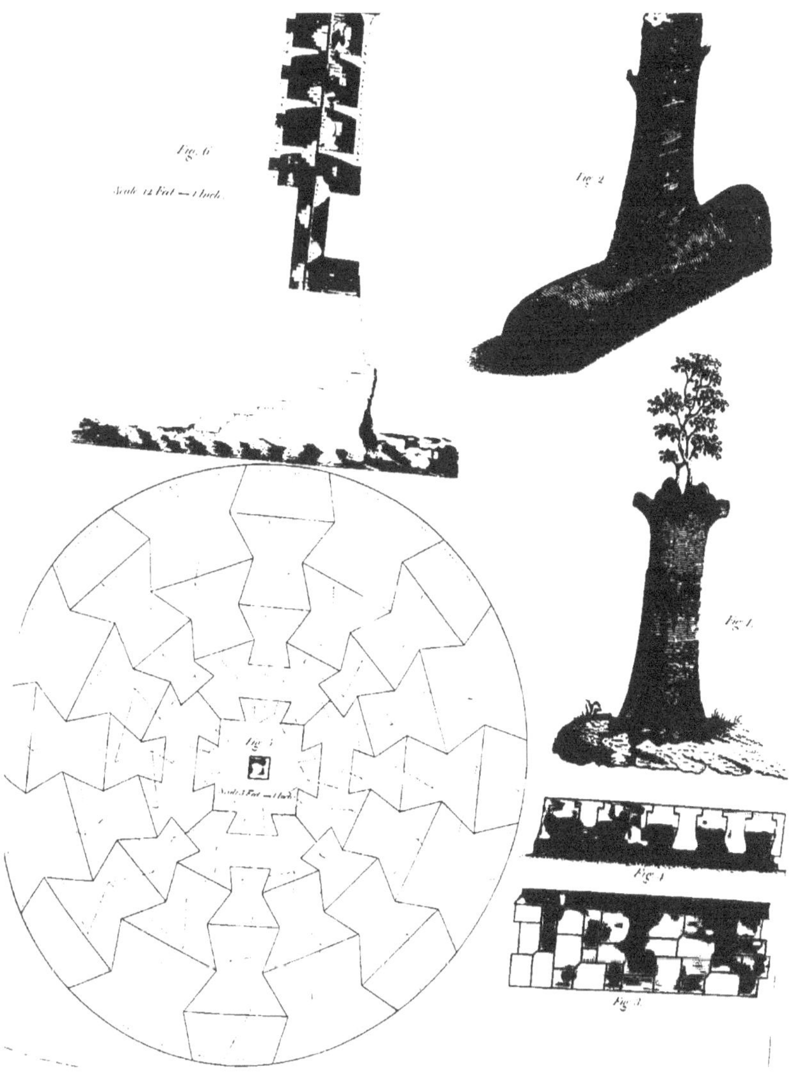

Fig. 6
Scale 12 Feet = 1 Inch.
Fig. 2
Fig. 1.
Scale 3 Feet = 1 Inch.
Fig. 4
Fig. 3.

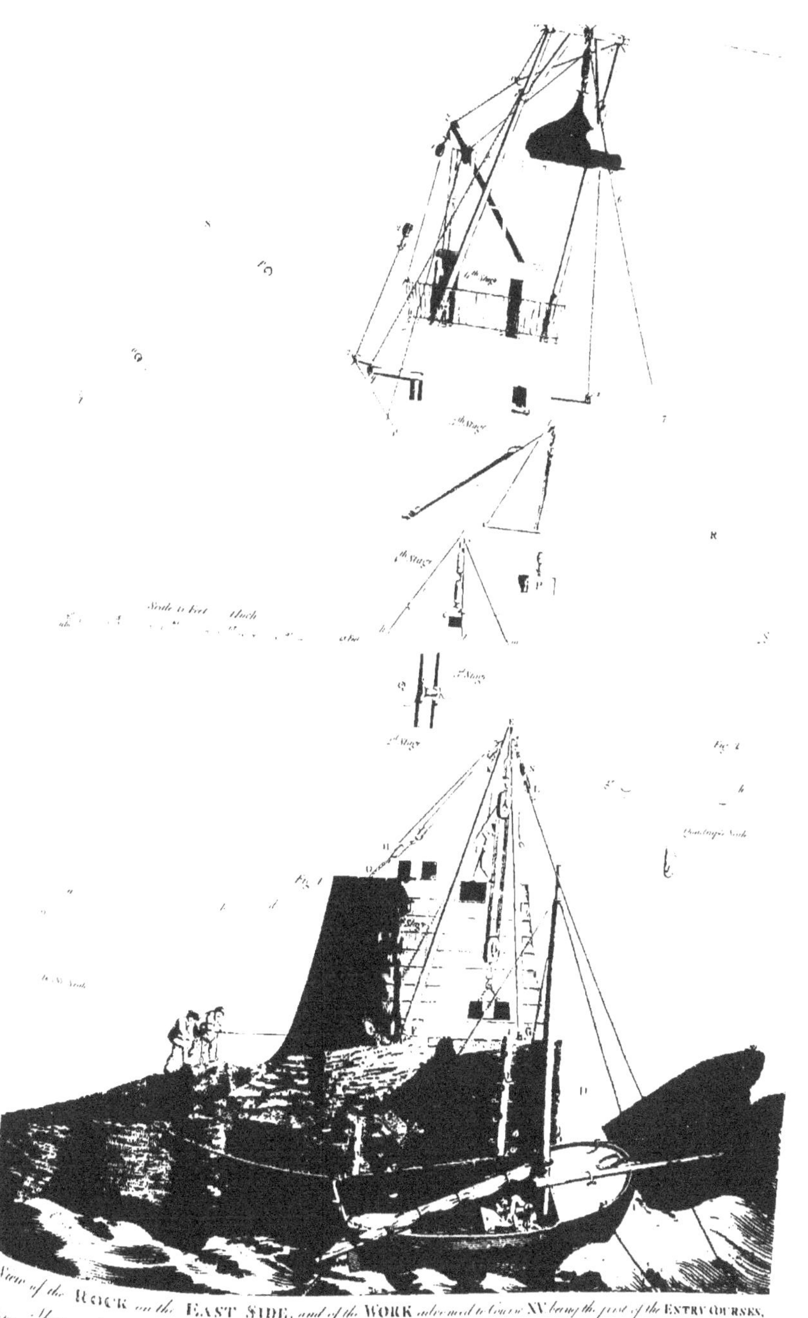

View of the ROCK on the EAST SIDE, and of the WORK advanced to Course XV being the first of the ENTRY COURSES, Shewing the manner of LANDING and HOISTING the STONES &c. in every Stage of the BUILDING.

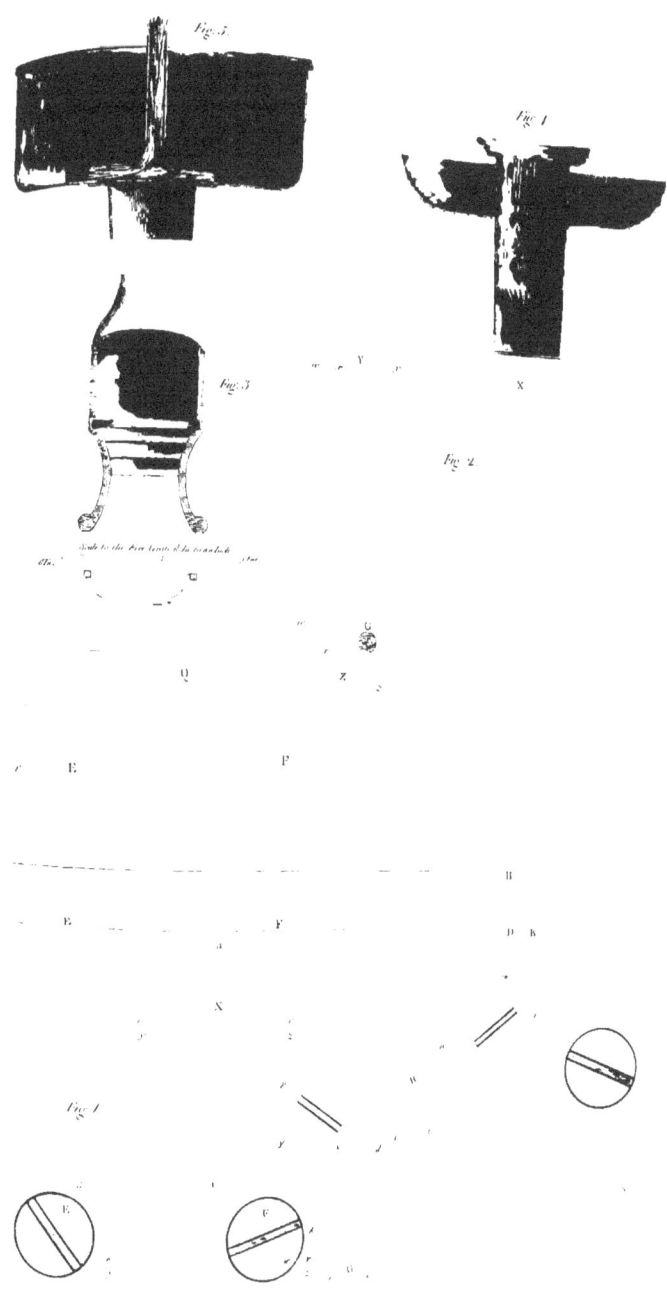

Scale of Feet

M^r. JESSOP's DRAUGHT *by which the* YAWLS *were built for the* EDYSTONE SERVICE.

J. Record sculp. 1786

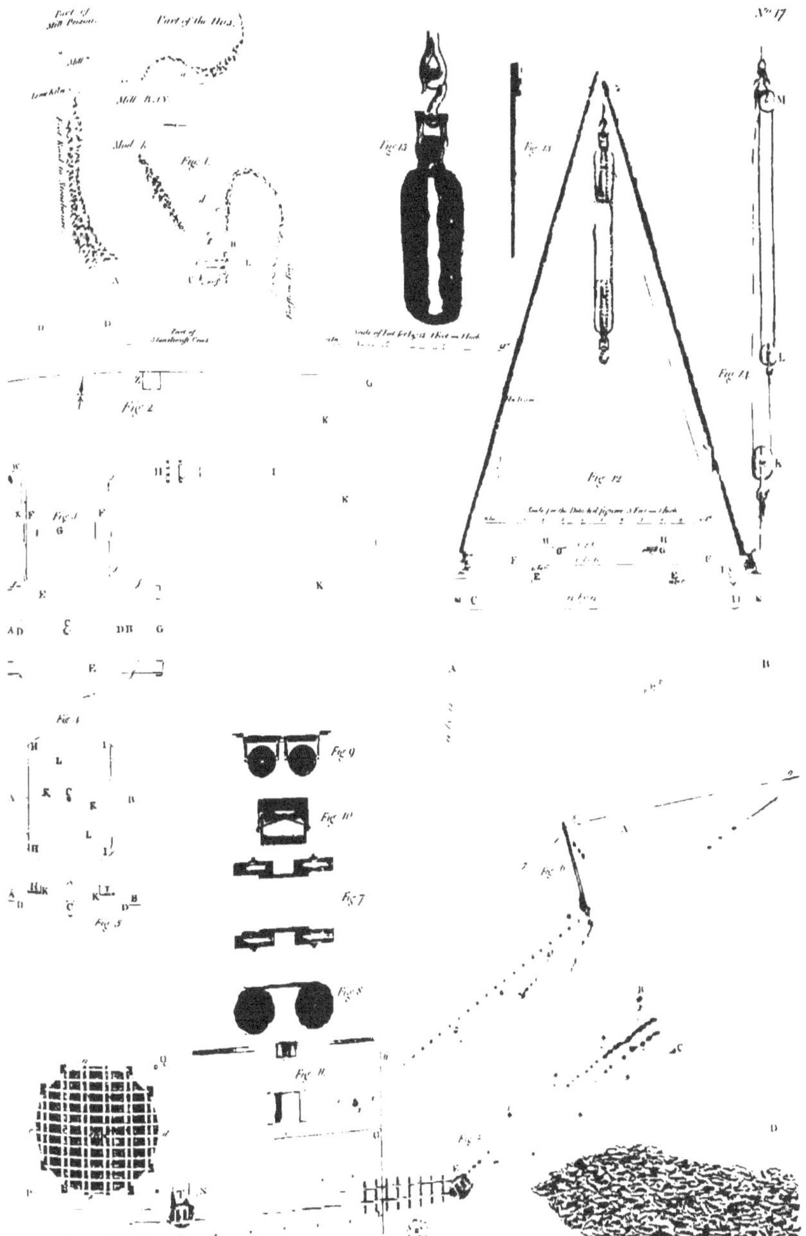

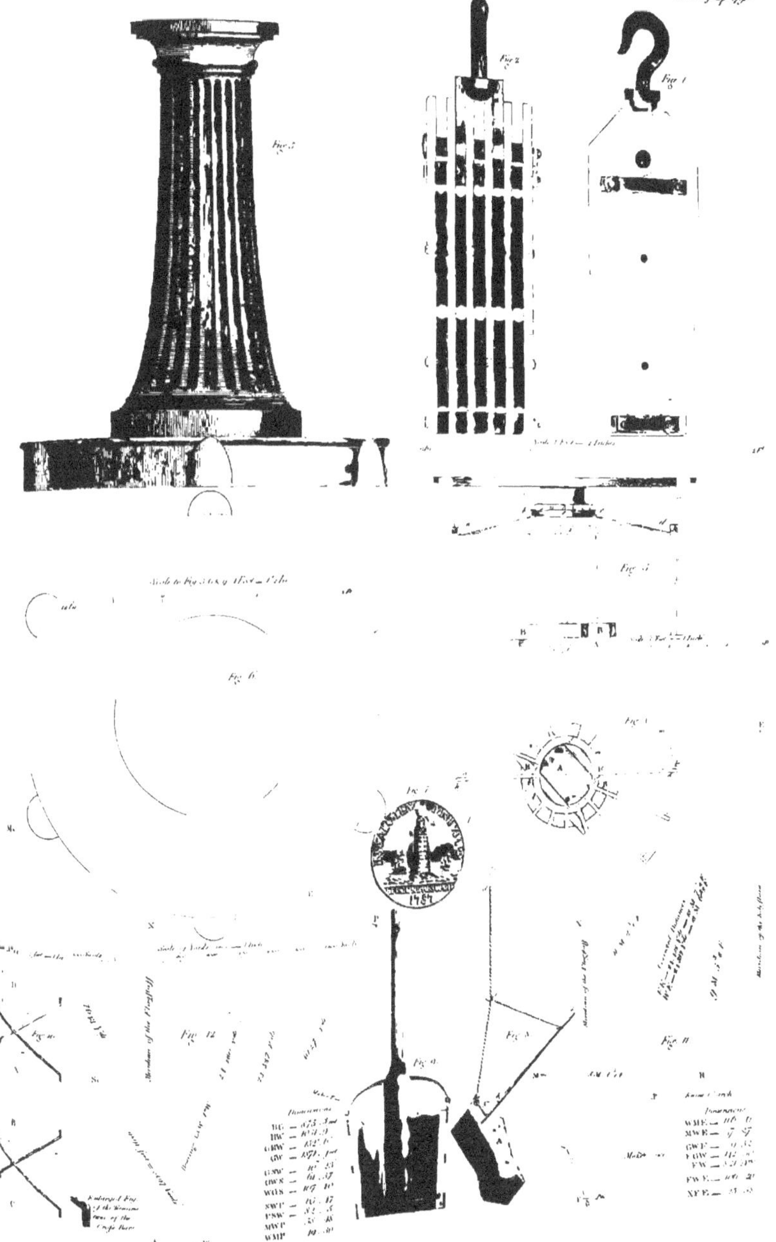

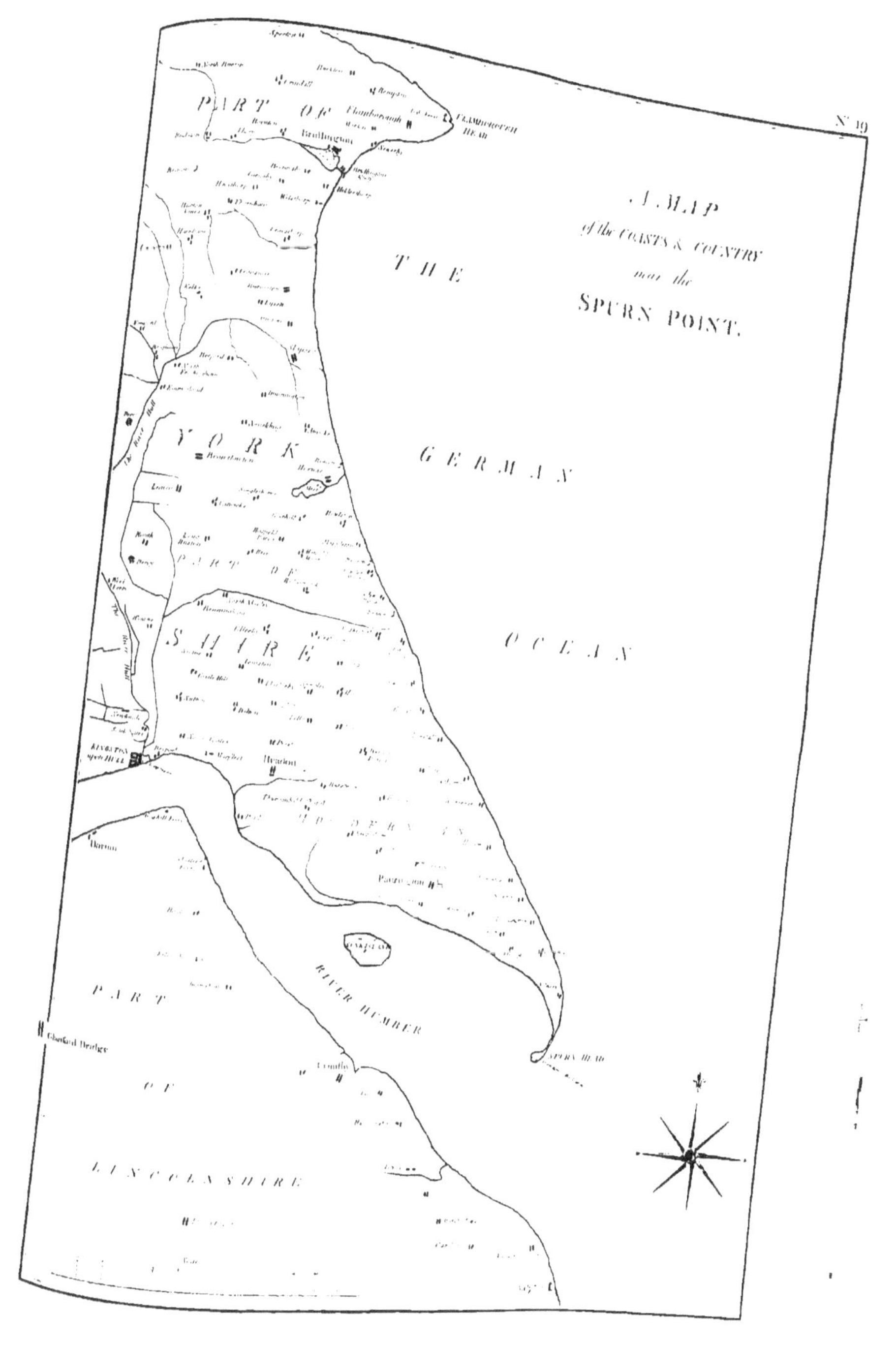
N° 19
A MAP
of the COASTS & COUNTRY
near the
SPURN POINT.
PART OF
YORK
SHIRE
THE
GERMAN
OCEAN
Flamborough
Bridlington
Headon
Patrington
RIVER HUMBER
PART
OF
LINCOLNSHIRE

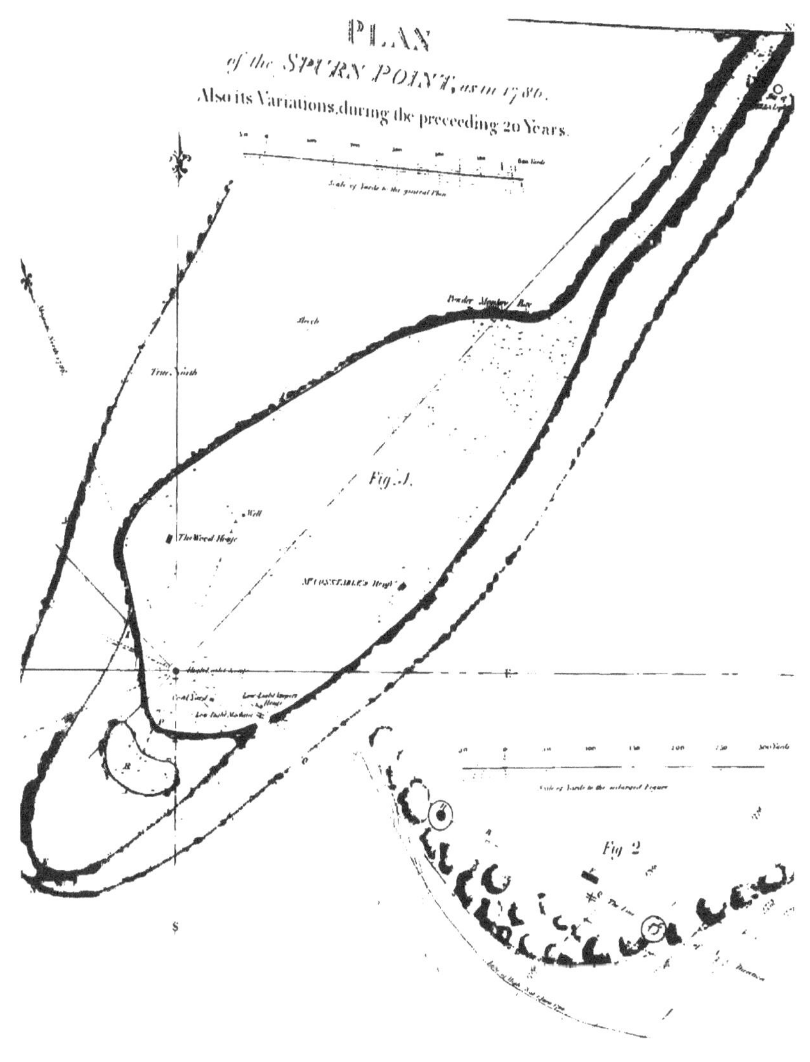
PLAN
of the SPURN POINT, as in 1786.
Also its Variations, during the preceeding 20 Years.
Scale of Yards to the general Plan
True North
Well
The Wood House
Fig. 1.
Fig 2

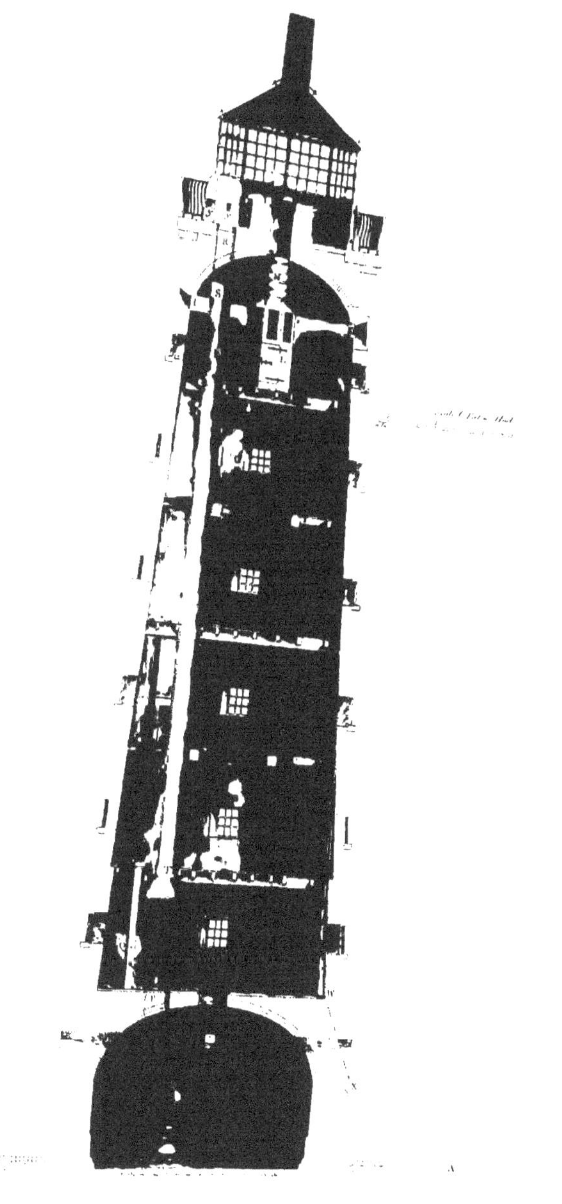

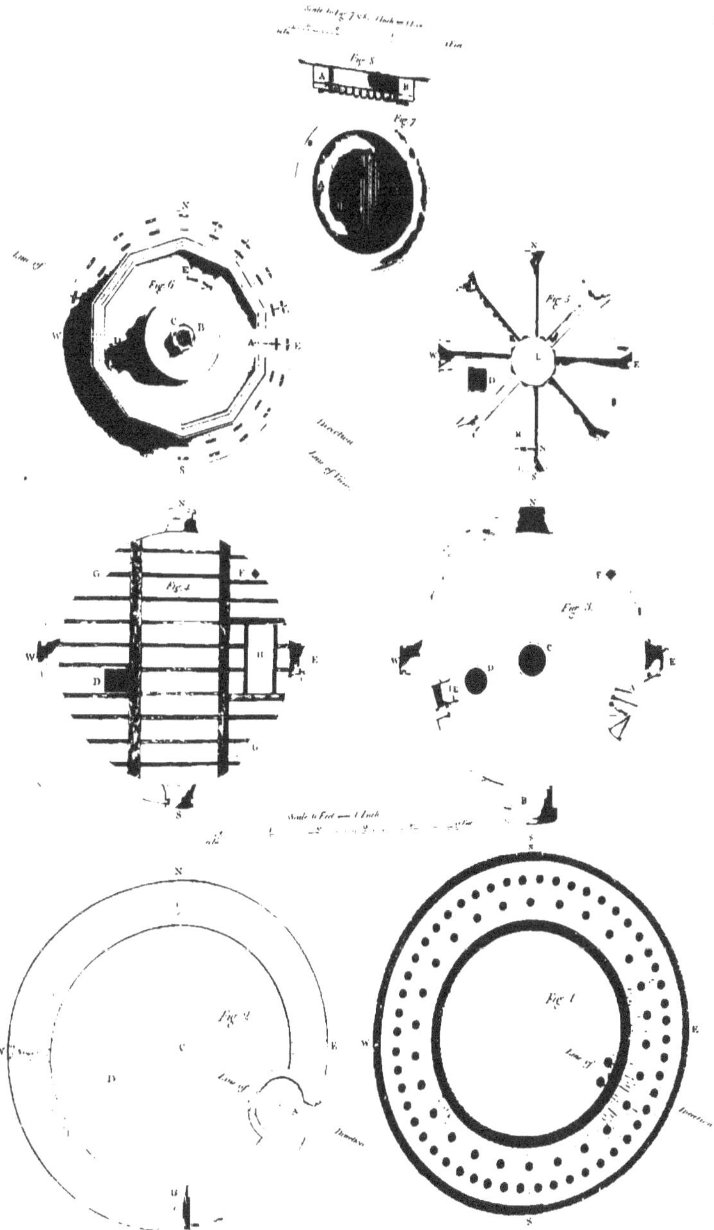
Fig. 8
A
B
Fig. 7
Fig. 6
N
W
S
E
C
B
A
Direction
Line of Vision
Fig. 5
L
D
N
S
W
E
Fig. 4
G
F
H
D
G
W
E
N
S
Fig. 3
F
C
D
E
W
E
B
N
Scale 6 Feet = 1 Inch
N
Fig. 2
W
E
C
D
Line of
A
Direction
B
S
N
Fig. 1
W
E
Line of
Direction
S

N° 23

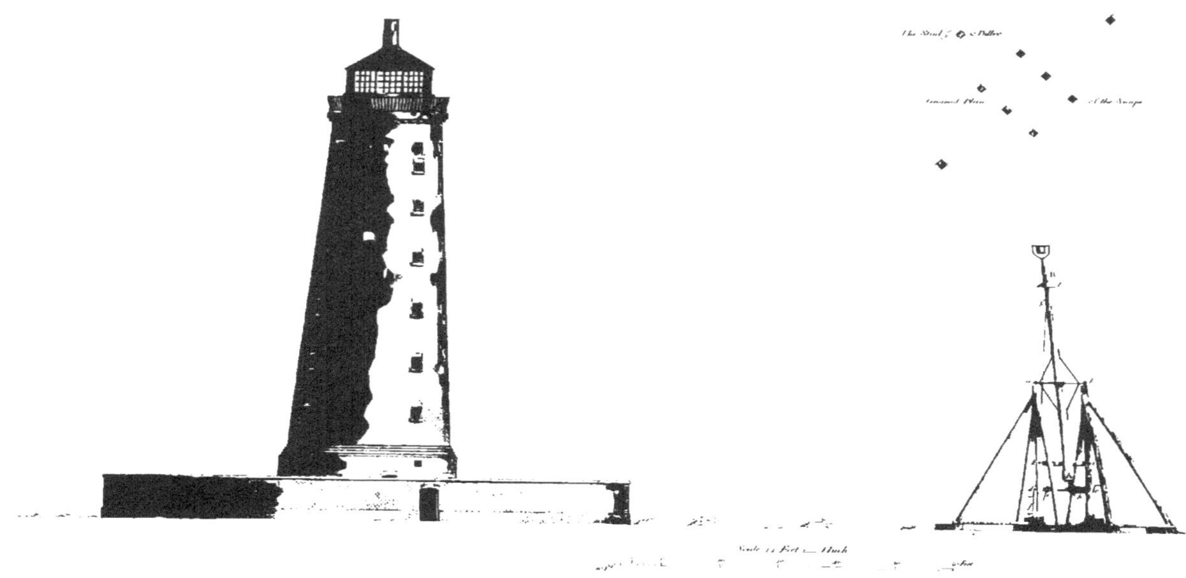

ELEVATION of the HIGH LIGHTHOUSE upon the SPURN POINT, & of the SWAPE by which the LOW LIGHT is Exhibited.

TECHNICAL REFERENCES TO THE PLATES.

THE VIGNETTE. *The* MORNING *after a* STORM, at S. W.

THE *Vignette*, as being placed in the title page, on that account claims priority: but in order of deſcription would have come in more naturally in a ſubſequent place. The intent of it is to give ſome idea of the nature of this ſituation in a ſtorm, and the violence of the ſeas upon this ſpot. The extraordinary ſwelling of the wave on the left hand, above the letter A, is doubtleſs owing to the gradual ſloping of the rocks underneath it, as will be more particularly explained in the ſubſequent *Plates*.——The wonderful riſing of the water, at B, by the ſtroke of it upon the building, which for the inſtant totally hides it from the eye, is certainly beyond what might be expected, or perhaps readily accounted for, from the reſiſtance of a round column; yet concurrent teſtimony from Mr. WINSTANLEY's deſcriptions (§ 17 and 21.) down to the preſent time leave no doubt of the height. This ſketch thereof, ſo far from being exaggerated is much reduced, both in height and bulk, in order that the idea of a building contained therein may preſent itſelf.——The *gathering* of the ſea at C is a natural conſequence of its being taken up by the ſouth *Reef* of rocks, which are fully deſcribed, Plate N° 3, to which I refer: as alſo to the Deſcription, § 301.

PLATE, N° 1. *A* GENERAL CHART *of the* SEAS *ſurrounding the EDYSTONE LIGHTHOUSE.*

The ſituation of the Lighthouſe in the chart will indicate its expoſure: for, if we ſuppoſe a line drawn from the point A upon the coaſt of *France*, to the *Lizard Point*, the diſtance being about 31 leagues, which may be eſteemed the width of the mouth of the *British Channel*, the *Edyſtone* will be found to lie only 15 leagues within this line; that is, leſs than half the width; and being expoſed to all winds from about S. by W. to W. by S. there will be nothing to hinder the *Ground Swells* of the *Bay of Biſcay* and of the *Atlantic Ocean* from coming home upon the Edyſtone Rocks uncontrouled, and even magnified, from the gradual leſſening of the ſoundings. See § 5 and 6.

PLATE, N° 2. MAP *of the* COASTS *and* COUNTRY *oppoſite the EDYSTONE ROCKS.*

This Map ſhews the general ſituation, and particular diſtances of the Edyſtone Rocks from the neareſt part of the coaſts of *Cornwall* and *Devonſhire*. The diſtance of the port of *Plymouth* being 14 miles, the *Mewſtone* or *Mayſtone* 11½, and the *Ram Head*, or perhaps more properly *Rame-head*, ſomewhat under 10.

PLATE, N° 3. *A* GENERAL PLAN *of the EDYSTONE ROCKS, as ſeen at low Water of a Spring Tide; comprehending every Thing liable to damage a Ship.*

From this Plan it appears from the ſoundings at low water, that the largeſt ſhips may ſail between the ſouth and the ſouth-eaſt *Reef*; upon a courſe between N. and N. N. E. or S. and S. S. W. by the compaſs, according to its preſent variation of two points weſt nearly; that is, in caſe of being inadvertently entangled; here being a clear width of 20 fathoms: but a veſſel ſailing up or down Channel upon any courſe from W. N. W. to N. W. by W. or the contrary; and giving the Lighthouſe a clear *birth* of 50 fathoms to the ſouthward, will be clear of the north end of the South Reef, full 30 fathoms, on one hand, and of the N. E. Rock as much on the other; in ſoundings of about 10 fathoms; and thus, a veſſel of any ſize, in moderate weather, may ſafely ſail within 50 fathoms of the Lighthouſe: but upon a S. W. or N. E. courſe, leaving the houſe on the eaſt, ſhe may ſafely paſs by the building at half that diſtance.

PLATE, N° 4. *South* ELEVATION *of the* ORIGINAL LIGHTHOUSE, *built upon the EDYSTONE ROCK, according to the firſt Deſign of WINSTANLEY. Taken from a perſpective Print drawn at the Rock by* JAAZIELL JOHNSTON, Painter.

A An *Eye Bolt* at the *Landing-place* for faſtening the Boats.——B The *ſloping ſurface* of the rock.——C The Foundation or *Baſement*, ſuppoſed to be of *ſtone*; and the horizontal joints of the courſes, to be bound round with *hoops of iron* or *copper*.——D The *Store Room*.——E The *State Room* (ſo called in the original) ſuppoſed alſo to ſerve as a lodging room.

F The *open Gallery* for looking out in fine weather, and ſuppoſed intended to let the ſeas go through in ſtorms.——G The *Kitchen*; ſuppoſed alſo to be uſed for lodging.——H The *Lantern*, about 8 feet diameter, corner and corner, and 7 feet high. N. B. The ornamental iron work appears to riſe near 18 feet above the uſeful part of the roof. See § 20.

PLATE, N° 5. *South* ELEVATION *of WINSTANLEY's LIGHTHOUSE upon the EDYSTONE ROCK; as it was finiſhed in the Year 1699. Drawn* orthographically *from a* perſpective *Print thereof, publiſhed by himſelf.*

A Repreſents the *Rock* at low water.——B The *Landing-place*, covered at half tide; and all the time the current runs eaſtward.

C The *Entry Door*.——DE The *Baſement*; which, in the fourth year's work, he deſcribes to have been added to the original one of 16 feet; ſo as to make an addition of four feet in thickneſs on every ſide. From the figure it ſeems, that on the weſt ſide at D, it has been a work of ſtone; the joints appearing to have been covered with *lead plates*, as before deſcribed of the original baſe; whereas the eaſt ſide E has the appearance of having been *wood*; and to have been bound together with *iron ſtraps*, as the whole of the ſuperſtructure evidently was.

F Is the *Store Room*, with a projecting cabin to the ſouth-eaſt.——G The *State Room*.——H The Kitchen.——I The open Gallery, or Platform.——K The *Lodging Room*.——L The attending or *Lanthorn* Room.

M The *Lantern* for the lights, ſurrounded by a Gallery or *Balcony*.——N The *Flag* uſed for making *Signals*.

PLATE, N° 6. *South* ELEVATION *and* SECTION *of RUDYERD's LIGHTHOUSE, completed in 1709. Repreſented as it ſtood previous to its* Demolition *by* Fire, *in the Year 1755.*

A Shews the *Rock* at low water of a ſpring tide.——B The *Landing-place*.

aa The *Steps* or Flats to which the rock was reduced. *bb* The *Branches*, &c. Floors of wood laid *lengthways* of the ſteps. *cd* Floors laid *croſswiſe* of the ſame. *ee* Courſes of *Compaſs Timber*.

D Five courſes of Moorſtone, which, with two courſes of wood marked E, completed the *entire ſolid*. To the top of which led

F The *Iron Ladder*, to G the *Entry Door*, and through G H the Entry or Paſſage, into H I the *Well-hole* for the ſtaircaſe.

K L The *Maſt*.——M Five courſes of Moorſtone, the height of which compoſed the entry or paſſage.——N Two beds of *Compaſs Timber*, making all good over the entry.

O Four beds of Moorſtone covered with two beds of Compaſs Timber; after which ſucceeded courſes of Timber alternately, *croſs* and *long*, with compaſs courſes interpoſed, as ſhewn in the ſection.

P Q Shew the upright timbers, or *Uprights*, as they appeared externally, being 71 in number.——*pq* the ſame in the ſection.

II The *Store Room* Floor; and R the Door of the Store Room; which was ſo much to the north of the entry, that when the caſks and ſtores were hoiſted up perpendicularly by a tackle, ſuſpended from above, they would clear the iron ladder.

S The *State Room*.——T The *Bedchamber*.——U The *Kitchen*.——W The *Balcony*.——X The *Lantern*.——Y The Lantern Door into the balcony.——Z The *Cupola* and Ball.

f Four curved Pipes for venting the ſmoke from the candles in the lantern.——*g* The top of the copper *Funnel* which paſſed through the lantern, from the kitchen fire place, which was of brick.

h The upper *Knees*, bent, or projection of the cornice, for throwing off the ſea, to prevent it from breaking the windows in time of ſtorms: which was neceſſary, though the panes were of *ground glaſs*, on account of ſtrength.

i *Knees* to ſtrengthen the junction of the *upright* with the balcony floor, and alſo in part to ſupport the weight of the lantern.

kkk The original *Knees* of compaſs timbers, to form the uprights to a circle, and ſupport the weight of the floors.——*mmm* *Knees* applied, of late years, for ſtrengthening the frame of the building.

nn The lower *Knees* at the foot of the uprights; and *oo* one of the *Stay bars* by which the knees were faſtened down.

p The place where a part of one of *Winſtanley*'s chains was jammed ſo faſt, on the deſtruction of that building, that it there remained, and was ſhewn as a curioſity of the place, during the time of the ſucceeding ſtructure.

q The natural *Cave* into which the lightkeepers retreated when the houſe was in flames.

N. B. The *technical references* to plates N° 4, N° 5. and N° 6, were inſerted in the body of the work; which the author thought it right no longer to encumber therewith; but are here inſerted, to preſerve the regularity of this part of the work.

The detached figure 2. ſhews the manner of jointing the five courſes of ſtone marked D (fig. iſt.) wherein K ſhews the *Maſt*, and *aa* the places of 8 upright Bars; *bb* being ſuppoſed two more of the ſame nature. The black lines ſhew the joints of the firſt courſe; the dotted lines those of the ſecond; and ſo alternately.

Fig. 3. Repreſents the manner in which the courſes of the bed of Moorſtone M (in fig. 1ſt) was jointed; wherein K is the *Maſt*, *abcd* the *Well-hole*, and *efgh* the *Entry* from the *Iron Ladder* into it. The jointing of the courſes in this [illegible] bed [illegible] were [illegible], according to the black and the dotted lines.—— T[illegible] may [illegible] courses of the bed of Moorstone O, if the passage [illegible].

PLATE, N° [illegible]. *A* PLAN *and* perspective ELEVATION *of the* EDYSTONE ROCK, [illegible] *from the* [illegible]. *Taken from the* [illegible] § 81, 175. [illegible] *the* THEODELITE.

The [illegible] on [illegible] the rock; *Fig.* 1. being the *Plan*, and *Fig.* 2. the [illegible] View. The same Letters refer to the same parts in both; the [illegible] upon the [illegible] answer to the [illegible] *Points*, E. W. N. S. according to the true [illegible].

[illegible] the [illegible], and C the *Summit* of the Rock; the general declivity being towards [illegible] S. W. [illegible] of the *laminated* moorstone that composes it being nearly [illegible] thereto. It has however, considerable irregularities: for upon the [illegible] Rock makes a [illegible] *drop* of 4½ or 5 feet (§ 7.); and by [illegible] westward, when there is a *ground swell* at S. W. the sudden [illegible] in an astonishing manner, even in moderate weather.

The [illegible] Rock is shewn, as supposed to have been for ages past; except [illegible] visibly altered by man's hand, chiefly within the circular area of the [illegible]. The flat *Treads* of the steps cut by *Rudyerd* are marked D; the [illegible] of the steps F; and E denotes the [illegible] parts, parallel to the [illegible] of the Rock.

[illegible] shew the remains of the cavities of eight of the 12 great irons fixed [illegible] which the stump of one only, viz. that at *a*, remained for my [illegible]; it was run in with lead, and had continued fast, till in planting a [illegible] there, it was cut out and found *club-ended*, see § 30. Which of the [illegible], that are left unmarked, make up the remaining four, I could not [illegible], as doubtless several of them appertained to the additional work that he [illegible] in the 4th year (§ 21).

Fig. 3. shews a pair of Rudyerd's iron *branches* (§ 36, 39) to a scale three times larger than that of the plan; wherein AB is the *main branch*, or *dove-tail* part; CD the [illegible], driven hard in, but without touching the bottom; their depth in the [illegible] the line EF its surface. The holes in the branches [illegible] timbers, by large bearded *spike bolts*.——Of those branches I traced 5th or 9th pairs, of different sizes; and two more modern: their places are shewn in the upright, *Fig.* 2. by inspection; and likewise in the plan, *Fig.* 1. at 1. 2. 3. 4. 5. and 6, 7, 8, 9, 10. &c. forming a double circle; also two pair of them at K [illegible] the mast, on two sides, to the center. The irons that remained [illegible] are distinguished in the plan by being hatched with *slant* lines, the empty [illegible] cavities by being black. Those that remained whole, whether [illegible] distinguished in *Fig.* 2. by their shapes.

X [illegible] the place of the [illegible] on the east side; and R a strong *Ring Bolt*, put into the Rock on the recommencement of the building in 1757, for fasten[illegible] of the *Sears*.

In *F*[illegible] 2. [illegible] shews the *three-legged* stool (§ 81) steadied with *cross* [illegible]. Upon [illegible] of the upper round plank [illegible] was screwed down the [illegible] T, to which [illegible] was screwed the long *horizontal Rule* TS, divided into [illegible] parts upon one edge, tending to the center.——Upon any [illegible] point of the Rock to be ascertained, suppose *x*, the rod *xy* was set upright [illegible] was preserved in an upright position by two small slips of [illegible] in two different directions. The divided edge of the [illegible] being brought against the upright rod, was shoved up by a short staff, [illegible] against the rod, till a *spirit level* laid upon the top of the [illegible] shewed it to be level. In this position the index would shew the degree and [illegible] of the [illegible], the upright rod would mark the distance from the center [illegible] the rule would mark upon the rod, how much the intersection was above its bottom at *x*, see § 81.

PLATE, N° 8. *South* ELEVATION *of the* STONE LIGHT-HOUSE *completed upon the* EDYSTONE *in* 1759. *Shewing a Prospect of the nearest Land, as it appears from the Rock in a clear calm Day.*

A The *Lantern-space*.——B The *Cove* in the east side of the Rock.——C The [illegible] cut to mount the Rock to the entry door.——D An Iron Rod, serving as a *Rail* to [illegible] by, in passing to the foot of the ladder, occasionally put out from the *Entry Door* at E.

Over the letter F [illegible] view of the land about *Whitsand-Bay*.——Over G the [illegible]——H [illegible]——I St. *Nicholas*, or *Drake's* Island.——K [illegible]——L [illegible] of Plymouth.——M Plymouth Town.——N [illegible]——O Mount *Batten*.——P Ships in *Catwater*.——[illegible] N. B. The *Cascade* shewn to the left of F must be [illegible] on the [illegible] of the water, the next moment to [illegible].

PLATE, N° 9. SECTION *of the* EDYSTONE LIGHT-HOUSE [illegible] *the East and West Line, as relative to* N° 8. [illegible] *the* LOW WATER *of a* SPRING TIDE.

[illegible] Rock, ABB [illegible] upright *Face* or *Drop*, marked with [illegible] BC shews the general direction of the [illegible] Rock [illegible] ward.

[illegible] of the [illegible] *first stone*. The black [illegible] of that is intersected by the [illegible] all course, [illegible] of the 2d. [illegible] 5 [illegible] the central [illegible] round Rock; *cd* [illegible] the ground

joint.——*f* Is the foot of the *temporary Ladder*; and there is shewn the manner in which the ground joint of the stone-work was sunk into the Rock, all round, at least three inches.——*h* Shews the first *marble Plug*, or central *Joggle*, that went through the 6th course, and reached half way through the 7th; and so on, in succession to the top of Course XIV.

ii In like manner shew, the place of the marble *cubic Joggles* inlaid between each two courses, which were in an octagon disposition round the center.——*l* Smaller cubes between the 5th and 6th course.

Course XIV. terminates the *entire solid*; as upon it is pitched the *entry* and *well-hole* for the stairs.——The temporary ladder *fg*, to the entry door D, is only put out when wanted; and then is lashed by eye-bolts to the stones; at other times, having a joint in the middle, it folds, and is laid along in the entry.

Above the top of the entire solid, the center stone being omitted to give space for the Well, the cubic joggles were of double the number, and half the size.——*Course* XXIV. terminated that part of the building called *the Solid*: and here the habitable part of the building began, whereof E is the *lower* Store-room.——F The *Store-room Door*.——G The upper *Store-room*.——H The *Kitchen*.——I The *Fire-place*, from which the smoke ascends through the floors and lantern, through a *copper funnel*, as per *section*, and through the *ball*.

K The *Bed Room*.——L The *Stone Basement* of the *Lantern*.——M The *Lantern Door* into the *Balcony*, and N the *Cupola*.

The ascent from room to room is by perforations through the middle or *Key-stone* of every floor; and the detached figure shews the means, by inclined step ladders, removable at pleasure.

PLATE, N° 10. PLANS *of the* ROCK *after being cut, and prepared to receive the* STONE BUILDING. *Shewing the Six* FOUNDATION COURSES.

Fig. 1. Plan of the Rock, as prepared for the stone-work, somewhat extended to shew how it applies to the plate N° 7. The line AB shews also here the place where the surface drops, as specified N° 9.

In this figure, *Course* I. appears in its place, as fixed with its *Trenails* and *Wedges*, § 222, 223. The part darker shaded, and marked DD, was not reduced to a *dove-tail* on account of fissures, but was sunk two inches lower than the rest of *Course* II. The stones laid therein would therefore be encompassed by a border, and held fast in every direction. The letters E. W. N. S. in all the figures denote the *Cardinal Points*; the same letters in every figure denoting the same parts.——The part of the Rock marked C, rises above the rest by an ascent or step of 15 to 18 inches, according to the line FDGE; which, laying somewhat without the general contour of the building, and affording a firm abutment, the advantage was taken; and the work of the 1st and 2d course carried against it, as shewn at G.

N° 1, 2, 3, 4, 5, 6 shew the level platforms, or *steps*, for the different courses, whose upper sides are even with these numbers in *Section* N° 9; N° 2 being upon the level of *Rudyerd's* lowest step.——X denotes a piece of stone engrafted into the Rock; serving as a bridge to cross a *Chasm*, opened by cutting down the top of the Rock to that level, into the *Cove*. Out of this stone is formed a part of the border that encircles the work.

Fig. 2. shews how the buttress G was terminated in the 2d *course*. It also shews the places of the *Trenails* and *Wedges*; which in all these figures are shewn in the same manner. The *dotted* lines every where refer to the course that is to come on; and shews how it will *break joint* upon the course supposed laid.

Fig. 3. shews how the space HIK, in *Fig.* 2. is filled up in *Fig.* 3. being confined in, by the rise of the step L at HI, and the *cramps a* and *b*; the ground proving here irregularly shattered by cutting the steps for the former Lighthouse.

Fig. 4. shews the structure of *Course* IV. where in this, as all the others, the stones lighter-coloured denote the *Portland*, the darker the *Moorstone*.

Fig. 5. shews the position of three *joggle holes* Y, betwixt this course and the next above.

Fig. 6. shews *Course* VI. complete, which brings the whole work to a level with the reduced Rock: it shews the joggle *holes* for the eight cubes; and the central *plug joggle*, fixed in place at O, ready for the reception of the center stone of the next *Course* N° VII.

PLATE, N° 11. PLANS *of all the different* COURSES *from the Top of the* ROCK *to the Top of the* BALCONY FLOOR *inclusive.*

Fig. 1. is the proper plan of Course VII. relative to the Section, Plate N° 9. As being the first entire course, the trenails and wedges are shewn; but afterwards omitted in the draughts, to prevent crowding the figures. The black lines and dotted lines shew the joints of the alternate courses. The center stones, and the four stones surrounding, were alternately of the same size to the top of Course XIV.——*a* is the center plug, first set: *bb* the square part of the center stone; from each of whose four sides a dove-tail projects, and thereon are fixed the four stones *cc*, by joint wedges and trenails, as per figure; which five stones united, make one stone, sufficiently large to receive eight smaller dove-tail stones *dd*; and whose projecting parts form dove-tails to receive another circle, or order of stones, fixed like the former. The cubic joggles are shewn at *ee*.

Fig. 2. gives the plan of the XIVth *Course*, ending the *fundamental solid*, and on which the entry and well-hole are begun. It also shews the diminution from *Course* VII. Upon this figure is shewn the distribution of the smaller cubic joggles, which take place upon the *entire* solid. The entry here appears to have a small *inclination* with the E. and W. line, which was not noticed in *Section*, N° 9, to avoid ambiguities.

Fig. 3. is the plan of Course XV. being the first of the entry door and well course.

Fig. 4. is the plan of *Course* XVIII. shewing the work of the entry closed in, and the solid reunited. Also the manner of *heat jointing* the four stones round the center to each other; which in the courses below the entry door, were united by by dove-tails to the center ſtone. Joint wedges were applied in the hook, as per *figure*. Thus the arrangement, in circles from the center, was again complete. In the entry courſes, as every piece had at leaſt one cubic joggle and two trenails, the work was ſecure againſt all ordinary attacks of the ſea; the weak-neſs being on the eaſt ſide: but when capped and bound together by this XVIIth *Courſe*, the whole was again conſidered as one *entire ſtone*, out of which the cavity had been cut.

Fig. 5. ſhews *Courſe* XXIII. ready for putting on the cap courſe of the ſolid.

Fig. 6. gives the *cap courſe*, making the *ſtore-room floor*, in its finiſhed ſtate; the firſt courſe of the habitable part of the building, viz. *Courſe* XXV. being upon it; and ſhewing the *ſtore-room door*, with its *joggles*, *joint ſtones*, and *cramps*.—— The detached figure, relative to it, ſhews a part of the top of the wall of *Courſe* XXV. to a triple ſcale; wherein *hhii* denotes one of the pieces of ſtone, whereof 16 complete the circle: *ſ* ſhews one of the *joggles* uſed in this part of the building; being ſlices of marble the ſize of a *common brick*, let half its thickneſs into the middle of the ſtone; ſo that the next courſe above, breaking joint upon the middle of this, according to the dotted line *p r*, half the joggles length will take one of the upper ſtones, whoſe joint comes upon it, and the other half joggle, the other: by which means every ſtone is fixed to its place, as it were, by two *ſteady pins*, one at each extreme. The black lines *hi* ſhewing the joint at each end of this ſtone; the ſmall *lozenge* figures *k* and *l* ſhew the ſhape of *grooves*, cut from the top to the bottom of each end of each ſtone, and which, when two are joined together, form that figure: *k* denotes the lozenge empty, or unfilled, and *l* the lozenge filled with a *joint ſtone*. See § 256, 257.—— *m n* ſhews the ſhape of one of the *cramps*, in upright; and *op* as ſeen upon the flat. The holes in the ſtones at *q r* are bored, to receive the round ſhanks of the cramp, and the rectangular cavities *q r* are ſunk, to bury the flat of the cramp *op*.

Fig. 7. gives the plan of the *Kitchen Floor*, and the upper bed of *Courſe* XXIX. that encircles it; ſhewing one of the *endleſs chains*, of which, as appears in *Section* N° 9. there are two to each floor. The *detached figure* ſhewing an enlargement of the chain, and groove that contains it, will need no comment, after peruſal of § 258. —— In the *principal figure* the dotted lines at *s* ſhew the place of the *fire grate*; *t t* the *ſink*; *v v* the *dreſſer*; *w w* the *ſettle*; *x* a place for a *clow table*; leaving a vacancy to the window between each. § 287.

Fig. 8. is the plan of the *Bedchamber*, taken upon the top of *Courſe* XLIII. which gives the horizontal ſections of the windows.—— *y y y* Shew the places of the three *cabin beds* for the lightkeepers, § *ibid.* *z* The hole in the floor for the *copper funnel* from the kitchen, and *a* ſhews the place of the *clock*.—— In the *detached figure*, *b b* ſhews how the cramps are diſpoſed in the *reduced jambs* of the windows. *c* Shews the plan of the *rabbet*, to receive the ſhutters or *ports* of the windows, whereof the uprights are ſeen in *Plate* N° 8 and 9. *d* Shews the *ſill* of the clear opening; againſt the ſolid of which, the window frame *ef*, and ſaſhes are lodged; the whole of which go in together, and are held in by wooden pins, two above, and two below, as ſhown at *g g*; the holes being bored in the ſolid ſtone. If thoſe pins are cut off, the whole can be drawn out and renewed, without injury to the ſtone work. The joint of the wood frame with the ſtone work, is ſecured againſt wet by white lead and oil.

Fig. 9. ſhews the *plan* of the *Cap* of the *main Column*, being in *Plate* N° 9. the XLVIth *Courſe*, and compoſes the *Balcony Floor*. *h h* Shews the *man hole* in the center correſpondent to the other floors: *i* the *funnel hole* accordant with *z* in the laſt figure. The dotted lines *k k* trace out the octagon *baſe* of the *lantern*. The place of the *under rail* of the balcony is ſhewn by the dotted lines *m m*; and *n n n* denote *ſections* of the *ſtuds* upon which thoſe rails are ſupported, correſpondent to the uprights of *Plates* N° 8 and 9.

PLATE, N° 12. *An enlarged* HORIZONTAL *and* VERTICAL SECTION *of the* EDYSTONE LANTERN, *more particularly deſcribing the* general Frame; *the* Windows *and* Apparatus *for moving and managing the* Chandeliers.

Fig. 1. is the horizontal, and *Fig.* 2. the upright *ſection* of the *Lantern*; the ſcale being three times larger than of *Plates* N° 8 and 9.

The eight corner *pillars* are of *caſt iron*, and, by large *claws* at top and bottom, are ſcrewed upon flat wrought iron bars, of one inch in thickneſs, and four inches in breadth; by which the whole frame is connected together, in a manner that will be more diſtinctly ſhown in *Plate* N° 15. what is peculiarly ſhown in this Plate is as follows:

The ſame letters denoting the ſame parts in each figure above mentioned: *a b* ſhews the *iron ring* of the *great chandelier*; 6 feet 4 inches diameter, and containing 16 candles: *c d* is the *ſmaller chandelier*, and contains 8 candles; diameter 3 feet 4 inches; their reſpective ſizes being ſuch as to diſtribute the candles as near as may be equally over the area of the lantern; ſo as to affect one another as little as poſſible by their heat. Theſe *two rings*, though of different ſizes, are of the *ſame weight*, and therefore a *counterpoiſe* to each other. The circumference of the great ring *a b*, is divided into four equal parts at the points *e f g h*; where four ſtaples or *eyes* are fixed, by which the ring being ſuſpended *horizontally* by cords, each quarter will be equally ſupported: and if two of theſe cords, as *e f* and *g h* are brought together, and reſpectively united into one, at a convenient height above the plain of the ring, ſo as to form an inverted V, then each *half* of the ring will become ſuſpended by a ſingle cord, in an horizontal poſition. In the *upright* let the points *i* and *l* be the two points of ſuſpenſion, after the union of the lines reſpectively; the cord *i k* being one of the ſuſpending lines, and *l m* the other. Now each of theſe cords paſſing reſpectively over the *pullies* AB, CD, and then turning downwards cloſe to each other, terminate each in an *hook* at *n o*; and there, each hooking hold of one and the ſame ſmall ring; and this ring having a ſufficient weight attached to it, will ſuſtain and balance the great chandelier, in an horizontal poſition.

The leſſer chandelier is alſo divided into four, and furniſhed with ſtaples, according to the letters *p r s q*, from whence proceed cords, as *p n*, *q n*, *r n*, *s n*, which all unite in the ſmall ring at *n o*; the leſſer ring being, as ſaid, as heavy as the larger, ſerves it for the *counterpoiſe required*.—— Again, if from the points of the *large ring e f g h*, on the under ſide, four cords are appendant, and are united, two and two, as above, ſo as each to form an erect Y, whoſe points of union are at *x z*; then the cords *x z*, *x 3*, *w* 1 be perpendicularly under the cords *i k*, *l m*, reſpectively. Alſo if from two oppoſite points underſide of the *leſſer ring*, two cords are affixed, as *t u*, *o v*, united at *v*, and thence dependant, then if the cord *w x* is pulled, it is evident that it hauls down the *leſſer chandelier*, and raiſes the *greater*; and if *either* of the cords *z* 2 or *z* 3 is pulled, it will haul down the larger chandelier, and raiſe the leſſer: and it will do it ſo as to be [illegible] *horizontal poſition* raiſe the leſſer chandelier: which giving leave to the hook at *o* to riſe, in effect gives leave to the rope *m l* to deſcend; and conſequently the whole circumference of the great chandelier falls or riſes together.

The upper works of the lantern having no affixture to the ſtone work but its own weight, I judged it proper to tie that, as well as the whole of the ſtone baſement down to the top of the building. E, F, G, H, ſhew bars in the angles of the lantern, whoſe *dog-heads* lay hold of the baſe of the iron work, and paſſing down the angle, form a *ſtirrup* as at K K, which is confined down by a ſcrew bolt paſſing through the arch. I, I, L, L denote air-holes of about 2 inches in diameter, which can be opened or ſtopped occaſionally, by a *kind of valve*.—— The *copper funnel*, fully ſhown in *Plate* N° 9, is here ſuppoſed not put up, except that part which paſſes through, and connects with the *ball*; the conſtruction whereof, ſo as to make a double ſet of vents, for the kitchen and for the lantern, without interference, will be beſt conceived by adverting to the *detached Fig.* 3. which is an horizontal ſection of the ball, and tubes, through the middle. The central tube (to which the funnel applies) being ſuſtained by *ſix partitions*, between that tube, and the neck of the *cupola*.—— The *ſtrengthening bars* of the cupola, the *crown*, the *angle pieces*, the *lantern door* into the balcony, and the *ſeat*, will appear ſufficiently plain by inſpection.

It is however to be noted, that the *croſs bars* of the ſaſh frames being an *afterthought*, they are here repreſented, rather as afterwards I would have wiſhed them, than as they really were, and which will be hereafter given. This figure ſuppoſes them caſt in one piece with the ſaſh frame; but yet ſo as not to interfere with the glaſs panes. The *detached Fig.* 4. is a ſection of a *window bar*, of its real ſize: the *croſs bars* are ſuppoſed to go no farther than the line *ab*, *a b* being on the inſide, and *c d* on the glaſs ſide.—I ſhall take this opportunity of remarking, that it would be unneceſſary to continue theſe croſs, or *diagonal* bars, over the *middle pane* of each ſaſh, as the *ſtrength* would be preſerved without it, and the *light* through each middle tier of panes *uninterrupted* for the exhibition of the lights.—— *p p* Shew *braſs pins*, two in each ſide of each pane, to keep the glaſs ſteady, independent of the *putty* neceſſary to render the panes *water-tight*.

PLATE, N° 13. *Original* IDEAS, HINTS, *and* SKETCHES, *from whence the general* Form *of the* PRESENT BUILDING *was taken.*

Fig. 1. ſhews the *Bole* of a *ſpreading Oak*, its ſide branches being lopped off, riſing out of the ground with a ſweep, its *waiſt* diminiſhing till the ſides become perpendicular; and on the inſertion of the great *boughs*, again ſwells, and overhangs. See § 65. p. 42.

Fig. 2. the manner in which the ſmaller *boughs* and *branches* are obliquely inſerted into the greater, with the *reverſing* curves that form the union. § *ibid.*

Fig. 3. A ſpecimen of *Paving* to be found in the *walking paths* of *London ſtreets*, being a mode of *dovetailing in flat*. See § 66. p. 43.

Fig. 4. A ſample of *dovetailing in the upright*, taken from *Belidor's Archit. Hydraul.* Part II. Tom. I. *Plate* 24. *Fig.* 2. See § *ibid.*

Fig. 5. A copy of the *firſt complete Deſign* made out for the *ſolid courſes* of the Edyſtone. The only material alteration afterwards was to diminiſh the ſize and weight of the outward circle of ſtones. § *ibid.* and alſo 77 and 82.

Fig. 6. Is a reduced copy to half the original ſize, of the *firſt laſt ſection* for a *Stone Building*, as exhibited to the proprietors § 68. p. 44. The principal difference afterwards, aroſe from finding leſs area upon the rock; and the neceſſity of *ſize* and *convenience* in the *habitable* [illegible].

PLATE, N° 14. *A* VIEW *of the* ROCK *on the* EAST SIDE, *and of the Work advanced to Courſe* XV. *the firſt of the* ENTRY COURSES: *ſhewing the Manner of* Landing *and* hoiſting *the* Stones, *&c. in every after Stage of the* BUILDING.

Fig. 1. ſhews the *Buſs* [illegible] in the *Gut*, delivering her cargo; PQ ſhew the two *fender Piles*, to prevent her rubbing againſt the rock. C The *Landing place*. X The *Cove*, here ſeen in front. D The Gut, through which a momentary caſcade makes its way; and which was propoſed to be ſtopped. § 84. EFG The *Sheers*; from the head of which are ſuſpended the *main tackle blocks* AB, whoſe tackle fall, after going to the *pulley* [illegible] E, paſſes to the [illegible]. [illegible] whole frame being of iron, is faſtened to the rock, as per *figure*.—— The enlarged *detached figure* [illegible], ſhews the *frame* and [illegible], as ſeen from the ſnatch block: *b* ſhews the ſide view thereof, the roll being ſeen endways: and *d* [illegible] ſhews the manner of coupling the [illegible] to the [illegible] ſhews, by a figure ſtill more enlarged, the upper end of the ſtanchions for receiving the *gudgeons* of the roll.

While the ſtone is hoiſting, the man repreſented at I is heaving-in the tackle fall, of the *runner and tackle* HK. [illegible] the ſtones are cleared of the boat, the ſheers lay out conſiderably, and the *back-bone guy* [illegible] M is fixed. This croſſes the *gut*, and is fixed by a ring bolt to one of the rocks of the [illegible]. By ſuch time therefore as the ſtone is hoiſted by the main tackle to the height of the entry door, the ſheers are got into the perpendicular; and then by eaſing the [illegible] The runner and tackle guy tackle L N the ſtone comes into the *entry door*.—— [illegible] HK is hooked to the *guy chain* O, which croſſes the work, and paſſes down to the ring on the weſt ſide of the rock; marked R in *Plate* [illegible].

In the *detached Fig.* 2. the [illegible] piece of iron by which the main tackle blocks are hung, is ſhewn to an enlarged ſcale at *e f g h*. This anchor being ſuſpended pen[illegible] that passes through the tops of the two shear legs, [illegible] and always putting itself in a perpendicular position, [illegible] upon them, without any unnatural strain or twist, [illegible] the greatest weight possible.——In like manner the two [illegible] the two guy tackles hooked to them, the action [illegible] and the feet of the shears turning [illegible] the rock, they are at liberty to conform themselves to the [illegible] upon the legs is always *constant*.

When the b[illegible] raised to the height shewn *Fig.* 1. the work was hoisted through [illegible] at the top of the *stairs*, by means of the *triangle* [illegible] wherewith the work was set; and are shewn as standing upon the [illegible] by the letters *i k l m*, being the 4th [illegible] But after that was completed, the [illegible] being too small, and the height too great, [illegible] was established, as shewn at the 3d *stage* [illegible] at Q, and a pair of [illegible] *shears*, the figure whereof is shewn at [illegible] the wall, at the *kitchen* floor; which, instead of [illegible] longer than the rest, whose bottom or foot being cut [illegible] internal angle of the opposite wall; and was long enough [illegible] sufficiently for the stone at P to clear the wall. The shears themselves were prevented falling over by a *Luff tackle* *, shewn upon the back leg, [illegible] lower block hooked upon a *Lewis*, in that stone the back leg [illegible] upon, by which it was brought tight and steady. When the stone was to be [illegible], this tackle being a little slacked, till the notch could be *disengaged*, and then [illegible] upon, the back leg would, by going over the wall, suffer the shears to come to the perpendicular, or beyond it.——The stones now become in general [illegible] tackle was employed at the shear head, which would go down [illegible] the entry door, and there met the stones hoisted by the great shears: the tackle fall of the moveable shears, being taken to the *jack roll* Q, the stones were got to the top of the building, in the same time they were raised from the [illegible] to the [illegible].——The [illegible] *figure* R is the *plan* of the *moveable* [illegible] where the [illegible] *rope* *n*, is shewn at the foot of the back leg. See § 2[illegible].

In this manner all the heavy materials were got up; the moveable shears rising [illegible] was to be let upon the *lantern*.——The 6th *stage* [illegible] for this purpose. *See* § 2[illegible]4. The great shears being now [illegible] and put through the windows of the uppermost room, [illegible] well steadied, served as *Booms*. The *detached figure* S being the [illegible] particular disposition; wherein *o p* shew the places [illegible] shears used for this particular purpose; also marked with [illegible] the relative *upright*. In this the rope *q r* shews a side *stay* to [illegible] the *pin* of the leg *p r*, each fastened to *q r*, the extremes of [illegible]——[illegible] each end of the [illegible] at the head of the *shear poles* pro[illegible] which [illegible] in one *guy rope* at [illegible], proceeds over a pul[illegible] the end of [illegible] timber at [illegible] from thence, with the intermediation [illegible] 1, 2, [illegible] proceeds [illegible] at the extreme end of the boom 3; and [illegible] principally lay on this *guy*, the *stay* or *fixed rope* [illegible] through the window of the room below, and is there [illegible] the tackle 1, 2 the shears can be let go over as [illegible] into the perpendicular; but to counteract this [illegible] and keep all steady, the rope 5, 6, 7, with a small tackle upon it, per[illegible] office of an [illegible] *guy*, fixing to the same ring in the rocks, as that of the main shears had before done. This apparatus enabled the *cupola* to be hoisted and set on whole without a *bruise*.

PLATE, N° 15. EXPLANATORY SKETCHES *of* particular Parts *comprehended in the foregoing* GENERAL DESCRIPTIONS.

Fig. 1. is the *plan* of the iron work, at each angle of the lantern, to its full size. A B B the line of the inside; and C D D that of the outside of the *groundsill*, of wrought iron; and the line D B shews the *mitre joint* of two continuous bars. [illegible] D shews the horizontal section of half of one of the *corner* [illegible] and *d* [illegible] shews the plan of the *claw* cast upon each side [illegible] the screws E F in each claw, serve to screw down the pillars [illegible] bars, and unite them all together; and are the same at top as [illegible].——The [illegible] *p q r s*, being screwed on before the pillars were fixed, served to unite the bars together; and the quadrangular space, [illegible] being sunk lower on the side [illegible] the opposite, shews that the *dog-head* of [illegible] upon the *fig.*, without danger of being displaced.——The [illegible] shew the inside, and *y z* the outside of an horizontal section of [illegible] being the rabbat in which they are lodged. *w*, *b*, 1, 2, [illegible] border, that goes round the circumference of each [illegible] by screws of *copper*, represented at G G, this border is fixed to [illegible] *e f g*, which surrounds the face of the pillars.——[illegible] and 5, 6 the outside contour, of the *ribs* or *sash bars*, [illegible] *t*, *u*, *x*, *o*, 6. The *detached figure* X, as in N° [illegible] of the window bars; the part 4 being supposed [illegible] *figure*.

Fig. [illegible] to the *Plan*, (*Fig.* 1.) wherein A B B is [illegible] C D D the [illegible] bars. D B X is the ele[illegible] D B X Y Z R S shews the *upright* of one of the [illegible] and the corresponding dotted line *y z r t* shews the [illegible] is marked *e f g* (in *Fig.* 1.) G G [illegible] copper bolts, that fix the border of [illegible] the pillars. E E, F F, the two [illegible] Shews the inside of the copper [illegible] the space P Q at top and bottom, [illegible] border, to make all good to the [illegible] the claws by the square bar [illegible] *P*[illegible] (*F*[illegible]) which is rivetted upon [illegible] screws.

Fig. 3. [illegible] venting the smoke, [illegible] to an enlarged scale. The *detached* *figure* below it, is the plan of the upper bar; the lowest being straight, and the intermediate ones reconciled to them.

Fig. 4. gives a *Section* of the *Socket* for the *Candles*; and

Fig. 5. that of the *Lamps*, both to their full size.

PLATE, N° 16. *Mr.* JESSOP's DRAUGHT, *by which the* YAWLS *were built for the* EDYSTONE SERVICE.

All that I think it necessary to remark upon this plate is, that the original drawing from whence this is copied, was sufficient for the direction of the *Boat-builder*; and that those *Yawls* answered well in a *short hollow sea*.

PLATE, N° 17. PLAN *and* DESCRIPTION *of the* WORK-YARD *at* MILL-BAY, *with its* FURNITURE *and* UTENSILS.

Fig. 1. The general *Plan* of *Mill-Bay*, wherein the dotted line *a b c* shews the line of *low water* spring tides. *d e* The *channel* dug from low water to convey vessels to the head of the jetty *f g*. *b i k l* The area of the *Work-yard*. Since the removal of this work, has been built L the *Long Room*; B the *Baths*; A C the *marine Barracks*; and D D new streets of *Stone-house*.

Fig. 2. *Plan* of the *Work-yard* and *Jetty*. A B C D is the line terminating the head of the Channel. Now any vessel laying against the two large piles B C, on which a pair of *shears* being erected, can be unloaded of her cargo of stone, and delivered upon a *wheel carriage*; that passing along the jetty to the *turn-rail* E, the carriage is there turned round till it becomes fair with the *rail-road* E F; and passing along it, enters the work-yard, whose boundary is marked by G G G G.——At T is another *turn-rail*, which enables the carriage to go on with its burthen; either in the streight line, or to turn there and go along the rail-road in the middle of the yard, and arriving at any destined point, suppose H, it is there met by a *roll-carriage*; for which, planks being temporarily laid, as at I; the burthen (being transferred on small rollers) will be easily moved thereon, to the extremity of the yard sideways; and thus stones can be deposited, as at K K (shewn *edgeways* upward) upon any point of the area of the yard, and returned by the same means. § 151. *Note* *, p. 94.

The area bounded by the line G G, and the dotted line L L, is the *Portland Workshed*. M denotes one of the *bankers*; to which, from the wheel carriage (supposed on the rail-road opposite) *strong joists* being laid, as shewn by the dotted lines, the pieces of stone are brought on *small rolls*; the bankers having notches sunk therein, to receive the ends of the joists.——In like manner, the area N O was the shed for the *Moorstone Workers*.

The square area P Q, denotes the extent of a *roof* supported by four posts covering the *Platform*; whereof *a b* represents the *platings* of rough stone walls; *c d* one of its principal *floor timbers*, 6 by 12; these being covered with three-inch *plank*, and brought to a *true level*, made a *flat floor*, upon which the *courses* were *brought together*, § 151.——R the *cabin* for the *foreman* of the yard. S a small *store-room* for tools and iron work. G W the *store-shed* for *Watchet lime* and *Puzzelana*. V X the shed for *bucking* or beating the larger parts of the *Puzzelana* upon W Y, the *bank* with three cast *iron bels* upon it.

Fig. 3. Supposed a *detached figure*, being the *ground plan* of the *turn-rail* at T, (*fig.* 2.) to an *enlarged scale*, wherein A B is a *dormant circle* of wood, well supported; of which C marks the *center pin* fixed in the transverse beam D D; E E being connecting studs. F F are portions of the *rails*, whereon the *wheels* move, which are kept in place by the *fillets f f*, nailed on each side. G G shew the *sleepers* for supporting the rails at about a yard's distance middle and middle; as is also shewn near E in *Fig.* 2.

Fig. 4. is the *Plan* of the moveable *turn-rail*, and *Fig.* 5. the relative *upright*; shewing also the section of the dormant circle. The three last figures having a mutual reference, the same parts are marked with the same letters: and furthermore, in *Fig.* 4 and 5. H, I shew the *rail part* of the turn-rail, correspondent to those parts marked F F, *Fig.* 3. in *width* and *height*. The *rail parts* H, I are strongly framed upon the *cross beam* K K, and connected by the pieces L, L. The whole being poized, with its burthen, upon the pin C, but without absolutely touching the dormant circle A B while turning; for bearing only upon the *flat shoulder* of the pin, it turns easily; but, when it is *bringing on* or *wheeling off*, the *equilibrium* upon the pin being destroyed, the ends H, I are then supported upon the dormant circle, and the wheels will move steady.

Fig. 7. shews the *Plan*, and *Fig.* 8. the *upright* view of the *wheel carriage* to the same scale as that of *Fig.* 3, 4 and 5.——Also *Fig.* 9. and *Fig.* 10. give the upright views of the *Roll carriage* in two directions to the same scale; which shew distinctly the manner of supporting the *axis* of the rolls on *iron frames*; and how the iron frames are kept upright by four pair of *cross bars*.

Fig. 11. gives the upright of the *Capstand roll*, *axis*, and middle part of the *bar* to the same scale.——At 1, 2 is shewn the capstand in full, to the *scale of the yard*; and 3, 4, 5 mark the *direction* of the rope; which, from a *snatch-block* at 5, ascends to the upper block of the *main tackle*, suspended from the top of the *shears*; as per *Fig.* 6. wherein the *in-hauler* guy-tackle is marked 7, being a *runner* and *tackle*; and the *out-hauler* marked 8, are *simple blocks*.——The guy-rope 7, 6 was attached to a *ring-bolt*, passing through a large rough stone, rammed into the ground; its place being shewn at 6, (*Fig.* 2.) the out-hauler guy 8, 9 being secured in the same manner.——The marble rocks marked 10, go round the point of the Bay.

Fig. 12. is the *elevation* of the upper part of the *jetty-head* in front, with the *shears* upon it, to an *enlarged scale*, more particularly to shew the smaller parts. A, B, the front pair of piles to which the *cross beam* C D is bolted; and in like manner to each pair of piles. E, E the ends of the longitudinal *half balks*; F F the *cross joists*; G, G the ends of the flat *rails* that the wheels of the carriage run upon; H H being a single *cross timber* serving as a *stop* to the carriage at the end. I, the snatch-block.——N. B. The *scantlings* are marked, because, this jetty or scaffold, erected *as slight as possible* for a temporary purpose, sustained the whole tonnage of the Edystone matter, in and out, without derangement.——The *detached Fig.* 13. gives a part of the top of one of the *shear legs*, shewing how they were *plated* on each side, to support the *bolt* of the anchor from bending, and

* A *Luff* [illegible] commonly consists of a pair of double blocks, being of the lighter kind for promiscuous uses.

and thereby from splitting the poles.——*Fig.* 14. is the enlarged figure of the *runner* and *tackle* (marked 7. in *Fig.* 6.) K, the *runner-block*, of one large single pulley; L M, the *tackle-blocks* of three pulleys each, making a purchase of twelve *equivalent* to the great blocks. (*See the Postscript.*)

Fig. 15. gives an upright *diagonal view* of the *main tackle blocks*; having six pulleys each upon two pins; the larger *tier* being ten, and the lesser eight inches diameter. This figure distinctly shews the method of *salvage strapping*, being *double*, that the pins being readily knocked out, they could be frequently greased without trouble.——N. B. The *shears*, *blocks*, and *tackles* used at *Mill Bay* were nearly the same as at the Rock; and *one pair* of main tackle blocks at each place, with the *same pulleys*, went through the whole service; but the pins were renewed each season, and sometimes oftener, being of *wood* on account of the *salt water*; but were frequently greased. The *main tackle-fall* at each place was no larger a rope than of three inches circumference; being a *white rope*, remarkable *soft* laid, *hawser-fashion* *; and which is of material consequence.

PLATE, N° 18. Descriptions *of* SUPPLEMENTAL MATTERS, *having* Reference *to the* EDYSTONE BUILDING.

Fig. 1. contains an upright *front view* of the *great tackle*, or *purchase-blocks* of twenty *sheaves* or pullies, mentioned § 126, 127.

Fig. 2. A *side view* of the same blocks, referring to *Fig.* 18. The *advantage* of this construction is, that the *tackle-fall* or *running-rope* may be *reeved* through the twenty sheaves, without a *cross* or interference; so that the standing part, or beginning, may be in the *middle* of the upper block, and the *ending*, hauling part, or *fall*, upon the *middle pulley* of the same block. The weight therefore being suspended by twenty ropes instead of six, as in common *triple* blocks, the *tackle-fall*, as relative to a *given* weight, may be *lesser* or of fewer *yarns* in the same proportion, which renders the whole much more *flexible* and *pliant*, and which, together with the advantage derived from the *mode* of *reeving*, occasions their *rising* and *falling* nearly upon a *parallel*.——The *uses* and *advantages* of these blocks, and also the *method* of *reeving*, are so particularly described in the *Philosophical Transactions*, *Vol.* 47, for the years 1752 and 1753, and are now so well known, that I shall but just touch upon the *principle* whereon the *reeving* is performed. Beginning in the middle, the *greater* sheaves are reeved as far as can be on them; from thence going to the first of the *smaller* sheaves, and reeving the *whole* of them throughout, you then go to the *first* of the *greater* sheaves, before left *unreeved*, ending upon the *middle sheave* of the upper block; and thus arises a *diminution* of the *friction* from the more *equal distribution* thereof.

Fig. 3. being an *upright section* of the *store-room* to an *enlarged scale*; in it is shewn the *center* whereon the *upper store-room floor* was turned; and in like manner the rest.

Fig. 4. is the *Plan* relative thereto, the *letters* being common to both. *a b*, *c d* Shew two of the sixteen *ribs*, formed to the circle of the [illegible] of the floors. These ribs are connected at their ends by two [illegible] *rings*, *e f g*, *h i k*; the *former* supported by four posts, three of which are shewn in their places; and the *latter* by [illegible] of which only one is shewn on the right hand, and one on the left, to avoid confusion. The *rings* are each made to take asunder, that after striking the center they might be got out of the room.——At *l k*, *m m*, two of the ribs are supposed taken out, to shew their bearings upon the rings; they were *open centers*, that it might be seen underneath when the joints were fair. *Fig.* 7. of *Plate* 11. shews how the 16 radii of stones would apply to the 16 *ribs*. In *this Plan*, *Fig.* 4. A shews the *well hole*, and B D the cross timbers for supporting the four middle posts, whose places are marked out by dotted little squares.

Fig. 5. is an *elevation*, and *Fig.* 6. the *relative plan* of a *Dial Stone*, taken professedly from the general figure of the Edystone Lighthouse; being the design of the late *James Duke* of QUEENSBERRY; and by him erected at *Amesbury*, *Wilts*, with a Dial upon it, by MR. RAMSDEN.——The drawing, of which this is a copy, was given me by the *Duke*; and is placed here as an instance, that the *Edystone column* may be applied to some uses of *Architecture*.

Fig. 7. represents one of the *silver medals*, given to the *seamen* as a *token* of the service, § 161.

Fig. 8. shews the *tool* wherewith the stones were got up from the *bottom* of the *gut*, mentioned § 212. A, one of the stones with two *trenail holes*, as per § 163.

Suppose this stone lying flat in the bottom of the gut, the side A uppermost. The tool has a *pole* or *staff* *b b* about twelve feet long, sufficient to reach to the bottom. The single *prong* *c* is forged to a very gentle *taper*, such as to be thrust eight or nine inches into a *trenail hole* (all of them being bored to a gauge) it can be driven by the pole, till *fast*; observing that the arm *c* corresponds to the *center of gravity* of the stone. The water is generally so clear as to see the bottom, and in case of any *ruffle* by the wind, can be in a great measure freed from agitation, by looking through a *speaking trumpet*, whose mouth is put down eight or ten inches into the water. The rope *d e f* being then *set upon* by the *main tackle*; instead of its drawing out, the length of the arm *g* causes the *prong* to *jamb* the faster in the hole; and the staff being quitted by the hand, with a cord to hinder its flying off too far, the whole assumes the position of the *figure*; and when brought above water, is lowered into a yawl.

Fig. 9. is a section of one of the *mortar buckets*, and in it the *beater*. This figure will need no further explanation, after what is said § 221.

Fig. 10. shews one of the *internal* faces of the lantern's *glass frames*, to the same scale as Plate N° 12, and therein the *cross bars* of *iron* as they were actually fixed according to § 290 and 291.——Besides the *flat* at each end of each bar, distinguished by a *darker shade*, and through which the *screws* passed; each end was also *cranked* about an inch, so as to set the transverse part of the bars, clear of the copper sash frame; and they were cleared of each other at their *intersection*, by one of them being made *straight*, the other *curved* in that part.——This figure, is less *regular* than what is shewn *Plate* N° 12, yet I do not look upon this assemblage as less capable of *resistance* to *external violence*, or less useful in regard to the *transmission* of *light*; for all the *panes* being taller than the *candles*, the *chandelier rings* are so hung, that when the candles are at *rest*, dispensing their light, that of *one chandelier* passes through the *range* of panes A, and that of the other through the *range* B; and when the candles are *snuffed*, one of the rings of lights being seen through the range C, the other mounts to D, and *vice versa*.

Fig. 11. shews the *Chain* of *triangles*, from the *Edystone* to the *Flag-staff* of the *Garrison* of *Plymouth*, for ascertaining their *distance* trigonometrically.

Fig. 12. is an *enlargement* of the work within the *Headlands* of the *Sound*, the same letters marking the same parts in both: whereof E denotes the *Edystone*.——R *Ramhead*.——M *Maker*, or *Mewstone*.——P the *triangular* stone on Point Penlee.——S *Stoddon Battery House*.——W the *western* *Beacon*.——G the *eastern*, upon the *Citadel*, near the *north* [illegible] turret.——B a *station* at the middle of the base.——F the *Garrison's flag-staff*.

The whole country about *Plymouth Sound* being very uneven, I could not readily obtain a *base* better, than by very carefully measuring the *two lines* BG, BW, taking the intercepted angle W B G; whence the right line W G was obtained, making a *base* of 1,674 feet, and which I cannot suppose to err more than half a foot.——Again, the nearest place from whence the *two beacons* W, G could be *commodiously* seen for the *purpose*, was the point S, and all the *three angles* of the triangle W S G being likewise carefully taken, I conclude the angle W S G, = [illegible] 23', taken *true* to a minute; that is to [illegible] part of the whole angle. The line S W could therefore be determined within [illegible] part; which being considered as a *new base* of *larger extent*, may be esteemed true within [illegible] part of the whole.——From this, and the angles taken as *marked* upon the scheme, the lines W P, W M, and W E, were successively determined; and finally E F, the distance of the *Flag-staff* from the *Edystone*, came out very near, but somewhat less than, 14 miles.——But the *interior* harbour of *Plymouth*, called *Sutton Pool*, being about 3 furlongs farther from the *Edystone* than the *Flag-staff*, the whole distance may be esteemed 14½ miles from *Plymouth Harbour*.

PLATE, N° 19. A MAP *of the* COASTS *and* COUNTRY *near the* SPURN POINT.

It appears that this Coast, from *Flamborough Head*, or at least from *Bridlington* to the *Spurn Point*, trending S. S. E. (*true Merid.*) and the tide of flood of the German *Ocean* setting strongly to the southwards; this will cause these flood-tides, when agitated by all winds from N. N. W. to N. E. to *bite* very hard upon this *stretch* of coast; and, no part of it being rocky, to *wear away*, the sand and matter dislodged to be driven towards the south, forming at the tail of the land, the *appendage*, called the *Spurn Point*, § 311. Doubtless this matter so brought would in time *choke* up the *Humber*, was it not for the *powerful reflux* of that river's *tide*, aided by the fresh water from the higher country. The *Spurn Point* being therefore the effect of a *struggle* between the *sea tide* of the *German Ocean* and the *reflux* of the *Humber*, we are not to wonder if the powerful effort of the sea by degrees drives the [illegible] the *Humber* southwards towards the *Lincolnshire* [illegible], thereby giving opportunity for the *Spurn Point* to *lengthen* towards the [illegible], as the coast wears away, to which it *hangs* as a *rudder*, to be also in a state of *travelling* [illegible], § 320, and 322.

PLATE, N° 20. PLAN *of the* SPURN POINT, *as in* 1786. *Also its* VARIATIONS *during the preceding twenty Years.*

Fig. 1. is the *Plan* of the *Spurn Point*, as taken in the year 1786, comprehending about 98 acres; upon which little needs to be said, after what is upon the *face* of it, and § 329 is considered.

Fig. 2. is an enlargement of the *extreme* point of the *Spurn*, wherein the boundary line of the *Sand Hammocks*, and its relative *high water line* is marked with the *year*. The space comprehended between these two lines was a kind of flat area or *fore shore* over which the sea beat in *rough weather*; and upon which (the whole being then considered as [illegible]) the *lower Light* was proposed to be built at A; ANGEL's *Light* [illegible] being at that time in use, and within the boundary of the [illegible] of the [illegible], § 329. B was the place marked out for the *high light*; and parallel to A B, the proposed *line of direction*, at the distance of 13 *yards* to south-westward, were the two points C, D marked out for the *temporary lights*, but for reasons that appeared before their erection, the point C was in *reality* carried to E.——F, a low building, containing two *cottages* for the temporary *Light-keepers* was erected at the same time. When the Lighthouses were begun in 1771, the high water line was as marked for that year. For *reasons*, § 318, the *low Light* marked at A was placed at G. The *high Lighthouse* was begun the latter end of the year 1772, and placed at H, § *ibid.*——In 1773 the high water line was as marked, and the boundary of the *Sand Hammocks* remained nearly the same for some time; but a *great storm* in *January* 1776 varied the high water line, as marked for that year, and described § 332. After this there was little variation of that line to the *conclusion* of the work in 1777.

On visiting the *Spurn* in 1786, the *high water line* ran as described for that year, approaching near to the *Low Light Machine* at Q.——I K L, *Fig.* 2. is the high water line, and M N O that of low water; from which it will appear, that the *Spurn Point* marked P, is advanced considerably to south-westward from the line of direction, and has considerably retreated to north-westward, or nearer [illegible] of the *high Light*.——Of the *island* R there were no traces in 1777; but now, being grown with the *bent grass* the *sand hammocks* had established themselves, and rendered the surface irregular.——It appears that *little* [illegible] has happened near the *high Lighthouse*, but that the *breadth of sand* was there *increased*.

PLATE, N° 21. SECTION *of the* HIGH LIGHTHOUSE, *upon the* SPURN POINT, *to the same Scale as the* Edystone.

A A The level of the *Pavement* of the *circular court-yard*.——B The *Coal Vault*.——C is a room for the *Smith's Shop*, and *Machine* for hoisting the coals.——D is a *vacant* room.——E, the *dwelling room*, having two opposite *fire places*, [illegible]——F and G *upper* chambers.——H The *Pipe Room*; wherein to be used as the wind suits.

* A rope laid *hawser* fashion is a rope consisting of any number of yarns according to the strength required, which divided into three *strands*, and each being twisted equally, are prepared to be *laid* into a rope. But if this, or any similar rope is further twisted, equally with two others, so as to make three *strands*, these will form a rope, said to be *cable laid*.

wherein I K, are two of eight *air pipes*, that convey air from the external *hopper-mouths*, to L the *receptacle*, which is lined with thick *plate iron*, the bottom being *shut*.——When the door is shut, the air ascends through the large *funnel* M, and the *hearth* N, to the fire grate. § 333.——The *flame* is seen in *every direction* through the windows of the lantern, and the *smoke* is collected in passing the *depressed conical roof*, composed of ten *Elland-edge flag stones*; and lastly, through the *upper funnel* O. The *coals* in the day-time are drawn up in a *tub* from the coal vault, through the opening P; by means of the *roll*, *wheel*, *pinion*, and *winch* at Q. A *rope*, from thence ascending through all the floors, goes over a large *pulley*, suspended from the roof, and thence downward through the hole in the arch at R, goes down the large *square wooden pipe* S T, which terminates at T in an *hopper-mouth*, proper for [illegible] in the bunkers.

The *ashes* and *hot cinders* passing through the grate, fall into the bottom of the *receptacle* L; and by heating the air therein, promotes a *sufficient draught* in the calmest weather; and which can be augmented and regulated, when there is a breeze; as any of the *air pipes* can be closed at pleasure.——Every morning when the receptacle is to be cleared, the ashes and cinders are thrown into the little *hopper* at V, and are conveyed down the square wood pipe V W, through W X, a pipe formed in the brick work, and from thence into a *Ring-stead* in the *court-yard*.

The *corner pillars* of the lantern are of *cast iron*, framed in a similar manner to what has been described for the *Eddystone*; allowing for difference in size and proportion. The *sash frames* are of *oak*. y y *Air holes* in the lantern, occasionally closed with a slider. z z Open holes in the *coal vault* to admit air and light. N. B. In 1780, this building was not sensibly out of upright.

PLATE, N° 22. PLANS *of the different* FLOORS *applicable to the preceding* SECTION.

Fig. 1. the ground plan. The outward circle, close piling. The stones in the interspaces of the bearing piles, were large *Elland-edge paving stones*, 12 inches depth, driven hard down, after the piling was done, with an heavy *two men's* [illegible]; intended, exclusive of the piling, to condense and consolidate the whole body of sand under the building, that the whole mass might *settle together*.

Fig. 2. an *horizontal section* of the *Coal Vault*. Wherein A is the *circular stair*, from the entry door to the stone floor of the first room.——B a Door into the coal vault; C and D the places of two *hatchways*, or openings through the vault. E. W. N. S. mark the *cardinal points* in all the figures; and also the places of the air holes of the vault in this.

Fig. 3. the plan of the *Stone Floor* over the coal vault. Wherein, A the *landing* of the stairs.——B An out door, having a *gibbet* for hoisting the coals to the stone floor, for their deposition after the lower door is blocked up.——C An *hatchway* in the middle for the equal distribution of the coals.——D The *hatchway* for the *coal tub*.——E The *roll*, *wheel*, *pinion*, and *winch*.——At E. W. N. are three windows; at S is the *gibbet* marked by dotted lines.——F is the *ash pipe*.

Fig. 4. shews the *framing* of the dwelling room floor. The place of the windows in this, as in all the rest, conform to the *cardinal points*.——G, G The *fire places*.——H The opening for the *step ladder*.——D The *coal pipe*.——F The *ash pipe*.——Besides this, there are four more timber floors, of similar constructions; the *girders* laying alternately E. and W. and N. and S.

Fig. 5. an *horizontal section* of the *pipe room*, *air pipes*, and *receptacle*; I K is one of the air pipes; their *hopper-mouths* being shewn at I.——One of the *sliders* is shewn in flat at M; as applied at N, which is the section of its groove. Each pipe having one, they can be regulated according to the *quarter* and *strength* of the *wind*.——D The *coal pipe*.

Fig. 6. *Plan* of the *Lantern* and *Balcony Floor*, ready for the reception of the iron work. The largest dotted circle shews the circumference of the top of the brick shaft of the *main column*. A The *Balcony Door*.——B The *Hearth*.——C The *Fire Grate*.——D The *falling door* closing the top of the *coal pipe*; and E the falling doors closing the top of the *man-hole*; to which the ascent is by a ladder from the *pipe room*.

Fig. 7. is the *plan*, and *Fig.* 8. the *section* of the *Fire Grate* to an enlarged scale.——It is chiefly of *cast iron*; the bottom made to take out. A, B circular bricks, of *fire clay*.

PLATE, N° 23. ELEVATION *of the* high LIGHTHOUSE, *and of the* SWAPE *for exhibiting the* low Light, *upon SPURN POINT*.

These structures are not supposed to be viewed upon the *line of direction*; in which case the *figure* of the *machine* would have fallen directly upon the *Lighthouse*. The line of view is marked in *Plate* 22. *Fig.* 6. being seen upon a *bearing* of N. W. by W. ½ W. in which position the two *structures* are seen *clear* of each other: and, to bring them into *one plate*, the *scale* is only *half* the size of the two former.——A person standing in the *entry door* of the *Lighthouse*, will see the low light machine, or *swape*, through the *door* of the *court-yard* wall; which is a circle of 93 feet diameter.

The *Swape*, including the walls whereon it stands, exhibits the light at the height of 56 feet.——The *fire basket* of iron turning upon an axis, always places itself *level*, in every position of the *mast* A B. This loaded with a *weight* at A, counterbalances the *iron work* and *fuel* at top; the whole being steadied, and clipped into an iron frame, that turns in *equilibrio* upon the *horizontal axis* a b; supported by *pillars* and *braces*, as *per figure*.——When the fire wants renewal, the attendant laying hold of one of the *winches* of the *roll* c d, turns it round, so as to wind the rope shewn at e upon it. This rope, after going obliquely towards the ground, passes a pulley in a *stud*, fixed therein, at some yards distance; and thence arising obliquely upward, as *f g*, it lays hold of the *mast* by a small chain. By the motion of the *roll* the *fire basket* is brought to the ground, where it is fed with a shovelful or two of coals. While the rope e was winding upon the *roll*, the rope *h* being coiled thereon the *contrary way*, was unwinding; and this being attached at A to the extreme of the lower end of the mast, and at equal distance, in rising it carries the rope along with it. The *fuel* being *renewed*, the *winch* is turned the *contrary way* round; by which, that end of the mast is brought down, and the *fire basket* carried up, into the position shewn in the figure. The lower end of the *mast* is steadied against the *cross piece* i i; the roll being then fastened.——The projecting part *l* is a small *umbrella* of sheet iron, serving to throw off the falling cinders from the rope.

N. B. The whole operation can be performed in a couple of minutes.

POSTSCRIPT.

IN the preceding references it is mentioned, in the explanation of Plate N° 17, *Fig.* 14. that the compound purchase, called the *Runner* and *Tackle*; which consists of one large pulley or sheave in the runner block; and which together with a pair of tackle blocks, of three pulleys in each; that altogether consist of *seven* sheaves; composes a purchase *equivalent* to that of the great blocks, which consisting of six sheaves each, makes the whole number *twelve*: this last, therefore, having a greater number of moving parts, and flexures of the *reeving* rope; being consequently less simple, and attended with more friction; it will naturally be enquired, by those of my readers who are not *seamen*, or versed in the *mechanic powers*, why the runner and tackle is not to be preferred in all cases?

The *Runner* and *Tackle* doubtless, working with less *friction*, is to be preferred wherever it can be properly applied; but many are the cases, in which it cannot be applied: for, it will readily be perceived, by inspection of Fig. 14. that while the tackle blocks L, M, are hauled together, or brought *block and block*; and one of them has moved through the space L M; the runner block K will only rise, or move, through *half* that space, on account of the runner rope being double. It therefore follows, that the weight can be lifted or moved only half the height or space, where a runner is applied, that it could be where the tackle alone is applied. In consequence, if a weight was to be lifted upon *Shears* by the *Runner and Tackle*, to a *given* height, the shears would be obliged to be *twice* as high, which would in most cases be very inconvenient: but where there is height enough; or in the case of a *Guy-rope* or guide rope, as in *Fig.* 6. marked 6, 7, there being a considerable length of Dead Rope, not engaged with any sheave; the runner may be of any length, to give the purchase the scope required.——The *Runner*, therefore, though it doubles the purchase of the tackle blocks, it reduces the height to which the weight could be hoisted by them alone, to *half*.——I shall conclude with observing, that if the *Great Purchase Blocks* of 20 sheaves (Plate N° 18, Fig. 1. and 2.) were worked with a *Runner*, they would form a purchase of *Forty* to *One*; and, of the size of Blocks described, would with security *hoist* a weight of [illegible] *Tons*.

THE END.

www.ingramcontent.com/pod-product-compliance
Lightning Source LLC
Chambersburg PA
CBHW021348230426
43666CB00006B/449